NURSE PRACTITIONER SECRETS

NURSE PRACTITIONER SECRETS

MARY JO GOOLSBY, EdD, MSN, APRN, ANP-C
Director of Research and Education
American Academy of Nurse Practitioners
Austin, Texas
Patient Care Research Specialist
University Health Care Systems
Augusta, Georgia

HANLEY & BELFUS, INC. / Philadelphia

Publisher: HANLEY & BELFUS, INC.
                  Medical Publishers
                  210 South 13th Street
                  Philadelphia, PA 19107
                  (215) 546-7293; 800-962-1892
                  FAX (215) 790-9330
                  Web site: http://www.hanleyandbelfus.com

Note to the reader: Although the information in this book has been carefully reviewed for correctness of dosage and indications, neither the authors nor the editor nor the publisher can accept any legal responsibility for any errors or omissions that may be made. Neither the publisher nor the editor makes any warranty, expressed or implied, with respect to the material contained herein. Before prescribing any drug, the reader must review the manufacturer's current product information (package inserts) for accepted indications, absolute dosage recommendations, and other information pertinent to the safe and effective use of the product described.

Library of Congress Control Number: 2002102757

NURSE PRACTITIONER SECRETS   ISBN 1-56053-520-2

Last digit is the print number: 9   8   7   6   5   4   3   2   1

DEDICATION

To the many nurse practitioners from whom I continue to learn daily, and to my husband, H.G., for his unwavering confidence and support in all that I do.

MJG

CONTENTS

CONTRIBUTORS

Louise A. Autio, PhD, FNP, BC, RN
Associate Professor, Texas A&M University–Corpus Christi School of Nursing and Health Sciences, Corpus Christi, Texas

Anna S. Beeber, MSN, RN, CRNP
University of Pennsylvania School of Nursing, Philadelphia, Pennsylvania

Vicki Ellison Burns, PhD(c), RN, FNP-BC
Assistant Professor, Department of Nursing, Cox College of Nursing and Health Sciences, Springfield, Missouri

Jill C. Cash, MSN, APRN, BC
Instructor, Department of Nursing, Southern Illinois University–Edwardsville, Edwardsville, Illinois; Southern Illinois Obstetrics and Gynecology, Carbondale, Illinois

Anne P. Ch'ien, MSN, FNP
Clinical Associate Professor, University of Tennessee at Chattanooga School of Nursing, Chattanooga, Tennessee

Valerie T. Cotter, MSN, CRNP
Associate Director, Adult Health and Gerontology Nurse Practitioner Programs, School of Nursing; Nurse Practitioner and Education Director, Alzheimer's Disease Center, University of Pennsylvania, Philadelphia, Pennsylvania

Carol E. Craig, PhD, FNP-C, RN
Associate Professor, Oregon Health and Sciences University School of Nursing, Klamath Falls, Oregon

Leslie L. Davis, MSN, RN, CS, ANP
Clinical Assistant Professor, University of North Carolina School of Nursing; Clinical Assistant Professor, Division of Cardiology, Department of Medicine, University of North Carolina Hospitals, Chapel Hill, North Carolina

Mary Jo Goolsby, EdD, MSN, APRN, ANP-C
Director of Research and Education, American Academy of Nurse Practitioners, Austin, Texas; Patient Care Research Specialist, University Health Care Systems, Augusta, Georgia

Laurie Grubbs, PhD, ARNP, ANP
Associate Professor of Nursing, Florida State University School of Nursing, Tallahassee, Florida

Tina Hackney, MSN, RN, CS, FNP
Nurse Practitioner, Congestive Heart Failure Clinic, Alamance Regional Medical Center, Burlington, North Carolina

Valerie A. Hart, EdD, APRN, BC
Associate Professor of Nursing, University of Southern Maine, Portland, Maine

Donna F. Haynes, PhD, RN, CS, WHNP, FNP
Nursing Instructor, Department of Nursing, Greenville Technical College, Greenville, South Carolina

Rodney W. Hicks, MSN, RN, FNP, CS, CCRN
Research Coordinator, U.S. Pharmacopeia, Rockville, Maryland

Deborah M. Judd, MSN, RN-C, FNP
Asthma Nurse Practitioner, Asthma-Chronic Obstructive Pulmonary Disease Clinic, University Hospital, University Health Care System, Augusta, Georgia

Sarah H. Kagan, PhD, RN, CS, AOCN
Assistant Professor of Gerontological Nursing, University of Pennsylvania School of Nursing;
Gerontology Clinical Nurse Specialist, Hospital of the University of Pennsylvania, Philadelphia,
Pennsylvania

Claudia R. Miller, MS, RN, NP
Anxiety Disorders Program, University of Michigan, Ann Arbor, Michigan

Karen Koozer Olson, PhD, FNP-CS
Professor of Nursing, Texas A&M University–Corpus Christi School of Nursing and Health
Sciences; Student Health Center, Texas A&M University, Corpus Christi, Texas

Arlene Pericak, FNP, MS
Assistant Professor, Department of Nursing, The Sage Colleges, Troy, New York; Albany Medical
Center, Albany, New York

Betsy Shank Pless, PhD, FNP
Associate Professor and Assistant Dean for Distant Programs, Department of Adult Nursing,
Medical College of Georgia School of Nursing, Athens, Georgia

Susanne A. Quallich, APRN, BC, NP-C, CUNP
Urology Nurse Practitioner, Department of Surgery, Veterans Affairs Medical Center, Ann Arbor,
Michigan

Ann Marie Ramsey, RN, MSN, CPNP
Adjunct Faculty, University of Michigan School of Nursing; Pediatric Nurse Practitioner, Section
of Pediatric Otolaryngology, University of Michigan Hospitals, Ann Arbor, Michigan

Katherine Russell-Lindgren, PhD, RN
Associate Professor of Nursing, University of Tennessee at Chattanooga School of Nursing,
Chattanooga, Tennessee

Theodore D. Scott, RN, MSN, FNP-C
Family Nurse Practitioner, Department of Primary Care, Kaiser-Permanente Medical Center, San
Diego, California

Lori Settersten, PhD, RN, WHNP, C, FNP, BC
Assistant Professor, University of Wisconsin–Milwaukee School of Nursing; Nurse Practitioner,
Riverwest Pierce Community Nursing Center, Milwaukee, Wisconsin; Nurse Practitioner, Planned
Parenthood of Wisconsin, Inc., Waukesha, Wisconsin

Lisa Theriault, RN, MSN, CS
Assistant Professor, Division of Nursing, University of Maine at Fort Kent, Fort Kent, Maine;
Horizons Health Services, Presque Isle, Maine

Mary Nell Waldrup, CPC
Chief Financial Officer, Compliance Officer, and Coding Director, Anesthesia Billing Associates,
Inc.; Chief Financial Officer, Compliance Officer, and Coding Consultant, MasterMed, a division
of Anesthesia Billing Associates, Inc., Augusta, Georgia

Paula J. Watt, PhD, FNP
Manager, Clinical Education and Practice, and Faculty Lecturer, Joseph F. Sullivan Center,
Clemson University School of Nursing, Clemson, South Carolina

PREFACE

Nurse Practitioner Secrets is written by nurse practitioners who are active in clinical practice both for their colleagues who are new to the profession and for those who are experienced but faced with new situations. This book is intended to serve as an easy reference for use on the job when nurse practitioners are faced with questions about issues such as practice management, selection or interpretation of diagnostic studies, differentiation and response to specific patient presentations, and collaboration with other disciplines. The unique combination of topics includes diagnostic studies, practice issues, clinical management, and collaborative practice relevant to nurse practitioners. The topics are suitable to practitioners with a wide range of interests and practice areas, including geriatrics, pediatrics, women's health, men's health, general adult health, and urgent care.

Although the subject matter is varied, this book is not intended to be a comprehensive or in-depth textbook on nurse practitioner practice. Instead, the emphasis is on pearls of wisdom and practical tips that generally are not detailed in larger texts. The content is provided in an easy-to-use question-and-answer format similar to the way a provider would receive information during an informal consultation.

The book has four major parts. The first part includes chapters on practice issues: contract negotiation, billing and reimbursement considerations, and the consultation and referral process. The second part addresses diagnostic issues. Several of these chapters answer common questions regarding the selection and interpretation of specific diagnostic studies, whereas others describe the assessment approach to special situations. The largest section of the book covers the diagnostic and management approach to a variety of common chief complaints such as chest pain, forgetfulness, and hematuria. Chapters also address the management of more complex chronic problems such as congestive heart failure and asthma. Several chapters address care issues of distinctive categories of patients in a primary care setting, such as patients with borderline personality disorder and women who are pregnant. The final portion of the book provides information that is essential to nurse practitioners who are considering whether or how to develop a more integrative practice. This section answers questions related to herbal and nutritional therapies, therapeutic touch, and when and how to collaborate with members of other disciplines. Although certainly not exhaustive, the information shared by the contributors exemplifies the diversity of nurse practitioner practice.

Mary Jo Goolsby, EdD, MSN, APRN, ANP-C

ACKNOWLEDGMENTS

I want to acknowledge my gratitude to each of the contributors to this work. Each readily shared his or her expertise and played a large role in designing the final work. Their suggestions for additions to the book, based on their years of experience, made the final product much richer. I am also grateful to Linda Scheetz, the Nursing Secrets Series® editor, for her confidence in my ability to edit this work and for her guidance in the process. I am indebted to Michael Zychowicz, for his thoughtful independent review of the work, and to Linda Belfus, the publisher, for her assistance in its development.

I. Practice Issues

1. NEGOTIATING A CONTRACT

Anne P. Ch'ien, MSN, FNP, and Katherine Russell-Lindgren, PhD, RN

1. What primary factors should a nurse practitioner (NP) consider when negotiating a contract of employment?

Every work agreement or contract is unique, and various factors should be addressed before negotiation. Two factors are essential: determining your needs and assessing the potential employer's needs. The first requires self-assessment and reflection. The second requires learning as much as possible about the employer. The following framework can be used for thinking about negotiable elements that the NP might want to include in a work contract. Examples are by no means inclusive.

1. **Compensation package**: salary; overtime compensation; other benefits such as personal/family health insurance, long-term disability insurance, life insurance, paid time off (PTO), retirement, various professional/journal dues, drug enforcement and malpractice insurance fees, profit sharing, and pension plan or 401 K. The NP should be knowledgeable about salary ranges and benefits in the geographical area where services will be rendered.

2. **Job obligations**: hours of work, on-call requirement, where duties will be performed, mileage reimbursement, and required meetings. Both parties should be clear about work conditions and work stipulations.

3. **Practice issues**: control over practice as an independent contractor vs. salaried employee, scope of practice and performance and peer review process. As an independent contractor, the NP has more control over practice. Independent contractors are responsible for their taxes, malpractice insurance, and health benefits. In an employee-employer relationship, more control can be exercised over the NP's practice, but the employer is bound to certain obligations such as withholding taxes and paying unemployment taxes.

4. **Employment course**: expected duration of contract and specific terms of termination, such as severance pay, restrictive practice clause, and process of resolving practice disputes in a timely and effective manner. The NP should be well versed in the conditions under which employment will and can be terminated. Generally, the length of time for the contract should be no longer than 1 year to allow review, renewal, or further negotiation.

2. What specific steps should the NP take when negotiating a contract?

Negotiation is a three-step process:

1. **Preparation**. Successful negotiation is achieved by being prepared to present the facts clearly and succinctly. Do your homework. One of the best ways to discover salary range and benefits is to network with other NPs in the area. Past and present employees are an excellent source of information about the employer's practice pattern, values and beliefs of care, and management style. During the preparation stage, write down optimal salary and benefits desired as well as your required bottom-line salary and benefits. This approach provides a reasonable reference salary range from which to bargain or negotiate.

2. **Bargaining**. NPs should market themselves as high-quality and cost-effective health care providers during the bargaining process. Negotiate for agreement, not for winning or loosing. Establish rapport and trust through avoiding one-sided gains. Therefore, it is necessary to take the time required for full discussion of each person's perspective. Listen actively

1

during the entire process. Ask questions and seek clarification when unsure or uncertain about what is said. Inattention by either party can foster miscommunication and a breakdown in the process. Avoid emotional outbursts; use reason and be reasonable when presenting your desires. Jotting down notes during the bargaining step can assist the NP in remembering exactly what agreements have been reached and assist with avoiding premature conclusion of the negotiation process.

3. **Finalizing**. If an agreement is reached that meets the NP's goal, the process should be finalized. All agreements should be written and the final contract signed as soon as feasible. Keep the contract simple. The NP should be active in drafting the contract. Seek the services of a competent attorney in the final draft, or have the attorney review the unsigned contract you have developed.

3. What should I do if a conflict arises during the negotiation?

During the negotiation process an honest difference of opinion can arise. Resolving the situation is wise and prudent behavior. An important principle in conflict resolution is to separate the issue from the person. Your mindset should reflect the following principle: "This is not about me and not about you, but rather achieving a mutually satisfactory outcome." Finding common ground and mutual understanding facilitates the refocusing of the process on what will be beneficial for both parties. The goal is to try to change the communication path that has contributed to the conflict to a path that leads toward a mutually satisfactory outcome. Clarifying misconceptions and centering on what has been achieved thus far can also be an effective strategy. If a win-win approach directed toward mutual goal achievement is used, both parties should be able to walk away from the process with positive feelings, even if a work relationship agreement is not reached.

4. How legally binding is a formal contract?

The law provides a remedy for any breach of contract or when a contract fails to perform what it states. For contracts to be enforceable, they must include several features:
- Competence and consent of the parties involved
- Purpose of the agreement
- Agreed terms or subject matter
- Mutuality of agreement and mutuality of obligations
- Completion of forms required by law

A contract lays out the rights and responsibilities of each party involved in a transaction and can be oral or written. Oral contracts are enforceable by legal action but more problematic to defend. A written contract provides a clearer basis for arbitrating disputes and is preferred over oral agreements. Contracts should be written if they are intended to last more than 1 year.

5. Should the contract include a clause that identifies the process by which the formal contract can be terminated?

All contracts should include a "termination" section to protect the NP's professional practice. The clause should define "just cause" for termination of the contract by the employer. Some employment agreements contain a "termination-without-cause" clause, particularly in states where employer can terminate employee "at will" without cause.

6. What does the term "restrictive employment covenant" mean?

A restrictive covenant is an agreement not to compete. The main types of restrictive covenants include noncompetition, nonsolicitation, "nonpiracy", "nondisclosure" and "return of property" clauses. A noncompetition agreement in an employment contract restricts one party from competing with the other party for a specific time and within a specific geographical area. The intent of the restrictive covenant is to prevent an employee from starting a competing business, working for a competitor, soliciting clients, recruiting current employees, or disclosing trade secrets or confidential information.

For NPs, a restrictive covenant restricts an employee from practicing within a set number of miles from an employer's business for a set period after the employee leaves the employer's business. The restrictive clause may specify the period of restriction and geographical boundaries. If the geographic boundary and term of restriction are significant, the NP may have to relocate to practice. To be enforceable, the restrictive covenant must be "reasonably" limited with respect to time and geographical location. If the restriction is too broad, thus restricting or inhibiting the NP from practicing in the profession, it is void. The restrictive covenant is considered "unreasonable," for instance, if the time frame is longer than 1–2 years. A restrictive covenant that restricts the NP from engaging in the professional practice under any and all circumstances in a broad geographical area for an unreasonable time is unenforceable. Specific state statutes and an attorney should be consulted before accepting the contract if the NP is unclear about the meaning of restrictive covenants.

7. Does a formal contract actually give an NP greater job security?

Many NPs practiced for years without employment contracts. In the past, an employer and employee negotiated salary, benefits, and hours of employment through conversation, and issues were handled when they arose. A primary advantage of a written employment contract is that the notice and condition of termination by either party to the contract are clearly stated. In addition a written contract gives incentive for parties to discuss issues and refreshes memories about original agreements. Thus, an employment contract can protect both employer and employee.

8. For NPs, what are the advantages to having a contract?

- Increased job security and greater control of professional practice
- Legal right to the job and economic and professional protection
- Upfront disscussion of issues to avoid potential future problems
- Identification of mutually agreed employment terms between employer and the employee
- Protection of employee from termination other than for just cause

9. For NPs, what are the disadvantages of not having a contract?

- In states where employment is "at will," employees can be terminated at any time for a good, bad, or no reason at all unless a contract states otherwise. Check your state law regarding "at will" employment.
- No due process for dispute is specified, and conflicts can go unresolved for an extended time.
- The NP has limited control of scope of practice and task assignments.
- The NP receives no additional pay for working overtime if salaried as an exempt employee.
- The NP has limited protection if physician office practices changes (e.g., physician decides to bring another physician and terminate the NP).

BIBLIOGRAPHY

1. Allen D, Ch'ien A, Trimpey M, Lindgren K: Employment contracts, negotiation strategies, and the nurse practitioner. In The 2001 Source Book for Advanced Practice Nurses, Springhouse, PA, Springhouse Corp., 2001, pp 12–17.
2. Black HC: Black's Law Dictionary, 6th ed. St. Paul, MN, West Publishing, 1990.
3. Buppert C: Nurse Practitioner's Business Practice and Legal Guide. Gaithersburg, MD, Aspen Publishers, 1999.
4. Ferreira VC: Encyclopedia of Georgia Law [Georgia attorneys and law school faculty members 1996 revision]. Norcross, GA, Harrison Co., 1996.
5. Greenberger D, Strasser S, Lewicki R, et al: Perception, motivation, and negotiation. In Shortell S, Kalunzy A (eds): Healthcare Management: A Text in Organizational Theory and Behavior, 2nd ed. New York, John Wiley & Sons, 1983, pp 81–141.
6. Mycounsel.com [on-line], (accessed September 2001). Available from URL: http://www.mycounsel.com/content/employment/contracts/.
7. NOLO law for all [on-line] (accessed September 2001): Available from URL: http://www.nolo.com/product/NCOMIC/summary.

8. Pulcini J, Vampola D: NPACE Nurse practitioner practice characteristics, salary, and benefits survey. Clin Excel Nurse Pract 4:366–372, 2000.
 9. Robinson D, Kish CP: Core Concepts in Advanced Practice Nursing. St. Louis, Mosby, 2001.
10. Rowland H, Rowland B: Nursing Administration Handbook. Rockville, MD, Aspen, 1997.
11. Sheeby CM, McCarthy MC: Advanced Practice Emphasizing Common Role. Philadelphia, F.A. Davis, 1998.
12. Swansburg R: Management and Leadership for Nurse Managers. Boston, Jones & Bartlett, 1996.
13. Tyson B: Practical aspect to protecting your client with restrictive employment covenants. Ga Bar J 7(1):8–14, 2001.

2. BILLING AND REIMBURSEMENT

Mary Jo Goolsby, EdD, MSN, APRN, ANP-C, and Mary Nell Waldrup, CPC

1. What must a nurse practitioner (NP) do before billing for visits?

Before billing a third-party payor, whether Medicare, Medicaid, or private insurer/managed care organization, you must:

- Obtain a provider number and/or panel membership, as necessary. A provider number is required by most third-party payors. You should contact the carrier for each payor and request information and provider application form.
- Familiarize yourself with the rules and policies of the third-party payor

Once you have received a provider number and/or panel membership and are ready to bill, you should:

- Include the appropriate diagnosis(es), using International Classification of Disease, 9th Revision (ICD-9) codes(s)
- Identify the appropriate type of encounter and/or procedures performed, using the Current Procedural Terminology (CPT) code(s)
- Identify any injectable drugs administered or medical supplies used, using the Health Care Financing Administration Common Procedure Coding System (HCPCS).
- Validate that your documentation supports the diagnosis and procedure code(s) selected, using the Evaluation and Management (E&M) guidelines, when appropriate

2. Why should NPs worry about billing and reimbursement criteria according to Medicare's E&M if they have a low or no Medicare base?

Although the E&M Documentation Guidelines were developed by the American Medical Association (AMA) and Health Care Financing Administration (HCFA) and are used by Medicare, other third-party payors use the same criteria for reimbursement decisions.

3. I am confused about the rate at which NPs are reimbursed. Is it 85% or 100%?

The rate depends on certain variables. NPs can be reimbursed directly at 85% of the amount determined by the Medicare physician fee schedule. NPs also may be reimbursed for services billed as "incident to" a physician's care at 100% of the physician's fee schedule.

The payment schedule is probably different for other third-party payors. For instance, Medicaid reimburses NPs at 70–100% the physician rate, depending on the state in which they practice.

4. What does "incident to" mean?

The term "incident to" has been used for some time by physicians to bill for services for varied personnel, performed in relation to (or "incident to") the care that the physician provided. Three major criteria should be met before billing for "incident to" services: (1) the physician must be available onsite to provide medical service (as opposed to purely administrative tasks); (2) the physician must have seen the patient previously and initiated care; and (3) the physician under whose direction the bill is made must have initiated the plan of treatment. The new guidelines further state that the physician should see the patient with ample frequency to indicate ongoing participation in the care provided. The person providing the service (the NP) must be an employee (i.e., not an independent contractor) of the physician/practice.

5. Can NPs alternate between direct and "incident to" billing?

Yes. The practice and NP may choose to use "incident to" billing whenever the criteria are met to receive the higher reimbursement. However, it is important to ensure that the service is billed directly under the NP's care if the physician is not on site and/or did not initiate the plan of care. It is also important to know the rules regarding if and when "incident to" billing is acceptable to payors other than Medicare. This policy may vary from state to state for Medicaid programs and private insurance companies.

6. How does Medicare know whether the "incident to" criteria have been met?

If the visit is audited, the physician's availability can be documented through clinic/practice records reflecting his or her presence in the clinic by patient schedule or administrative tasks. The physician could cosign the records at the time of visit, indicating his or her presence. Absence from the site is reflected by factors such as scheduled vacation, continuing education registration, and surgical or hospital round documentation. The record should reflect who initiated the patient's care for the problem addressed.

7. What is an ICD-9 code?

This code is used to identify the patient's diagnosis(es) or reason(s) for seeking care, based on the International Classification of Disease. The codes cover specific illnesses or diagnoses as well as a range of signs and symptoms and other reasons for encounters with a health care provider. Each code includes three to five digits, depending on the degree of specificity. The newer ICD-10 version should be available in 2003 or soon after and should be used as soon as available.

8. What is the link between the diagnosis and care provided at the payor level?

The selection of the correct diagnosis(es) is an important aspect of the reimbursement process. Only certain procedures are appropriate to specific diagnoses. If the diagnosis does not support the selection of a test or consultation, for instance, the requested reimbursement will not be allowed. Medical decision making, one variable used to determine the level of visit, is also influenced by the number and complexity of the problems addressed during a visit.

9. Should I check the list of diagnoses that are allowed for a particular diagnostic study to ensure that I select a diagnosis supportive of the procedure?

No. You should work the other way around. You are not supposed to decide the tests/procedures for which you wish to bill and then pick a diagnosis to justify your plan. Linking of a particular ICD-9 code with a CPT code for reimbursement purposes rather than the true clinical reason can be construed as fraud. You should definitely check to make sure that the diagnosis/problem that you have identified justifies a specific test or procedure. For instance, you should not routinely order an electrocardiogram (EKG) or chest x-ray, without some supportive rationale. Some reason should trigger consideration of an EKG and may be listed as one of the criteria supporting the procedure. If none of your patient's diagnoses or findings support the selection of the procedure, you may be selecting the wrong procedure. If you believe that the test is necessary but not clearly supported by the diagnosis, you should discuss the situation with the patient and ask him or her to sign an Advance Beneficiary Notice/Waiver (ABN). The ABN documents that you and the patient have discussed the possibility that the patient may be responsible for the cost of the service.

10. What is an ABN?

An ABN is a waiver that you may choose to ask the patient to sign before performing services that you believe may be denied by Medicare, Medicaid, or a third-party payor as "not reasonable and necessary." Blanket waivers are not acceptable; waivers should be used only when you legitimately believe that a specific service may be denied as not medically reasonable and necessary. There are reasons for denial of payment other than the failure of the diagnosis to support a service. The carrier may limit the number of times a treatment or service will be reimbursed within a specific time frame or the extent of the service provided, or the carrier may consider the service experimental. In any case, when the patient signs an ABN, it is necessary to add the HCPCS level II modifier GA to your CPT code to indicate to the carrier that you have an ABN on file. Without the GA modifier, the claim will be denied as provider responsibility and you will not be able to seek payment for the service(s) from the patient.

11. How specific should the diagnosis be?

The code should be as specific as possible. A "diagnosis" need not be a medical diagnosis or specific illness. If you have not yet determined or confirmed the cause of th epatient's problems, list the presenting symptom or physical finding as your diagnostic statement. For instance, if the patient indicates that he has had chest discomfort and you have not completed your evaluation, do not choose the ICD-9 code for angina (413.0) or myocardial infarction (410.0). Instead, designate "chest pain" as the diagnosis. There are codes for many types of chest pain, and you should select the one that best describes the patient's presentation. Make sure that your documentation always supports the diagnosis/problem that you list.

12. How many diagnoses or ICD-9 codes should I list for an encounter?

The HCFA 1500 claim form allows four diagnostic codes. One diagnostic code is linked to each CPT code. List the code(s) that directly relate to the patient's reason(s) for seeking care and any evaluation or management performed during the visit. Your clinic note should include a list of diagnoses (or codes) for any active problems that you have considered during the diagnosis or management because of their potential impact on the disease process, outcome, or therapeutic regimen.

13. What is a CPT code?

This code, from Current Procedural Terminology, describes the services and/or procedures for which reimbursement is sought. CPT codes are available for specific types of encounters (e.g., new and established visits, outpatient visits, consultations and referrals, inpatient observations) and a myriad of procedures, therapeutic measures, and diagnostic studies. This chapter describes codes related to outpatient visits.

14. How do I locate the appropriate CPT code from the many possibilities?

CPT codes are categorized into six sections (evaluation and management, anesthesia, surgery, radiology, pathology and laboratory, and medicine) in the CPT book. The placement does not imply that a code found in the surgical section is performed only by a surgeon; its placement is a matter of convenience, because it is believed to be most often used in a surgical practice or setting. The categorization was chosen to assist persons in finding the appropriate code/procedure. You can use the index to locate specific entries.

15. The CPT codes differentiate whether a patient is a new or established patient. Does the term "new" mean simply that patient has never been seen by the billing provider?

No. A new visit code should be chosen if the patient meets the following criteria: he or she has not been seen in the past 3 years by the billing provider *or* another provider in the same practice with the same specialization. An established patient, by contrast, may have been seen at some point in the past 3 years, either by the billing provider or another provider in the practice with the same specialization.

16. What components of care/service are used for reimbursement decisions related to office visits?

The seven measurement components include history, examination, medical decision-making, counseling, coordination of care, presenting problem, and time. These components are included in the Evaluation and Management (E&M) Guidelines for each type of visit covered in the CPT code book.

17. Are all seven components equally weighted?

No. The three main components on which an encounter is evaluatedare history, physical exam, and medical decision-making. The other criteria are considered "contributing factors."

18. How is the history used in reimbursement decisions?

The history, with other variables, is used to determine the work performed/level of care provided during a visit. The E&M guidelines address four major components of the history, which are considered in determining the level: (1) the reason for seeking care, (2) history of present illness (HPI), (3) review of systems (ROS), and (4) past, family, and social history (PFSH). All visits require a clear statement of the patient's reason for seeking care. In addition:

- Problem-focused histories require only a brief HPI.
- Extended problem-focused histories require a brief HPI and problem-pertinent ROS, but no documentation of pertinent PFSH.
- Detailed histories include extended HPI, extended ROS, and pertinent PFSH.
- Comprehensive histories require an extended HPI, complete ROS, and complete PFHS.

19. How do I determine whether the HPI is brief or extended?

The guidelines identify eight aspects of symptom analysis explored during the HPI, specific to the patient's reason for seeking care: duration, quality, severity, timing, location, context in which the complaint occurs, any modifying factors, and any associated symptoms. A brief HPI need only include three of the eight components. An extended HPI includes at least four of the components or statements about the status of at least three chronic illnesses.

20. How do problem-pertinent, extended, and complete ROS differ?

The E&M guidelines identify 14 areas that the ROS can address: constitutional, eyes, ENT (ear, nose, throat), cardiovascular, respiratory, gastrointestinal, genitourinary, musculoskeletal, integumentary, neurologic, psychiatric, endocrine, hematologic/lymphatics, and allergic/immunologic systems. The recent 2000 draft revisions also list functional status in this section.

Problem-pertinent ROS includes information about the system(s) involved in the presenting problem; usually one system is involved; two systems may be involved for some complaints.

Extended ROS includes 2–9 systems, including the one directly related to the complaint (the draft 2000 guidelines suggest 3–8 systems).

Complete ROS includes at least 10 systems, including the related system (draft 2000 guidelines suggest at least 9 systems).

21. Is it necessary to document the presence or absence of each possible symptom in each of the systems explored, or can I just say the "ROS–negative" and receive credit?

You cannot use a blanket statement about a negative ROS. For systems directly related to the chief complaint, you should list all positive findings as well as the pertinent negatives. For the other systems that you explore, you should list each system and then document that it was negative. Of course, you should document any positive findings for each system.

22. How do I decide whether the PFSH is pertinent or complete?

A pertinent PFSH, as the name implies, addresses only the history related to the specific problem(s) acknowledged in the HPI. A pertinent PFSH must document at least one of the three PFSH components (past health, family, or social history). A complete PFSH differs depending on whether the visit involves a new or established patient. For established patients, at least one item must be addressed from any two of the three components. For new patients, at least one item must be addressed from each of the three PFSH components.

23. What if a thorough history has already been obtained at an earlier visit? Is it necessary to repeat the history at each visit?

Absolutely not. However, the documentation should reflect that the history was reviewed and verified during the visit and that any necessary additions or other changes were made. The mere presence of an initial detailed history in the record does not confirm its consideration.

24. Must the patient provide the history for it to qualify under the E&M guidelines?

Whenever possible and appropriate, the patient should be the source of the history. At times, however, the history also should include information from family members, friends, or others who are familiar with the history. This approach is acceptable as long as the source is identified.

25. How is the physical documentation used to determine the appropriate E&M code?

A physical examination can be either organ-specific or multisystemic. Determination of the detail with which an examination is performed and whether it should focus on one or a few organs or adopt a more generalized multisystem approach is made by the clinician, based on the patient's presentation and history. The major components addressed by the latest draft guidelines are listed in the table below.

Body areas	Organ systems	
• Head/face	• Ophthalmologic	• Genitourinary
• Neck	• Otolaryngologic	• Hematologic/lymphatic
• Chest/breasts/axillae	• Respiratory	• Allergic/immunologic
• Abdomen	• Cardiovascular	• Integumentary
• Genitalia/groin/buttocks	• Endocrine	• Psychiatric
• Back/spine	• Musculoskeletal	
• Each extremity	• Neurologic	
Constitutional	**Special examinations/test/assessments**	
• Each vital sign	Three or more special examinations/tests/	
• General appearance	maneuvers/assessments are equivalent to 1	
Three or more from this category	body part/organ system.	
is equivalent to 1 body part or		
organ system.		

The earlier 1999 guidelines breakdown the examination components slightly differently. Become familiar with the set of guidelines used in your practice setting.

26. How do I determine which type of examination best fits what I have performed and documented?

Types of Physical Exam

Problem-focused (brief)	Limited evaluation of the body part or system implicated in the reason for contact or HPI; usually involves one system/part.
Expanded problem (focused, brief)	Limited evaluation of the implicated body part or system, as well as other symptomatic or related system(s); usually involves 1 or 2 systems/parts.
Detailed	Extended evaluation of the implicated part or system as well as other symptomatic or related systems; usually includes documented findings from 3–8 body areas or systems.
Comprehensive	Involves either a general multisystem examination or a complete examination of one organ system; usually includes findings from at least 9 of the body areas and/or systems.

27. How is the intensity of medical decision-making determined?

The guidelines describe four levels of medical decision making: straight-forward, low complexity, moderate complexity, and high complexity. The four levels are differentiated by the following factors:

- Number of problems addressed, diagnoses considered, and treatment options that must be considered
- Level of control or degree of exacerbation associated with the problems
- Amount and complexity of information that must be reviewed in medical records/studies and any other information that must be obtained and considered
- Potential for complications, morbidity, and mortality
- Patient's comorbidities that must be considered as the presenting problem is addressed, investigated, or treated.

Summary of Decision-making Levels

TYPE OF DECISION-MAKING	DIAGNOSES	INFORMATION*	RISKS†
Straight-forward	Minimal (1 minor problem)		Minimal (self-limited problems and/or treatments with well-established safety profile—both with little likelihood for complications, noninvasive diagnostic tests)
Low complexity	Limited (≥ 2 minor, 1 stable chronic, or 1 uncomplicated acute problem)	Limited (limited number of considerations in differential diagnosis, few diagnostic studies and treatment options to consider)	Low risk (multiple self-limited, minor problems or at least one chronic problem that is currently controlled, but has the potential for change, studies with small risk potential—superficial biopsies, arterial punctures, contrast medium)
Moderate complexity	Multiple (≥ 1 mildly exacerbated chronic, ≥ 2 stable chronic, undiagnosed new, acute/systemic, acute/complicated problems)	Moderate (more information must be considered in developing/narrowing differential diagnosis, diagnostic studies to be reviewed and treatment options offer higher complexity)	Moderate risk (acute or chronic progressive illnesses with increased likelihood for complications, treatments with higher side effect profiles, diagnostic studies associated with increased numbers of potential risks—performed under stress)
High complexity	Extensive (≥ 1 severely exacerbated chronic problem, unstable/threatening chronic problem, or problem with abrupt neurologic change)	Extensive (differential diagnosis requires review of an extensive amount of information, including status of comorbidities, complex diagnostic studies, or the design of complex therapeutic regimen including multiple therapeutic options)	High risk (illness with severe exacerbations, high potential for complications, treatments with great potential for adverse effects, diagnostic studies performed with identified risk factors, cardiovascular tests with contrast and/or stress)

* Lab values, old records, added history from relatives, diagnostic tests, interpretation of images, etc.
† Associated with diagnostic procedures, presenting problem, treatment options.

27. Summarize the documentation requirement for the three key components.

Brief Overview of Documentation Requirements for 3 Key Components

HISTORY (Hx)		PHYSICAL EXAM (PE)		MEDICAL DECISION-MAKING (MDM)	
Problem focus	Brief HPI	Problem focus	1 body part/ area/system	Straight-forward	Minimal diagnosis and information, risk
Expanded PF	Brief HPI, problem-pertinent ROS	Expanded PF	1 or 2 body parts/areas/ systems	Low complexity	Limited diagnosis and information; low risk
Detailed	Extended HPI and ROS, pertinent PFSH	Detailed	3–8 parts/areas systems	Moderate complexity	Multiple diagnoses, moderate risk
Compre-hensive	Extended HPI and ROS, complete PFSH	Compre-hensive	General multi-system exam or complete exam of 1 system	High complexity	Extensive diagnoses and information and high risk

29. How is the time involved in an encounter used in determining the level of care?

Although the guidelines identify an estimate of the amount of time spent face to face with patients at each level of visit, this estimate generally is considered as a determining factor only when over 50% of the encounter is spent in counseling, teaching, and case management functions. At such times, you should identify the type of visit based on the time involved. If this method is appropriate, you should still document any history, physical exam, and plan developed during the visit. In the record, document the total encounter time and the specific amount of time spent in counseling. You also should document adequately to indicate the involved decision-making.

30. How is all of this information used to select the specific CPT code?

The information discussed in response to the previous questions has been specific to general outpatient visits and does not apply to consultations, inpatient visits, or other types of encounters. The CPT codes that correspond to outpatient visits include 99201-99205 (new patients) and 99211-99215 (established patients). The "billing web" below summarizes the defining criteria of each code, based on the E&M guidelines, and serves as a "cheat sheet" you may use to remember the criteria for established outpatient visits.

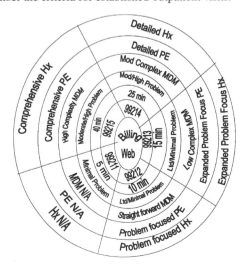

31. Because specific components are required to be documented for each level of visit, must a NP or other provider use a standardized documentation format to ensure each criteria is met?

No—there is no mandated format. However, the record must be legible and complete. It must clearly identify the date of service and the health care provider seeing the patient. The note may be in "SOAP" format, a checklist, or any combination of styles as long as all necessary components are addressed. The documentation should be adequate to support the selected diagnosis, the visit level, and any further procedures or diagnostics.

Support of bills/claims is only one purpose for the clinical record. Use a format that allows you to track your patients' problems, response to care, and preventive health needs and documents the standard of care. You may need to develop a record format that allows easy incorporation of information into a major database. Make sure that your format also complies with the expectation of third-party payors.

32. Can NPs bill only for certain level visits?

NPs can bill for any level of visit/care that they are educated, trained, and licensed to perform. There is no limit to the level of visit as long as the documentation supports the charges and they are reasonable and medically necessary.

33. Do the recommendations specify what level of history and physical exam should be performed and documented based on specific complaints or illnesses?

No. The guidelines leave the level of examination and history to the clinician's discretion/clinical judgment.

34. Is a particular provider or practice expected to submit bills that are relatively uniform in billing level (i.e., consistently at level 3 or 4)?

No. In fact, third-party payors expect to see somewhat of a "bell curve" in billing, with the more moderate levels documented most often and the lower and higher levels less frequently.

35. Why would a bill be rejected by a payor?

There are many reasons, including failure to document an ICD-9 or CPT code, lack of agreement between the documented ICD-9 and CPT code, or failure to provide adequate information about the provider. Sometimes the payor simply makes an error. It is important to follow-up promptly on any rejected or questioned claims.

36. How can I ensure that I am meeting the guidelines related to billing and reimbursement?

It is recommended that each practice develop an individualized compliance plan that best suits its needs and facilitates self-monitoring while allowing timely and appropriate response to any identified concerns. The basic components of a compliance plan include establishment of the following elements:

- Internal auditing system
- Standards and procedures specific to the practice
- Compliance officer within the practice to oversee the plan
- Education of all employees about the compliance plan
- Prompt responses to any detected offenses with appropriate corrective actions
- Open lines of communication
- Standards enforcement

37. What should be monitored during the compliance audit?

The major concerns that should be addressed include determining whether services provided were reasonable and necessary and whether the documentation supports the codes on the HCFA 1500 billing form. During the audit, billing should be specifically scrutinized in relation to the following major risk areas:

- Billing for services not provided
- Billing for services that were not medically necessary
- Submitting duplicate bills
- Clustering billing codes (i.e., choosing mid-level codes consistently)
- Upcoding

38. If a compliance plan is in place, does it relieve me of responsibility?

Even when a compliance plan is in place, each provider should examine his or her documentation, performing self-appraisal. When comparing the billing with the medical record, an individual provider can look at the same items that would be determined by an auditor. Some of the items that should be addressed include the following:

- Is the record complete and legible?
- Does it include the necessary components? (Examples include reason for contact, history, examination and tests, assessment and diagnosis, and treatment plans, among others.)
- Does it identify the provider and date of care?
- Does it include the rationale for diagnostics or testing?
- Does it note past and present diagnoses or problems?
- Does it identify risk factors?
- Does it identify the appropriate ICD-9 and CPT codes?

BIBLIOGRAPHY

1. American Medical Association: Current Procedural Terminology: CPT 1999. Chicago, AMA, 1999.
2. American Medical Association: Principles of CPT Coding. Chicago, AMA, 1999.
3. Artz C: Physician compliance plan risk areas. Physician's news digest. Available on-line: URL: http://www.physiciansnews.com/law/1200artz.html (accessed August 2000).
4. Buppert C: Avoiding medicare fraud: Part 1. Nurse Pract 26(1):70, 72–75, 2001.
5. Buppert C: Avoiding medicare fraud: Part 2. Nurse Pract 26 (2):34, 36–38, 41, 2001.
6. Buppert C: Reimbursement for nurse practitioner services. Nurse Pract 23(1):67, 70, 72–74, 76, 81, 1998.
7. Burke M: Overview of the OIG's MD compliance guidance. Physician's news digest. Available on-line: URL: http://www.physiciansnews.com/law/1200burke.html (accessed August 2001).
8. Health Care Financing Administration: Draft evaluation and management documentation guidelines (June 2000 with December revisions). Available on-line: URL: http://www.hcfa.gov/medlearn/2000emd2.doc (accessed August 2000).
9. Health Care Financing Administration: 1997 Documentation guidelines for evaluation and management services. Available on-line: URL: http://www.hcfa.gov/medicare/master1.wpd (accessed August 2001).
10. Moore K: Billing for NP services: What you need to know. Family practice management 1998. Available on-line: http://www.aafp.org/fpm/980500fm/billing.html.
11. Rapsilber L, Anderson E: Understanding the reimbursement process. Nurse Pract 25(5):36, 43, 46, 51–52, 54–56, 2000.
12. St. Anthony's Updatable ICD-0-CM Book for Physician Compliance. Reston, VA, St. Anthony Publishing, 1998.

3. REFERRALS AND CONSULTATIONS

Mary Jo Goolsby, EdD, MSN, APRN, ANP-C

1. What is the difference between a consultation and a referral?

A **consultation** is a request for direction or guidance on a diagnosis or treatment from another provider. In informal consultations, the request for guidance may be made during rounds, at a professional meeting, or by telephone/e-mail. In formal consultations, the patient is sent to the other provider for a more in-depth evaluation.

A **referral** is a request that another provider accept the ongoing treatment of a patient, at least in regard to one specific health problem. The terms are sometimes confused. Some providers use the term *referral* when scheduling a patient to visit another provider for assessment and guidance. However, a consultation does not imply the continued treatment that is part and parcel of a referral.

2. How do you determine who should be consulted for a specific problem?

First, you should determine what specialty or experience would best prepare a provider to answer your question, provide the desired service, or otherwise meet your patient's need. It is important that you select an appropriate consultant. Consultations with or referrals to inappropriate providers delay desired outcome, may result in unnecessary service, and can result in related problems.

3. When should a referral or consultation be sought?

There are many reasons for referrals and consultations. When you are uncomfortable with a patient's care, it is time to seek assistance through a consultation or referral. All providers must be able to recognize the need to involve other providers in the care of their patients and to do so at an appropriate time (i.e., before it is too late for the patient to derive the most benefit from the other provider's expertise).

4. What are the most common reasons for consultations and referrals?

- Advice (on a diagnosis or treatment, for medicolegal reasons)
- Specialized skill (nonsurgical technical procedure, surgery, mental health counseling, specialized medical treatment, failed conventional treatment)
- Patient or third-party request (by patients or specialist, for insurance guidelines)

5. Is it acceptable to ask other providers to provide a consultation on an informal basis?

Yes. Many providers are happy to provide direction or share their opinion and consider it an opportunity to provide professional development for their colleagues. Informal consultations are quite common and are often called "curbside consults."

6. What sort of problems is best suited to informal consultation?

The topic of an informal consultion should be a well-defined, well-focused problem so that the consultant can respond briefly but adequately. If you ask a question that is too broad, the consultant probably will suggest that you arrange a formal consultation. It is important to pose a "good question."

7. What constitutes a good question to ask of a consultant?

The question should ask the consultant's advice or opinion about a diagnosis, prognosis, or treatment. It must include adequate detail on which an opinion can be based. For example, you may inform the consultant of a specific laboratory or physical finding, supply a brief description of the patient, and ask the related diagnosis or prognosis. An example of a poorly worded, inadequate question is "Should I put my patient with diabetes on an angiotensin-converting enzyme inhibitor?" Alternatively you could ask: "I am treating a 36 year old with type 2 diabetes who has had good control on oral agents, with a hemoglobin A_{IC} of 7–7.5. He has recently had mild elevations of blood pressure. Should I consider using an ACE inhibitor as the initial antihypertensive therapy?" The consultant has adequate information to consider responding to the second question.

8. What is the procedure for a formal consultation?
The consultant should be supplied with all relevant information about the patient and the problem of concern, including:
- Name and age
- Summary of the current problem
- Related health history
- List of medications
- Summary of pertinent family and social history
- Summary of related physical findings
- Results of any diagnostic studies
- Results of previous consultations
- Clear specification of the problem that you wish to have evaluated/treated
- Urgency of the information
- Specifics about the patient's preferences and values

9. Is there a specific format by which a consultation should be transmitted?
No specific form is universally used. Some practices with computerized records are able to automate the consultation process somewhat, using relational databases to import standardized information into a request, supplemented as the provider sees fit. Others include a cover letter, with copies of recent records, that specifies the service sought. Regardless of the format, the consultant should be provided with hard copies of all necessary information. Although urgent requests for consultation can be made over the phone, written materials should be provided by mail, courier, or fax or, when necessary, hand-carried by the patient.

10. Why is the detail supplied to a consultant so important?
The consultant requires adequate information on which to determine how to approach the problem. By supplying adequate details and records, the provider avoids unnecessary duplication of effort, needless tests, or adverse reaction. Duplication is not only redundant but also wastes time, energy, and financial resources. Failure of the consulting provider to provide adequate detail is a common complaint from consultants.

11. Is there a recommended method through which the consultant should respond?
The consultant should convey promptly the findings and/or recommendations to the referring provider. Even when you receive the information over the phone, a written report should follow. Failure of the consultant to provide written feedback is a common complaint of primary care providers.

12. What specific information should be received in the consultant's formal report?
The more clearly your consultation request is written, the more detailed and applicable the consultant's response is likely to be. Ideally, the written report should include:
- Statement of the purpose of the consultation, as understood by the consultant
- Findings of the consultant's history and physical exam
- Results of any diagnostic studies
- Any treatment provided

• Patient's response to any treatment
• Consultant's diagnosis or assessment of the problem
• Any further treatment recommended
• Any consultations recommended
• Statement about the urgency of any recommendations
• Summary of any instructions or guidance given to the patient
• Statement about whether the consultation is considered to be completed or any plans to see the patient in the future

13. What is the patient's role in a consultation or referral?

The patient should be involved in the initial decisions about the consultation or referral. A frequent reason for incomplete consultation is the patient's belief that the consultation was not needed. The patient must understand the purpose of the consultation and be satisfied with the consultant chosen. The patient should be informed of any procedures anticipated during the consultation and any expected costs. Once the patient has agreed to the consultation or referral, he or she should agree to share relevant information with the consultant. On occasion, the patient may be asked to hand-carry certain records.

14. What is the typical turn-around time for a consultation?

The period between the time that the need for a consultation is recognized and the patient is seen by the consultant varies. It depends on many factors, including the availability of the needed specialty, any third-party procedures required, and clinic scheduling procedures. You should have your staff inform you if there is going to be a delay in fulfilling a consultation; as you may need to contact the consultant personally to expedite evaluation or treatment. Personal contact with consultants has been shown to minimize the turnaround time.

15. How do the procedures differ for a referral?

The procedures for requesting a referral are similar to those requesting a consultation. The accepting physician should be supplied with the same details, including pertinent history of current and previous health problem(s), medications, family, and social history. Copies of records such as pertinent diagnostic studies and previous consultations should be provided. The referral should clearly state the problem to be addressed, with a clear request that the receiving provider assume responsibility for care related to that problem.

16. What documentation should I expect after a referral?

The accepting provider should provide the same type of information that is expected after a consultation, including adequate detail to ensure the referring provider that his or her request was understood, the accepting provider's assessment of the problem, the details on which the assessment is based, and plans for further evaluation or care. The accepting provider/specialist should make any recommendations for further follow-up that he or she believes the referring provider should pursue as part of the overall primary care management of the patient.

17. What should I do if a patient specifically requests a consultation with another provider?

If you have not detected a reason for referral or consultation, you should seriously explore the patient's reason for the request. A request for a consultation or referral may indicate problems that the patient has not shared, symptoms that have not been identified, or recent changes in known problems. Something may have happened to trigger concern about the patient's health. Sometimes a discussion with the patient identifies the need for further diagnostic studies. At other times, they may identify patient misconceptions that can be corrected. You should provide the patient with an honest assessment of the situation, whether a consultation or referral is appropriate, and, if so, which type of consultant can best meet the identified needs. When a patient desires a consultation, it is generally advisable to follow through with the request.

18. What about the patient who continues to request consultations with specialists, even after all initial problems have been addressed?

Some patients persist in desiring consultations, even after the provider is comfortable that all necessary consultations have been made and that access to care has been adequate. In this case, you should share your perception with the patient and consider whether there is some problem with the relationship between you and your patient. At this point, it may be necessary to refer the patient to another provider for ongoing care or to obtain one last consultation in which another provider reviews all previous efforts and determines whether he or she agrees with your assessment and assessments of the other providers. You should reflect carefully on whether your consultations have been appropriate and the patient's complaint and/or condition adequately evaluated and/or treated. Consider the role of any emotional disturbances that may require attention and are responsible for the patient's request. Requests may result from anxiety, depression, or other disturbances.

19. What are the specific responsibilities of a primary care provider in coordinating the care of patients during the consultative or referral process?

During consultations or referrals to specialists, the primary care provider must take care to coordinate the patient's care. When several providers are involved in a specific patient's care, coordination can be complex. The primary care provider must document not only the care activities that he or she provides but also any communications with the specialist(s). A system must be identified through which patients' movement across settings can be tracked so that they do not "fall through the cracks."

20. What is the rationale for having the primary care provider assume responsibility for coordinating the patient's care when multiple providers are involved?

Close coordination is necessary to avoid delays in treatment, iatrogenic morbidity, and risk of litigation.

BIBLIOGRAPHY

1. Bergus G, Randall C, Sinift S, Rosenthal D: Does the structure of clinical questions affect the outcome of curbside consultations with specialty colleagues? Arch Fam Med 9:541–547, 2000.
2. Borowitz X, Wyatt J: The origin, content, and workload of email consultations. JAMA 280:1321–1324, 1998.
3. Keating N, Zaslavsky A, Ayania J: Physicians' experiences and beliefs regarding informal consultations. JAMA 280:900–904, 1998.
4. Kuo D, Gifford D, Stein M: Curbside consultation practices and attitudes among primary care physicians and medical subspecialists. JAMA 280:905–909, 1998.
5. Royal College of Physicians and Surgeons of Canada and College of Family Physicians of Canada: Guiding Principles in the Referral Consultation Process. 1996. Available on-line: URL: http://www.rcpsc.medical.org (accessed August 2001).
6. University of Iowa. FPInfo: Email consult service. Available on-line: URL: http://fpinfo.medicine.uiowa.edu/ecstutorial/htm (accessed August 2001).

II. Diagnostic Issues

4. DEMYSTIFYING RADIOLOGY

Rodney W. Hicks, MSN, RN, FNP, CS, CCRN

1. What is the purpose of radiology?

The purpose of radiology is the evaluation of bones and soft tissue to support the diagnostic evaluation of patient care. Radiology complements the history, physical examination, and other diagnostic tests in reaching a diagnosis.

2. What general considerations relate to radiologic exams?

When considering whether to select specific radiologic exams, you should take into account the complexity and severity of the patient's illness or injury and compare the potential benefits, costs, and risks. Consider the degree to which the test will help to narrow the differential diagnosis or to confirm specific findings/diagnosis. Consider the financial and time costs associated with the study and how they will be offset by savings in arriving at a diagnosis in a more timely manner or in savings or decreased risks associated with more focused and accurate diagnosis and treatment.

Once you decide to proceed with a specific study, the local radiology department will provide a practitioner guide to help ensure that you properly prepare the patient for the exam. This manual should include the required patient preparation (e.g., when and what medicines to hold or give, whether oral ingestion is permitted, whether the patient has a full or empty bladder), scheduling procedure, and result reporting guidelines. As a courtesy, you may inform your patient that many exams require complete disrobing. Shielding clients of reproductive age offers protection from scatter radiation.

3. What are the most common radiology exams with which I should be familiar?

Your ordering of exams depends on patient presentation and practice guidelines. The most common radiology exam types are as follows:

- **Plain films**: films that vary by density and anatomic location. Common examples are chest x-rays and bony structures in extremities.
- **Fluoroscopy**: the technique that allows real-time visualization. An example is the intravenous pyelogram looking at renal structures.
- **Angiography**: imaging of the vascular system.
- **Computed tomography (CT)**: cross-sectional slice radiographs of the body such as head, abdomen, or chest.
- **Ultrasound**: recording of the reflection of sound against organs and structures, such as an obstetric and gallbladder ultrasound.
- **Magnetic resonance imaging (MRI)**: enhanced scanning to produce images from multiple planes or axis, especially in areas of soft tissue. Examples include brain and spine.
- **Radioisotope scanning**: visualization of specific organs or tissue, such as bone or lung perfusion scans.
- **Bone densitometry**: an accurate means of measuring bone mass and predicting risk of fracture.

4. Why do I have to fill out a lengthy requisition to get a simple x-ray?

Requisitions serve many functions. *All* diagnostic tests must have a purpose. The Health Care Financing Administration (HCFA) requires that all tests be relevant to the patient's condition.

Completion of the requisition gives the clinician time to think about what type of study is needed and what will be gained from the study. The requisition communicates patient's age, sex, and coexisting medical conditions to the radiology technologist who performs the exam and to the radiologist who interprets the final film. Both are valuable consultants in your delivery of patient care and rely on your judgment and the information you supply.

5. What major factors should be considered in the selection of specific radiology tests?

You should consider the purpose of the particular exam (what are you looking for?), the anatomy/structure of which you wish to have an image, and the radiodensity of the structure when deciding on the positioning and alignment that will provide the desired image. Once you receive the image, you should practice a systematic approach to studying the image and consideration of recommended follow-up studies or consultations/referrals.

6. What are the anatomic considerations?

You should review normal gross anatomy from calvaria to phalanges (head to toe) and be familiar with all bony structures and organs in the area that you plan to x-ray. Radiographic examination of the body is concerned primarily with internal anatomy and secondarily with physiology of that region. The body is divided along imaginary planes that describe central locations and show the relationship of body parts.

Anatomic Landmarks

Planes

Sagittal	Vertical plane from front to back, creating right and left portions
Midsagittal	Vertical plane through midline, creating equal right and left portions
Transverse	Horizontal plane passing through body at a right angle to sagittal plane
Coronal	Vertical plane dividing body into anterior and posterior portions

Relative positions

Anterior (ventral)	Forward or front part of body part
Posterior (dorsal)	Back part of the body part
Inferior	Direction below a point of reference
Superior	Direction above a point of reference
Medial	Direction toward the median plane
Lateral	Direction away from the median plane
Proximal	Point closest to the origin
Distal	Point furthest from the origin
Plantar	Posterior (bottom) surface, generally related to the foot
Dorsum	Anterior surface (top), generally relates to the foot
Palmar	Palm side of the hand
Ipsilateral	Same side of the body part
Contralateral	Opposite side of the body part

7. What variables are to be considered in selecting specific imaging views?

The radiology technician takes into consideration the patient position (as well as the patient's medical condition), the projection (the path of the central ray indicating the entrance and exit points of the x-ray beam), and the intensity of the x-ray beam to produce the image. Views are used to describe the patient's placement with both entrance and exit points of the central ray that are not otherwise defined. Schematically, it may look as follows:

(Anatomy) + position + projection + view = findings

ANATOMY	POSITION	PROJECTION	VIEW

Part examined	Erect
	  Upright or standing
	Recumbent
	  A reclining position
	Supine
	  Lying on back
		AP (anterior to posterior):
		  from front to back
		PA (posterior to anterior):
		  from back to front
			Lateral: named by the side
			  closest to the image
			  receptor
			Oblique: a patient rotation
			  somewhere between
			  frontal and lateral position
			Decubitus: a patient is
			  recumbent when the
			  radiograph is taken with
			  a horizontal beam

8. What determines the visibility of a radiologic image?

The guiding principle of radiodensity determines what you see on the image. The less dense the object is, the darker in color it will be on the film. Therefore, air is less dense (blacker) and bone is more dense (whiter). Organs, soft tissue, and body fluid have varying densities and often appear gray on plain films.

9. How many views are necessary for adequate information from plain film?

Plain films produce single-dimension pictures of multidimensional structures. Having more than one picture (view) of the structure is essential. Multiple views increase the chance of capturing abnormalities. At a minimum, the examination should include at least two projections, taken at right angles to one another. If a joint is involved, then at least three projects are warranted. A common principle is that *one view is no view*.

10. Once I have a radiologic image, how should I go about studying it?

A systematic approach must be used. A one-glance, quick view may miss subtle changes. Picture the patient mentally; sometimes a physical representation is helpful. What complaint or problem led you to order this x-ray? What were your physical exam findings? With these issues in mind, approach the x-ray view box. Always match the x-ray by name, sex, and age of the patient. Now position the x-ray in the proper position on your viewbox because you are examining it as you would examine your patient.

Structures generally have smooth margins or borders. Disruption of the smoothness may indicate pathology. Disruption on a bone, may be a fracture. Whenever possible, compare the affected area with the unaffected area. This approach may require additional films known as **comparison views**. Alignment is often useful in judging symmetry.

11. What are the most common plain film views in a chest x-ray?

The projection for chest x-rays varies. They may be PA projection (most common) along with a lateral view. In some instances, a portable chest x-ray (AP view) is taken. Less common but still important are the lateral decubitus, oblique chest, and dorsal decubitus positions.

12. What should I expect to see on the PA chest x-ray film?

- Lung apices
- Aortic arch
- Cardiac silhouette
- Costophrenic angles
- Clavicles
- Trachea (air-filled)
- Hilum
- Air bubble in stomach
- Scapulae
- Vertebral bodies
- Pulmonary markings
- Hemidiaphragms

13. What are the recommended steps in viewing a PA chest x-ray?

Using a systematic process, consider each of the following "normal" findings:

- **Rotation**: the sternoclavicular joints should be equidistant from vertebral column and form a cross. The distance between the vertebral column to the outer rib cage should be equal on each side.

- **Inspiration** should be sufficient to identify at least 10 ribs, and both costophrenic angles should be seen on the films.
- **Cardiac diameter** is less than half the distance across the chest at the widest point.
- **Hilar markings** are vascular marking passing from the mediastinum to the lungs.
- **Lung markings** are normal and extend to the edge of the film. Absent markings may indicate serious pathology.
- A **gastric bubble** is often seen on the left, confirming that the right diaphragm is slightly higher than the left.

14. In comparison with the PA view, what should be seen in the lateral film?

The lateral chest demonstrates anatomy of lungs, heart, great vessels, mediastinum, and presence of chest lesions. It is shot 90° from the PA film and shows a different view of the same anatomy (see above).

15. What pathologic findings may be seen on chest x-rays?

- **Pneumonia**: a bacterial or viral condition that may affect one or more pulmonary lobes. The findings are generally described as a consolidation by location (anatomic region). Follow-up or repeat x-rays often are done to document resolution or patient progress.
- **Emphysema**: a chronic disease resulting in overinflation of the lungs, which leads to the barrel chest phenomenon. Radiographic findings inlcude loss of lung markings and flattened diaphragm and may include increased air trapping.
- **Pneumothorax**: the presence of free air in the thoracic cavity, evidenced by a pleural line indicating that long tissue has been pulled away from the thoracic wall. There may be a loss of lung marking and a noticeable change in the density. A pneumothorax may cause a shift in the mediastinal architecture.
- **Congestive heart failure**: characterized by an enlarged heart silhouette and distinctive fissure markings between lung lobes. Follow-up or repeat x-rays often are done to document resolution or patient progress.
- **Pulmonary nodules**: round radiopaque shadows of various sizes that can occur anywhere in the lung fields, including on bony structures. They may be benign or metastatic. *All* pulmonary nodules require further evaluation, which generally is accomplished with CT of the chest.
- **Pleural effusions**: characterized by a fluid level that "blunts" or obscures the costophrenic angle. Effusions may be recognized more easily on the lateral decubitus view.
- **Tuberculosis**: a disease of the pulmonary system that often affects the apices of the chest. A lordotic view (which removes the clavicular shadows) highlights the apices.
- **Fracture** of any bony structure, such as ribs, sternum, clavicles, or scapulae. These bones are smooth, and disruption of smoothness indicates a fracture.

16. When should you order more than a plain film of the chest?

The answer depends, of course, on what you are evaluating and/or what the plain film images show. When evaluating a pulmonary nodule, you would probably order a chest CT next. If concerned about skeletal changes, you might request a bone scan. It is always appropriate to contact the radiologist by phone and request consultation and guidance regarding which diagnostic imaging studies are needed for a particular problem.

17. Discuss the practitioner's responsibility regarding structures seen on a film that are not related to the presenting problem.

The radiologist and any other provider looking at a film has a responsibility to the patient to observe each structure carefully. For instance, when studying a chest x-ray ordered for hemoptysis, you must closely scrutinize not only the lungs themselves, but also all of the bony structures, which may demonstrate bone changes consistent with malignancy. Although you were not concerned primarily with the ribs or clavicles, they must be examined with the other structures.

18. What is the purpose of abdominal x-rays?

The purpose of ordering abdominal x-rays is to satisfy your concern about the organs and structures of the abdominopelvic cavity. Indications may include abdominal pain of any etiology, trauma, or foreign bodies. The plain radiograph also gives information about gas patterns, constipation, soft tissue shadows, and organ and skeletal structures. Generally, abdominal x-rays include the supine and upright view or an acute abdomen series.

Specialized views of abdominal x-rays may include contrast media for enhanced details. If contrast media is indicated, the practitioner must be familiar with allergies (especially to iodine), renal function tests (blood urea nitrogen and creatinine), and other co-existing diseases (e.g., diabetes, heart failure).

The CT scan is often used for appendicitis, renal calculi, diverticulosis, or aneurysms and when plain films are inadequate to confirm a diagnosis.

The intravenous pyelogram is generally used for renal evaluation of urine flow or obstruction.

Ultrasound is useful in evaluation of pelvic masses and gallbladder disease and for evaluation of pregnancy status.

19. What anatomic structures are seen on plain abdominal films?

Anatomy seen on the various abdomen x-rays includes bones (lower ribs, lumbar vertebral body, transverse and spinous processes of lumbar vertebra, iliac crests, or pelvis), organs (right and left hemidiaphragms, kidneys, stomach, bowel, liver, and spleen) and gas patterns. Bones are more dense and appear lighter on the films. Organs are often evident as various shades of grey, and only portions of their margins may be easily visualized. If the structure of interest is not distinct on the plain film, you may consider a study with contrast—for instance, a barium enema or contrast-enhanced CT scan.

20. How do I determine which of the available views to select?

- The supine/kidneys-ureters-bladder (KUB) view is an AP projection valuable for visualizing abdominal masses, calcifications, foreign bodies, and obstruction.
- The upright AP view is most valuable for demonstrating free intraperitoneal air and air-fluid levels.
- The lateral decubitus position is valuable for air-fluid levels.
- The acute abdomen series includes supine and upright abdominal views and a chest x-ray.

21. How should I study a set of abdominal films?

Use a systematic approach:

1. Alignment is adequate when the iliac crests are on the same horizontal plane and the spinous processes of the vertebral bodies are in the center of the film.

2. Look first at bony structures for any abnormalities: first the vertebrae, then the ribs, and finally the pelvis.

3. Examine soft tissues in each of the abdominal quadrants, beginning with the upper left quadrant and moving across. Note border irregularities, masses, fat lines, calcification, or shift in placement. A prominent gastric (stomach) bubble should be easily identified.

4. Examine the colon for distention or dilation. The causes may be excessive feces or excessive air.

22. What are common reasons for ordering plain films of the extremities?

The purpose for most x-rays involving the upper extremity is trauma, seeking evidence of fracture, sprain, or dislocation. Films are often ordered for postoperative evaluations of appliances. Other reasons include joint diseases such as arthritis, gout, bone degeneration, or localization of foreign bodies.

23. What anatomic structures are visible in extremity films?

The structures depend on what portion of the upper extremity is requested. Your requisition should specify for what reason the imaging study is requested to ensure that the placement is adequate to visualize the structures of interest. Films of a long bone, such as the radius, or region, such as the forearm, routinely include both distal and proximal joints to ensure that a complete image of the long bone or region is included. When the structure of interest also includes one of the joints, it is important to order those views specifically, because the views provided as part of a long bone film are inadequate to assess the joint carefully.

24. How should I study films of extremities?

Begin with projection (which is generally anterior to posterior), then position (generally oblique with corresponding lateral views). Use a systematic approach to analyze the smoothness of the bone. Tracing the bone cortex into the bony shadow helps to isolate interruption of the continuity. There may be subtle (nondisplaced) or obvious radiolucent (displaced) fracture lines.

25. What are common reasons for ordering plain films of the spine?

The primary purposes for obtaining radiographic examination of the spine are trauma and degenerative disease. Films should be ordered in an appropriate setting (e.g., trauma should be evaluated in an emergency care facility). An outpatient setting may be appropriate for evaluation of degenerative diseases of the spine (e.g., osteoarthritis), ankylosing spondylitis, compression fractures, and spondylolisthesis.

26. What structures are seen on plain films of the spine?

Various structures are evident on spine films, depending on the level at which the film is taken. For instance, in cervical films, a portion of the skull is visible as well as the trachea and first two ribs. In lumbar films, portions of the pelvis and the lowermost ribs are visible. A certain number of vertebral bodies from the group just above or below the region of interest also are visible but not with the quality that they should be used diagnostically. You should be familiar with the basic structural differences in vertebral bodies by region as well as the anticipated spacing of vertebrae and their relationship to one another.

27. I need additional assessment of the bony structures/orthopedic system. What exams should I order? Why?

The skeletal system is composed of multiple joints. Disruption of the function of a joint (muscle, tendon, or ligament) requires an emphasis on the soft tissue structures. An MRI is usually ordered, although it is common to order a plain film first and follow up with an MRI. If the concern is a potential stress fracture, a bone scan may be required.

Similarly, decisions about subsequent studies must be individualized for assessing neck and back complaints. For instance, if plain films are either equivocal or positive after trauma, CT is the next appropriate image. A helpful set of guidelines for the section of radiologic studies can be found at the American College of Radiologists site listed below. Again, when in doubt about the specific type of study that will be most efficient and cost-effective in identifying the problem and have the best risk-to-benefit ratio, you should consult a radiologist. Alternatively, if the patient will be referred to an orthopedist or neurologist, the specialist may be consulted about which, if any, other diagnostic studies would be helpful at the time of the initial consultation.

28. List electronic resources that further understanding of radiology.

The world-wide web has brought many resources to your fingertips. Many prominent universities have published teaching files that are available through your browser. The purpose of these teaching files is to introduce you to the concepts of viewing films and working through case studies.

Sites may change their address. Become familiar with key search words (e.g., radiology).
• http://www.urmc.rochester.edu/smd/rad/
• http://www.rad.washington.edu/

- http://www.radiology.co.uk/xrayfile/xray/indes.htm
- http://www.vh.org/Providers/Lectures/icmrad/Opening.htm
- http://www.mamc.amedd.army.mil/WILLIAMS/index1.htm
- http://www.radiology.com/edures1a.htm
- www.octet.com/~mikety/list.html (Cases of Michael Tobin, M.D.)
- www.indyrad.iupui.edu (Indiana University)
- www.omed.pitt.edu (University of Pittsburgh)
- www.rad.washington.edu (University of Washington Department of Radiology)
- www.sbu.ac.uk (South Bank University, United Kingdom)
- http://sprojects.mmip.mcgill.ca/radiology (radiologic anatomy)
- http://gentili.net (A. Gentili, UCLA Department of Radiological Sciences)
- http://www.acr.org (American College of Radiologists)

BIBLIOGRAPHY

1. American College of Radiology: The ACR Appropriateness Criteria. Available on-line: http://www.acr.org/cgi-bin/fr?tmpl:appcrit,pdf:introduction.pdf (accessed September 2001).
2. Greathouse JS: Delmar's Radiographic Positioning and Procedures. Albany, NY, Delmar Publishers, 1998.
3. Novelline RA: Squire's Fundamentals of Radiology, 5th ed. Cambridge, MA, Harvard University Press, 1997.
4. Rothenberg MA: Understanding X-rays. A Plain English Approach. Eau Claire, WI, Professional Education Systems, 1998.

5. CARDIOVASCULAR DIAGNOSTIC STUDIES

Laurie Grubbs, PhD, ARNP, ANP

1. What are the uses and limitations of electrocardiography (EKG)?

Uses:
- Assistance in diagnosing coronary artery disease (CAD), particularly in the case of acute myocardial infarction (MI)
- Detection of hypertrophy of the chambers of the heart
- Assistance in detecting electrolyte imbalance
- Detection of rhythm disturbances

Limitations:
- Cannot evaluate cardiac function
- Cannot detect congestive heart failure
- Cannot by itself rule heart disease in or out
- Cannot determine the etiology of shortness of breath
- A normal EKG does not exclude heart disease; an abnormal EKG alone does not establish heart disease
- Cannot by itself determine cardiac status
- Does not substitute for clinical evaluation

EKG as a screening tool in asymptomatic clients yields little useful information. EKGs are done routinely as a preoperative screen but usually are not useful in detecting silent heart disease. Nonspecific ST-T–wave changes do not predict silent heart disease. If a client has chest pain and ST-segment elevation, suspect MI; if the client has chest pain and new-onset ST-segment depression, suspect unstable angina.

2. What parameters should be evaluated on the EKG and what are their reference values?

PARAMETER	REFERENCE VALUE*
Rate	60–100 beats per minute; may be lower in patients taking beta blockers or athletes.
Rhythm	P-P and R-R intervals should be regular; the exception is sinus arrhythmia.
P wave	Regularity and configuration. Absence of P waves may indicate atrial fibrillation or an idioventricular rhythm.
P-R interval	0.12 –0.20 seconds, measured from the beginning of the P wave to the beginning of the QRS. Prolongation of the P-R interval indicates a conduction delay producing first-, second-, or third-degree heart block. A shortened P-R interval is seen in Wolff-Parkinson-White and Lown-Ganong-Levine syndromes.
QRS duration	0.08–0.12 seconds. A wide QRS is seen in conduction delays in the ventricles (i.e., bundle-branch blocks and complete heart block) and in ventricular ectopic beats such as premature ventricular contraction (PVC).
QT interval	Should be < 0.05 seconds. Prolongation may result in syncope and sudden death.
QRS complex	The amplitude of the R wave is decreased in myocardial infarction due to altered depolarization and in pericardial effusion.
S-T segment	Should be isoelectric. Myocardial injury causes elevations in the S-T segment in the leads that reflect the area of injury and reciprocal S-T depression in the leads opposite from the area of infarct.

(Table continued on next page.)

PARAMETER	REFERENCE VALUE*
T wave	Configuration should be upright. Myocardial ischemia, injury, and necrosis cause inversion of the T wave due to altered repolarization. Hyperventilation also may cause flipped T waves.
Q wave	Represents death (infarction) of the muscle and is due to the absence of depolarization current from dead tissue. A pathologic Q wave measures > 0.04 seconds and is $> \frac{1}{3}$ the height of the QRS.

* Each small block on the EKG represents 0.04 seconds; each large block represents 0.20 seconds.

3. How is axis determined on an EKG?

Axis can be determined using the Hexaxial Reference Wheel. There are four axis quadrants: right axis, left axis, normal axis and "no man's land." Axis is determined by looking at whether the QRS complex is positive or negative in leads I and aVF. In right axis, the QRS in lead I is negative, and the QRS in lead aVF is positive. In left axis, lead I is positive and lead aVF is negative. In normal axis, leads I and aVF are positive (between 0° and 90°). In "no man's land," leads I and aVF are negative.

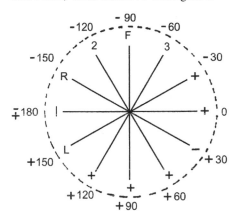

Hexaxial reference wheel.

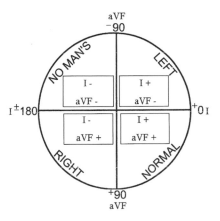

Axis quadrants.

4. What causes left axis deviation?
- Normal variation
- High diaphragm (pregnancy, ascites, tumors)
- Left anterior hemiblock
- Left bundle-branch block
- Congenital lesions
- Wolff-Parkinson-White syndrome
- Emphysema
- Right ventricular paced or ectopic rhythms

5. What causes right axis deviation?
- Normal variation
- Emphysema
- Right ventricular hypertrophy
- Right bundle-branch block
- Left posterior hemiblock
- Dextrocardia
- Left ventricular ectopic rhythms
- Wolff-Parkinson-White syndrome

6. When the axis is not "normal" or deviated in either the left or right quadrant, what is its significance?
- Ventricular ectopic rhythms
- Right ventricular paced rhythms
- Less common: multiple myocardial infarctions and cardiomyopathies

7. How is the area of injury determined from an EKG?
- The lateral wall is reflected in leads I, aVL, V_5, V_6.
- The inferior wall is reflected in leads II, III, aVF.
- The anterior wall is reflected in leads V_1, V_2, V_3, V_4.
- The posterior wall is reflected in leads V_1, V_2, V_3. Reciprocal EKG changes can be seen in the area of the heart opposite the injured area.

8. Which areas of the heart are affected by blockage in specific coronary arteries?

1. Blockage in the right coronary artery (RCA) results in damage to the posterior/inferior area of the heart. Blockage in the left main coronary artery (LCA) results in damage to the atrial, apical, lateral, and septal areas and is usually fatal.

2. Blockage in the left anterior descending artery (LAD) results in damage to the anterior portion of the heart.

3. Blockage in the circumflex branch (CFX) results in damage to the posterior and lateral areas.

9. How often should a routine EKG be ordered?

On healthy clients under the age of 40, routine EKGs give little information. Preparticipation sports physical exams may require an EKG, although routine EKG may not show typical causes of sudden death in athletes except in the case of idiopathic hypertrophic subaortic stenosis (IHSS).

In clients between the ages of 40 and 50 years or preoperative clients, it is prudent to get a baseline EKG to have as a reference for future comparison. In asymptomatic clients over 50 years, EKGs may be helpful in detecting abnormal rhythms and conduction delays, all of which occur more commonly in this age group. In the absence of ischemia, however, impending MI is not detected by routine EKG.

10. Other than for suspected MI, when should a diagnostic EKG be ordered?

An EKG should be performed on clients who complain of chest pain with activity or at rest, dyspnea on exertion, shortness of breath, palpitations, irregular heart rate, syncope, weakness, or dizziness.

11. What is the significance of a prolonged QT interval?

There are two types of prolonged QT syndrome. One is idiopathic and is thought to be caused by pathology of the sympathetic nervous system. It is characterized by recurrent syncope, a long QT interval (usually 0.5–0.7 seconds), ventricular arrhythmias, and sudden death. The familial syndrome is characterized by deafness, syncope, and sudden death.

The second type is acquired and is due to the use of antiarrhythmic agents or antidepressant drugs, electrolyte abnormalities, myocardial ischemia, or significant bradycardia. Anti arrhythmic agents that prolong the QT interval for > 0.5 seconds should be discontinued.

12. What factors determine ordering a 12-lead vs. a limb-lead EKG?

A limb-lead EKG, commonly called a rhythm strip, can be used to detect arrhythmias. For other purposes, a 12-lead EKG should be ordered.

13. When should a graded exercise test (GXT) be ordered?

A GXT should be ordered for clients with new-onset angina or suspected angina, especially if they have any cardiovascular risk factors such as age > 50 years, hyperlipidemia, history of smoking, family history of CAD, diabetes, obesity, hypertension, sedentary lifestyle, or hostile behavioral attributes.

In clients older than 50 years with any two cardiovascular risk factors, especially diabetes, smoking, hyperlipidemia, or severe hypertension, a GXT is prudent even in the absence of any anginal complaints.

For complaints of exertional angina, a GXT is reasonable and helpful. If a client complains of chest pain at rest, an emergency department visit rather than a GXT is warranted. Pain at rest signifies either unstable angina or MI.

As a screening test for asymptomatic and low-risk clients wanting to start an exercise program, positive yield is low and is used mostly to reassure clients. In a client with more than two risk factors, a preexercise GXT is advised.

14. What is the clinical significance of ordering a nuclear GXT?

A nuclear stress test is useful if the baseline EKG is abnormal (ST-segment depression, left ventricular hypertrophy, left bundle-branch block) and is commonly used to determine ischemia, which appears as a perfusion defect, and to determine ejection fraction. Nuclear stress testing is helpful in distinguishing transient ischemia from infarction. Cardiolyte or dual isotope imaging with cardiolyte and thallium are used most often because of greater accuracy and fewer false positives. Because nuclear tests carry a significant additional cost, they should be reserved for situations in which ordinary exercise testing is not indicated or needs confirmation.

15. What other imaging modalities are used?

Radionuclide angiography (RNA) is usually performed at rest and provides measurement of ventricular ejection fraction to assist in prognosis, especially after MI. The RNA is helpful in determining left ventricular function.

Echocardiography (ECHO) is the old stand-by for determining ventricular size, function, and wall thickness. It also provides information about valvular function. There are several choices, including M-mode, two-dimensional, Doppler ultrasound, transesophageal, and stress echocardiography. Stress ECHO is not widely used because of difficulty in obtaining accurate imaging results when the client is exercising.

Cardiac magnetic resonance imaging (MRI) provides excellent anatomic definition for assessment of pericardial disease, cardiac neoplastic disease, myocardial wall thickness, chamber size, congenital heart defects, and dissection of the aorta. It provides high resolution without radiation exposure or use of contrast media. MRI is not commonly used and not recommended for acute chest pain because it does not give information about coronary artery disease.

Heart catheterization is used for assessing valvular function and coronary artery blood flow for diagnostic and interventional procedures such as angioplasty, stent placement, and other techniques of clot ablation.

Electrophysiologic testing is useful for detection and treatment of significant arrhythmias and for evaluating recurrent unexplained syncope.

Computed tomography (CT) scan uses high temporal resolution and gives assessments of cardiac structure and function. It is not commonly used in hospitalized clients.

Ultrafast CT is advertised by and performed in mobile units to detect calcium in the coronary arteries. Clients targeted for this test are older than 60 years. The problem is that most clients older than 60 years have *some* calcium in the coronary arteries, even in the absence of significant CAD, thus giving a high rate of false-positive results. It is not a particularly useful test and is not recommended for determining CAD.

16. What is the best method for imaging the heart?

There is no "best" method for imaging the heart. The method depends on the suspected problem and the information necessary for diagnosis and prompt, appropriate treatment. For suspected CAD, GXT and/or nuclear GXT is the best place to start. For valvular heart disease, ECHO is an inexpensive, noninvasive starting point. If there are questions or dilemmas about the appropriate test, a referral to the cardiologist may be the best option. It may be more cost-effective for the cardiologist to determine which testing is appropriate.

17. What is a nonstress test?

A nonstress test is used for clients who cannot exercise on a treadmill because of physical limitations such as paraplegia, hemiplegia, multiple sclerosis, Parkinson's disease, arthritis, orthopedic problems, or other musculoskeletal/neurologic diseases. Dipyridamole (Persantine) and adenosine are used to cause vasodilation and introduce differential flow as if the client were exercising. The nonstress test has a lower sensitivity and specificity compared with nuclear testing but is recommended if no other diagnostic choices are available. Stress tests can be performed with the patient doing only arm exercises if the walking stress test cannot be performed and yield better results than a nonstress test. Exercise testing, from a diagnostic standpoint, is always preferable.

18. What serum laboratory studies are helpful in evaluating cardiovascular health?

Helpful laboratory studies include complete blood count, electrolytes, glucose, lipids, and renal function tests. To determine the presence of MI, a troponin level and/or MB-creatine phosphokinase (CPK) should be ordered. Both the CPK and troponin levels rise 4–6 hours after injury, but the troponin level stays elevated much longer (up to 4–7 days). If the client had pain 3 days ago, it may be more helpful to order a troponin rather than a CPK test. Troponin levels also may be slightly elevated in unstable angina. The downside of a troponin level is that it is not quantitative and, therefore, cannot determine the size or severity of myocardial damage. A normal MB-CPK or troponin level does not rule out MI if the test is done in less than 4–6 hours after injury.

19. How are lab tests interpreted?

Complete blood count: important in evaluating anemia, which, if severe and long-standing, can put stress on the heart resulting in ventricular hypertrophy.

Electrolytes: important for proper functioning of the electrical conduction pathways in the heart.

- Potassium: Hypokalemia can cause electrical instability and increased automaticity, which may result in ventricular arrhythmias. EKG changes consistent with hypokalemia are the appearance of a U wave and T-U fusion, which can be confused with a prolonged Q-T. Excessive diuresis is the most common cause. Hyperkalemia can cause cardiac depression, ventricular arrhythmias, and asystole. EKG changes seen are peaked T waves, QRS widening, and disappearance of the P wave. Excessive potassium supplementation is the most common cause.
- Calcium: its main role is in contractility. Hypocalcemia results in decreased contractility of the heart and a prolonged S-T segment. Hypercalcemia results in increased contractility and a shortened S-T segment.
- Sodium: its main role is in fluid volume regulation. An imbalance can be a contributing factor in congestive heart failure and dehydration.

Glucose: diabetes is a significant risk factor for cardiovascular disease, and maintenance of normal blood glucose levels can decrease the lifetime risk of developing coronary heart disease.

Lipids: elevated cholesterol, particularly elevated low-density lipoprotein (LDL), is an independent risk factor for cardiovascular disease. Lipid-lowering drugs have been shown to decrease cardiovascular morbidity and mortality.

Renal function tests: important in maintenance of normal blood pressure and fluid and electrolyte balance.

MB-CPK: indicative of cardiac muscle injury. Levels elevate 4–6 hours after MI.

Troponin level: slightly more sensitive for cardiac muscle injury but only qualitative, not quantitative.

20. What medicines affect the EKG?

Many medicines can affect the EKG, particularly the antiarrhythmics and digitalis preparations (e.g., quinidine, ethmozine, pronestyl [all three are rarely used]), diltiazem (Cardizem), isoptin, verapamil (Calan), and diuretics (which may decrease potassium).

21. What is a tilt-table test? When is it indicated?

A tilt-table test is used to evaluate recurrent syncope when no associated heart, neurologic, or endocrine disease can be found. Syncope can be neurocardiogenic in origin, mediated by excessive vagal stimulation or an imbalance between sympathetic and parasympathetic autonomic activity. In a standing position, venous pooling in the legs causes a subsequent increase in heart rate and vasoconstriction. In some clients, instead of the normal response, a sympathetically mediated increase in myocardial contractility activates receptors to trigger reflexive bradycardia and vasodilation. The result is a sudden drop in blood pressure, which leads to syncopal episodes. Head-up tilt-table testing can identify such clients. Tilting the table to at least 70° for 10–40 minutes induces hypotension and syncope in approximately one-third of patients with recurrent syncope. Treatment includes beta blockers and educating clients to maintain sodium and fluid intake.

22. Should a Holter monitor be ordered whenever an irregular heart rate is detected?

Most people have occasional ectopic beats, whether it be with activity or at rest. If the irregular rate is detected by EKG and found to be benign and the client is asymptomatic, Holter monitoring is not necessary.

23. What are the indications for Holter monitoring?

Holter monitors are worn continuously for at least 24 hours. Clients complaining of palpitations or irregular heart beats that cannot be captured by EKG in the office should wear a Holter monitor. Usually the palpitations are found to be benign in nature, but bursts of supraventricular tachycardia, atrial fibrillation, atrial flutter, bigeminy, trigeminy, and ventricular tachycardia may be discovered. For a recording that lasts up to 1 month, an event recorder is the correct diagnostic method.

24. Which noninvasive studies are used for the evaluation of peripheral vascular disease?

The ankle-brachial index (ABI) is currently the easiest, least expensive, noninvasive method for diagnosing peripheral vascular disease (PVD) and is particularly helpful in the office and home settings. The ABI is obtained by the following steps:

1. Obtain brachial systolic pressure
2. Use Doppler stethoscope to obtain systolic pressure in the dorsalis pedis or posterior tibialis vessel.
3. Divide ankle pressure by brachial pressure.
4. The index should be 1.00 or higher. If it is less than 0.5, impairment to blood flow is significant. An abnormal ABI indicates the need for a vascular consult.

ABI may be falsely elevated in diabetic patients because calcification of the vessels raises the pressure, especially in the ankle.

Doppler ultrasound is the other widely used noninvasive test for evaluation of PVD. Arteriography is the next choice, but it is invasive and requires inpatient postprocedural monitoring.

25. When should ambulatory blood pressure monitoring be ordered?

Ambulatory blood pressure monitoring should be recommended for all clients taking antihypertensive medication and all clients with borderline hypertension (blood pressure > 140/90 mmHg). Tight control of both systolic and diastolic hypertension significantly decreases coronary and cerebrovascular events. Ambulatory blood pressure may be helpful for "white-coat syndrome," but it is necessary to ascertain that the home blood pressure monitoring equipment is properly calibrated.

26. What controversies exist in cardiovascular diagnostics?

Cardiovascular diagnostic studies such as EKG, ECHO, or GXT for athletic clearance remain controversial. These tests have low yield in detecting future cardiovascular events in young athletes, except in the case of IHSS. IHSS is known to cause sudden death in young adults, especially during exercise. EKG changes include left ventricular hypertrophy and occasionally a septal Q wave in the absence of infarction. ECHO shows septal and ventricular hypertrophy.

Marfan's syndrome may be seen on ECHO with valvular changes but usually can be suspected with a good history and physical exam. Signs of Marfan's syndrome include tall, thin stature with long limbs; large narrow hands and narrow, flat feet; slender chest wall and pectus excavatum; narrow jaw and palate; abnormal joint flexibility; and usually heart murmur and/or aortic bruit.

Other causes of sudden death, such as coronary artery spasm and spontaneous arrhythmia, probably go undetected by routine cardiovascular diagnostics.

ACKNOWLEDGMENT

A special thanks to Dennis Williams, M.D., for his expert cardiology advice.

BIBLIOGRAPHY

1. Sokolow M, McIlroy MB: Clinical Cardiology, 6th ed. Los Altos, CA, Lange Medical Publications, 1996.
2. Tenenbaum A, Motro M, Fisman EZ, et al: Clinical impact of borderline and undiagnosed diabetes mellitus in patients with coronary artery disease. Am J Cardiol 86:1363–1366, 2000.
3. Tierney LM, McPhee SJ, Papadakis MA: Current Medical Diagnosis and Treatment, 38th ed. Stamford, CT, Appleton & Lange, 1999.
4. Vinsant MO, Spence MI: A Commonsense Approach to Coronary Care: A Program, 6th ed. St Louis, Mosby, 1994.

6. HEMATOLOGIC STUDIES

Theodore D. Scott, RN, MSN, FNP-C

1. How often should a patient have a routine complete blood count (CBC)?

Routine ordering of CBCs is not indicated in asymptomatic adults, but a CBC should be ordered when a specific condition, such as an infection or hematologic disorder, is suspected. Some individual blood tests are routinely indicated in certain patients, however—for example, hemoglobin or hematocrit determinations are recommended for pregnant women and high-risk infants. There are no current recommendations for healthy adults to have a CBC as part of a routine, preadmission, or preoperative physical exam if little or no blood loss is anticipated.

2. What are the indications for ordering red blood cell studies?

Red blood cell studies (RBC count, hemoglobin, hematocrit, and indices) are indicated in the diagnosis and management of acute blood loss, anemias, and hemoglobinopathies (thalassemia, sickle cell disease).

3. What are the normal values for standard red blood studies?

The **RBC count** measures the number or RBCs per cubic milliliter of blood. The average adult count is 4.3–5.9 million per cubic milliliter for males and 3.5–5.5 million for females. Because of variation in laboratory methodologies, you should refer to the normal values reported by your testing lab.

The **hemoglobin (HGB) level** is reported as grams per deciliter and correlates to the oxygen-carrying capability of the blood. The normal range is 14–18 gm/dl for adult males and 12–16 gm/dl for adult females.

Hematocrit (HCT) is expressed as the percentage of the blood that is made up of the packed red blood cells. Normal ranges are 42–52% for males and 37–47% for females.

For pediatric patients, the normal values vary significantly with the age of the patient. The laboratory doing the testing should provide the normal value for pediatric patients, which depend on the method used.

4. What is the significance of the RBC indices?

The RBC indices are useful in the evaluation of anemias, polycythemia, and other hematologic and nutritional disorders. Depending on the method used by the laboratory, the indices are either measured directly or calculated from the RBC, HGB, and HCT values.

Mean cell volume (MCV) indicates average size of individual RBCs. Normal range (normocytic) is 76–96 femtoliters. The MCV is increased (macrocytic) in megaloblastic anemias (vitamin B_{12} deficiency, folate deficiency) and liver disease (alcohol abuse) and by some drugs (e.g., zidovudine). The MCV is decreased (microcytic) in iron deficiency anemia, defects in porphyrin synthesis (lead poisoning), and hemolytic anemias and after splenectomy

Mean cellular hemoglobin concentration (MCHC) indicates the average amount of hemoglobin in each deciliter of RBCs. The normal range (normochromic) is 27–32 grams per deciliter of RBCs. The MCHC is rarely increased (hyperchromic) but is decreased (hypochromic) in iron deficiency anemia, defects in porphyrin synthesis (lead poisoning), and hemolytic anemias.

Mean cell hemoglobin (MCH) indicates the average amount of hemoglobin in each RBC expressed as picograms. The normal range is 30–35 picograms. MCH is of little use clinically. Values of the MCH parallel those of MCV.

5. What CBC values are indicative of anemias?

The primary screening tests for amenias are measurements of hemoglobin concentration and hematocrit. In adult men, anemia is defined as an HGB level < 13 gm/dl or HCT < 41%. For adult females, an HGB < 12 gm/dl or HCT < 36% indicates anemia. For pediatric patients, anemia is defined as HGB or HCT levels below the normal range based on age.

6. What is the significance of the reticulocyte count?

The reticulocyte count indicates the percent of newly maturing red blood cells released from the bone marrow. The study determines the percent of circulating RBC that still have remnants of endothelial reticulum, which the RBC loses as it matures. The normal range is 0.5–1.5% in adults and children.

The reticulocyte count is elevated in hemolytic anemia (as the body tries to replace loss), hemolysis or acute blood loss, response to anemia treatments (e.g., iron, folic acid, vitamin B_{12}), and bone marrow disorders (immature RBCs are displaced by other proliferating cells). The reticulocyte count is decresed in aplastic anemia (bone marrow has shut down production of all cell types), poisonings and toxins, drug therapy, and disorders of red blood cell maturation (e.g., iron deficiency anemias).

7. If the red cell studies are abnormal, what further diagnostic studies are indicated?

Follow-up testing is usually determined by the classification of the type of anemia based on indices. The following tests are indicated based on the classification of the anemia:

Microcytic, hypochromic anemia ($\downarrow$MCV, $\downarrow$MCHC)
• Serum iron and total iron binding capacity (TIBC)
• Serum ferritin

Normocytic, normochromic anemia (normal MCV, MCHC)
• Reticulocyte count (if reticulocyte count is low, consider referral; bone marrow studies may be required [i.e., aplastic anemia], and/or hemoglobin electrophoresis)
• Direct Coomb's test (autoimmune hemolysis)

Macrocytic anemia ($\uparrow$MCV, normal MCHC)
• Serum vitamin B_{12} (B_{12} deficiency)
• Serum folate (folate deficiency)

Consultation with a hematologist is recommended if a frank anemia is detected *without* an easily explained physiologic reason (e.g., iron deficient diet, recent blood loss, occult gastrointestinal bleeding, or medication therapy that may produce anemia as a side effect).

8. What are the indications for ordering a white blood cell count? When should you request a differential?

The white blood cell (WBC) count is useful in the diagnosis and management of infection, inflammatory disorders, bone marrow disorders and the body's response to drugs and toxins. It is indicated when one of these conditions is suspected and for monitoring the patient's response to treatment. A differential is indicated when the relative or absolute numbers of each of the WBC types are needed. Most labs automatically perform a differential when the WBC is abnormal. Conversely, most labs require a separate request for a WBC differential if the WBC count is normal.

9. What is the clinical significance of the WBC differential?

The WBC differential gives the relative percentages of the various lines of WBCs and is usually based on the first 100 WBCs found on a blood smear. The relative relationships between the major WBC types (granulocytes, lymphocytes, and monocytes) can be indicative of different states of health or some disease processes. The differential is reported as percentages of cells present. To calculate the absolute count, multiply the percent by the WBC count (for example, WBC count = 8,600/cubic milliliter, eosinophils = 2%, absolute eosinophil count = $8600 \times .02 = 172$/cubic milliliter).

10. What are the normal values for the WBC count and differential?

In adults, the normal WBC count is 4.5–11.0 thousand per cubic milliliter. As with RBC values, the normal values for pediatric patients vary with the age of the patient. For the differential, the normal value for each cell line is given below, with the most common reasons for increased or decreased percentages.

Granulocytes

• Neutrophils (polymorphonuclear [PMNs] or segmented [segs]): 50–70%; and band neutrophils (immature forms of neutrophils, "bands"): 0–5%. Increased in acute bacterial infections, some viral infections, parasitic infections; acute inflammation (acute rheumatoid arthritis, rheumatic fever); myelocytic leukemias. Decreased in some bacterial infections (typhoid, paratyphoid, gram-negative septicemia), viral infections (hepatitis, mononucleosis), and overwhelming bacterial infections of any kind.

• Eosinophils: 1–5%. Increased in parasitic infections (malaria, trichinosis, ascariasis), allergic diseases (asthma, allergic rhinitis), and skin diseases (eczema, atopic dermatitis, urticaria).

• Basophils: 0–1%. Increased in chronic hypersensitivity reactions (foods, drugs, inhalants), myeloproliferative disorders (polycythemia vera, chronic granulocytic leukemia).

Lymphocytes: 20–40%. Increased in viral infections (hepatitis, infectious mononucleosis, cytomegalovirus, herpes zoster), lymphocytic leukemias, some bacterial infections (pertussis, brucellosis). Decreased in immunodeficiency disorders, corticosteroid therapy, debilitating diseases (lupus erythematosus, Hodgkin lymphoma).

Monocytes: 1–6%. Increased in bacterial infections (tuberculosis, syphilis, subacute bacterial endocarditis), viral infections (hepatitis, mumps), monocytic or myelomonocytic leukemias.

11. What is the meaning of the term "shift to the left" or "left shift"?

A shift to the left indicates an elevated WBC count and a relative increase in segmented and band neutrophils. Clinically, it indicates that the body is responding to an acute need before the neutrophils can fully mature in the bone marrow. Left shifts usually are seen in acute bacterial infections such as acute sepsis or appendicitis. The term originated from the Shilling hemogram, which charted the maturation of the granulocytes from the least mature (blasts) on the left to most mature (segmented neutrophils) on the right. A line was drawn between the band neutrophils and segmented neutrophils to represent the border between the bone marrow and the circulating blood. When the body releases immature cells into the circulation (i.e., in response to an infection), there is an increase of cells in the circulating blood from the left of the line ("left shift"). In the early hand devices for counting cells in a differential, the keys were lined up in this fashion so that technicians had to move their hand to the left to hit the keys for the more immature granulocytes.

12. What are the indications for ordering a platelet count?

Platelet counts are usually ordered when a bleeding disorder is suspected, when patients present with petechia or purpura, or when patients with leukemia are monitored. Platelet counts are not routinely ordered as part of preadmission or preoperative studies, unless clinically indicted by physical exam or history. Platelet counts are almost always reported as part of an automated CBC.

13. What is the clinical significance of the platelet count?

The platelet count in normal adults should be between 150,000 and 400,000 per cubic milliliter. Platelet counts below 20,000 to 50,000 per cubic milliliter can cause spontaneous bleeding; the patient may present with petechia, epistaxis, or gingival bleeding. The most common causes of decreased platelet counts are as follows:

• Decreased production (aplastic anemia, radiation and chemotherapy, leukemias)
• Increased destruction (idiopathic thrombocytopenic purpura, systemic lupus erythematosus [SLE], infectious mononucleosis)

• Coagulation disorders (disseminated intravascular coagulation, septicemia, eclampsia)
The most common causes of increased platelet counts are as follows:
• Myeloproliferative disorders (leukemias)
• Polycythemia vera
• Splenectomy

14. When is it appropriate to order a prothrombin or partial thromboplastin time?
Prothrombin time (PT) and partial thromboplastin time (PTT) are used to monitor antico-agulant therapy and to evaluate coagulation disorders. These tests are not routinely ordered for preoperative screening in asymptomatic adults unless the patient has s specific clinical indica-tion (e.g., family history of bleeding disorder, active bleeding, liver disease, malnutrition).
PT: normal value is 10–13 seconds. The time of a pooled normal human serum control is reported as the normal value for the laboratory's method. PT is prolonged in oral anticoagu-lant therapy (warfarin), defects of the extrinsic coagulation pathway (factors I, II, V, VII, and X), liver disease (hepatitis, cirrhosis, poisoning), and inadequate dietary vitamin K.
PTT, also known as activated partial thromboplastin time (aPTT): normal range is 20–34 seconds. PTT is prolonged in heparin therapy, defects of the intrinsic coagulation pathways (factors I, II, V, VIII, IX, X, XI, and XII) (hemophilia A is deficiency of factor VIII, hemo-philia B is deficiency of factor IX), and circulating inhibitors of clotting factors (i.e., lupus an-ticoagulant in SLE).

15. Should you order an international normalized ratio (INR) when ordering a PT?
Yes—if you are monitoring a patient on oral anticoagulant therapy. The INR corrects for the differences in method and control serums used in PT testing. Without calculating the INR, comparing PT results from lab to lab or even week to week is like comparing apples to or-anges. It has become standard practice for all labs to report INRs along with PT results. The therapeutic range of INR in orally anticoagulated patients is 2.0–3.0. (2.5–3.5 in patients with artificial heart valves).

BIBLIOGRAPHY

1. Bakerman P, Strausbauch P: Bakerman's ABC's of Interpretive Laboratory Data, 3rd ed. Myrtle Beach, SC, Interpretive Lab Data, 1994.
2. Guide to Clinical Preventive Services: Report of the US Preventive Services Task Force, 2nd ed. Baltimore, Williams & Wilkins, 1996.
3. Lee G, Foester J, Lukens J, et al: Wintrobe's Clinical Hematology, 10th ed. Baltimore, Williams & Wilkins, 1998.
4. Tabas GH, Vanek MS: Is 'routine' laboratory testing a thing of the past? Current recommendations re-garding screening. Postgrad Med 105:213–220, 1999.

7. SERUM CHEMISTRIES

Donna F. Haynes, PhD, RN, CS, WHNP, FNP

1. When is it advisable to order a profile instead of an individual test?

In most laboratories, a profile is less expensive than selecting multiple individual tests. Frequently, when a patient's lab status is followed, multiple values need to be assessed. For instance, in assessing a diabetic client, it is important to measure fasting blood sugar as well as the blood urea nitrogen (BUN) and creatinine. In this case, the clinician should order a chemistry profile.

When the clinician is following a specific lab value after an intervention, it is appropriate to order the individual test. For example, potassium level should be obtained after prescribing supplements in a patient with hypokalemia. The potassium level is less expensive than the complete chemistry panel.

2. How often should I routinely order electrolyte tests?

There is no established recommendation for routine monitoring of electrolytes. The frequency depends entirely on the client's diagnosis, status, and medications. Certainly, when a client is undergoing frequent medication changes or is critically ill with many medical problems, such as renal insufficiency and/or congestive heart failure (CHF), the frequency is greater than for a client on routine medications for hypertension. In the acute stage of illness, electrolytes may be ordered as often as every 6 hours to monitor potassium levels after IV potassium supplementation. In hospitalized patients with CHF who undergo aggressive diuresis and inotropic management electrolytes with BUN and creatinine should be ordered daily. After the patient is discharged home, electrolytes may be ordered weekly until the patient's condition is stabilized and then every 4–6 weeks.

3. What is the clinical significance of the various proteins measured with lab studies?

Proteins make up about 75% of the body's solid mass and are important in the transport of amino acids, vitamins, hormones, and lipids. Proteins regulate osmotic pressure, tissue maintenance and repair, and the body's buffering system. Routinely measured values include total protein, albumin, globulin, and albumin-to-globulin ratio. Electrophoresis studies also are performed. Serum proteins are altered in malnutrition, renal disease, liver disease, connective tissue disorders, and hemorrhagic diseases. Patients with severe allergies have decreased gammaglobulins, such as IgG, IgA, IgM, IgD, and IgE antibodies.

Disease Entities and Abnormal Protein Results

DISEASE	ABNORMAL LAB	SIGNS
Cirrhosis	↓ Albumin	Ascites
	↓ Total protein	Edema
	↓ Vitamin K	Bleeding
	Abnormal liver function tests:	Bruising
	↑ Bilirubin	
Chronic renal failure	↓ Albumin	Edema
	↑ BUN/Creatinine	Uremia
	↑ Potassium	Arrhythmias if potassium significantly increased
Allergies	↓ IgE	Hayfever
	↓ IgM	Rashes
	↓ IgG	Urticaria
	↓ IgA	Hives

4. What studies are routinely considered to be tests of liver function?

Liver function tests consist of alanine aminotransferas (ALT), alkaline phosphatase (ALP), aspartate aminotransferase (AST), bilirubin (total, direct, and indirect), gamma-glutamyl tranferase/transpeptidase (SGGT/GGTP), lactate dehydrogenease (LDH), and protein electrophoresis. Other liver function tests specific to the disease process include hepatitis profiles.

5. What is the clinical significance of liver function studies?

Abnormal liver function tests can be attributed to multiple causes. It is the practitioner's responsibility to determine the underlying pathology related to these tests and the client's physical findings. When patients are symptomatic, it is easier to determine the cause of abnormal lab tests because the patient's symptoms help guide the practitioner in deciding which specific laboratory and/or diagnostic tests need to be ordered.

Clinical Significance of Liver Function Tests

SYMPTOMS	DIAGNOSIS	ABNORMAL LAB. VALUES
Right upper quadrant pain penetrating into right shoulder Nausea Fever with or without jaundice Fatty food intolerance	Cholescystitis with or without obstruction	↑ Lipase ↑ Amylase ↑ Bilirubin Normal ammonia
Nausea/vomiting Right upper quadrant or diffuse abdominal pain with or without ethanol history Clay-colored stools	Pancreatitis	↑ Amylase ↑ Lipase ↑ Alkaline phosphatase Normal liver function tests (unless due to obstruction)
Jaundice Ascites with or without confusion Nausea/anorexia	Cirrhosis	↑↑ Liver function tests ↑↑ Ammonia ↑ Total bilirubin
Nausea/vomiting Anorexia Fever Diarrhea	Hepatitis	↑ Liver function tests Abnormal hepatitis series

6. When a patient's liver function tests are abnormal, what further studies are warranted?

When a patient has abnormal liver function tests and is completely asymptomatic, the first avenue to pursue is personal medication history. History of prescription medications as well as all over-the-counter medications and herb usage should be ellicted from the patient. Although many patients may feel reluctant to disclose use of herbal remedies, many herbs are hepatotoxic, including several of the popular weight loss formulas currently used in the United States. Acetaminophen is one of the key medications that may contribute to abnormal liver function tests. All of the statin medications are hepatotoxic, and routine liver function monitoring should be performed as described above.

If medication-induced hepatitis is unlikely, further investigation into other causes, such as viral infections, biliary disease processes, and alcohol, should be pursued.

7. When should a hepatitis panel be considered?

Hepatitis panels should be ordered in suspected viral infections. The table below summarizes the results found in the three most common types of hepatitis.

Hepatitis

TYPE	A	B	C
Early	Anti-HAV + Total anti-HAV + (infectious)	HbeAg +	Anti-HCV + ALT ↑
Acute	Anti-HAV + Total anti-HAV + (infectious)	HbeAg + HbsAg + Anti-HBc IgM + Anti-Hbe + (infectious)	Anti-HCV + (false-negatives) RIBA + confirms
Recovery	Total anti-HAV +	Anti-HBc + Anti-Hbe + Anti-HBs + (infectivity unknown)	
Immune	Total anti-HAV +	Anti-Hbc + Anti-Hbe + Anti-Hbs +	
Carrier	NA	HbsAg + Anti-HBc total + Anti-Hbe + can be HbeAg +	Anti-HCV + RIBA + ALT ↑

HbsAg = hepatitis B surface antigen, Anti-Hbc = total antibody to hepatitis B core antigen, Anti-HbcIGM = IGM antibody to hepatitis B core antigen, HbeAg = hepatitis B e antigen, Anti-Hbe = antibody to hepatitis B e antigen, Anti-Hbs = antibody to hepatitis B surface antigen, Anti-HAV = total antibody to hepatitis A virus, Anti-HAV IgM = IgM antibody to hepatitis A virus, Anti-Hd = antibody to hepatitis D virus, ALT = alanine aminotransferase, Anti-HACV = antibody to hepatitis C, RIBA = recombinant immunoblot assay (potentially infectious), HCV RNA test confirms hepatitis C but is expensive and not used much.

8. What studies help to assess jaundice?

Symptomatic patients with an abnormal liver function test may have associated jaundice. The chart below summarizes the abnormal tests involved with the specific types of jaundice.

Specific Laboratory Values in Jaundice

	TYPES OF JAUNDICE		
	HEMOLYTIC	HEPATOCELLULAR (CIRRHOSIS)	OBSTRUCTIVE (BILIARY STONES AND/OR TUMORS)
RBCs	↓	N	N
Unconjugated bilirubin	↑		
Urobilinogen	↑	↑	↓
Total bilirubin	↑↑	↑	↑↑
AST, ALT, SGGT	N	↑↑	↑
Alkaline phosphotase	N	N	↑
Ammonia	N	↑↑	N

AST = aspartate aminotransferase, ALT = alanine aminotransferase, SGGT = serum gamma-glutamyl transferase.

9. Which patients are candidates for lipid profiles?

The practitioner should keep risk factor analysis in mind in trying to determine when a lipoprotein analysis is indicated. The National Heart, Lung, and Blood Institute (NHLBI) expert panel recommends that total cholesterol (with high-density lipoprotein [HDL], if available), be measured every 5 years for all persons over 20 years old. According to the U.S. Preventive Services Task Force and the U.S. Department of Health and Human Services, routine cholesterol screening in persons with normal values should be performed every 5 years, beginning at the age of 18. This initial lab sample can be drawn regardless of time of day or fasting status. Any patient with a total cholesterol ≥ 200 mg/dl should have a complete lipid panel analysis after at least a 9-hour fasting period (8–12 hours is optimal). In patients with two or more risk factors, a complete lipoprotein analysis should be performed routinely. In determining the type of cholesterol measure to order and in interpreting the lipid profile results, the practitioner should stratify the patient's risk for cardiovascular disease. The risk factors identified by the Second Report of the Expert Panel on Detection, Evaluation and Treatment of High Blood Cholesterol in Adults are as follows:

1. Male > 45 yr or female > 55 yr of age or menopausal without hormone replacement therapy
2. Smoker
3. Hypertension
4. HDL cholesterol < 35 mg/dl
5. Diabetes
6. Primary relative with premature heart disease

10. What are the key elements of lipid profiles?

Lipid panels should be ordered with the patient fasting for at least 12 hours before the test is performed. The ideal amount of time is 16 hours. The key elements are total cholesterol, triglycerides, LDL, HDL, very low-density lipoproteins (VLDL), and HDL-to-LDL ratios. The LDL level is the most important level for determining risk for cardiovascular disease.

11. What does the cholesterol ratio indicate?

The ratio of total cholesterol to HDL levels indicates risk for developing coronary artery disease:

$$Ratio = Total\ Cholesterol/HDL$$

For example, a client with a total cholesterol of 250 and a HDL of 25 has a ratio of 10. Another person may have a total cholesterol of 250 and a HDL of 80, which equate to a ratio of 3.1. The first person's risk is almost tenfold that of the second person, if all the other risk factors are the same. Ratios are useful in the determination of risk as long as LDL is the final determining factor for risk and intervention stratification.

12. What are the recommendations for LDL levels?

LDL (mg/dl)	> 2 RISK FACTORS	RECOMMENDATIONS
< 130	NA	1. Lipid panel in 5 years 2. Nutritional counseling 3. Increase exercise 4. Smoking cessation
130–159	No	1. Annual lipid panel 2. Educate as above
> 160	Yes	1. Clinical work-up 2. Risk education 3. Step I to step II diet 4. Add medication

Goals: known CAD: LDL < 100; no CAD but high risk: LDL < 130.

13. What should I know about ordering and interpreting thyroid function tests?

When a client complains of symptoms that may indicate thyroid disease, the clinician may want to order thyroid function tests. Currently Medicare will reimburse the patient only for assessment of thyroid-stimulating hormone (TSH) level when the clinician is screening for thyroid disease. If the client has an abnormal physical finding, such as thyroid nodules or a goiter, or prior diagnosis of thyroid disease, a panel may be ordered. TSH is the most specific screening tool in thyroid disease. If the TSH is abnormal or the client has abnormal physical findings, a complete thyroid profile should be ordered, including triiodothyronine (T_3), thyroxine (T_4), T_3 uptake, and free thyroxine index (FTI). Most laboratories have a specific profile that is much less expensive than the individual tests. Multiple medications and diseases either increase or decrease T_4 levels. Therefore, T_4 alone cannot exclude or diagnose thyroid disease without other thyroid function test abnormalities. T_4 is used to confirm hypo- or hyperthyroidism in combination with an abnormal TSH level.

14. How are specific thyroid tests interpreted?

See chart for interpretation of thyroid function tests.

Thyroid Function Tests

	TSH	T_4	T_3	T_3U
Hypothyroidism	↑	↓		↑
Hyperthyroidism	↓	↑	↑	↑
T_3 toxicosis	↑	N	↑	
Normal	N	N or ↑ or ↓	N	N

N = normal, ↑ = increased, ↓ = decreased, $T_3U = T_3$ uptake.
A patient taking estrogen can have increased T_4 and T_3 uptake due to increased thyroxine-binding globulin (TBG) production. However their TSH should be normal.

15. What are the indications for the measurement of blood levels of drugs or other potentially toxic substances?

Patients receiving medications that have a low therapeutic index, such as digoxin, often require serum drug levels. Therapeutic indexes are defined as a small range between toxicity and therapeutic levels. In other words, patients can quickly and easily become toxic with small change in the medication. The low therapeutic threshold requires close monitoring by the practitioner, and the patient should be made aware of the *first* symptoms of toxicity. The first symptom of digoxin toxicity is nausea and/or anorexia. The medications that require serum blood tests are easily found in the *Physician's Desk Reference* (PDR). These medications also require the practitioner to write "no substitution," because even the smallest variation between companies can cause blood levels to become either nontherapeutic or toxic.

16. If a patient's blood glucose is abnormal, should I automatically obtain a glucose tolerance test or hemoglobin A_{1C}?

Hemoglobin A_{1C} provides the patient's glucose levels over the past 8–12 weeks. It is the most accurate assessment of the average glucose levels and is crucial in considering changing dosage of insulin or oral hypoglycemic agents. The hemoglobin A_{1C} also aids the practitioner in determining patient compliance/adherence. The disadvantage of this test is the cost. The table below summarizes specific guidelines outlined by the American Diabetes Association.

Glucose tolerance tests are no longer readily used in diabetic clients. The hemoglobin (HGB) A_{1C} is the gold standard for following the diabetic client's progress.

Glucose tolerance tests are routinely used to diagnose gestational diabetes and to detect hypoglycemia. The glucose tolerance test is ordered in prenatal patients with an abnormal random glucose > 200 mg/dl.

17. How do you interpret the HGB A_{1C}?

An HGB A_{1C} of 7% is associated with an average glucose of 150 mg/dl. For each 1% increase in HGB A_{1C}, the glucose average is approximately 30 mg/dl higher. Rough estimates follow:

8% = 180	10% = 240	12% = 310	14% = 370
9% = 210	11% = 280	13% = 340	

18. How is the level of control determined by glucose and the HGB A_{1C}?

Blood Sugar Goals in Diabetes

Poor control	FBS: 180–380 mg/dl	HGB A_{1C} > 8%
Good control	FBS: 140 mg/dl	HGB A_{1C} < 7%
Excellent control	FBS: 80–110 mg/dl	HGB A_{1C} < 6%

FBS = fasting blood sugar.

19. What tests should be ordered when the client is anemic?

The determination of the cause of anemia is a step-wise process. A discussion of red blood cell indices and differentiating between macrocytic, normocytic, and microcytic anemias can be found in the preceding chapter. The table below summarizes the abnormalities that are noted in patients with the specific types of anemia and aids the practitioner in determining the cause of the anemia and recommendations for further diagnostic evaluation.

Common Anemias

IRON DEFICIENCY	THALASSEMIA	VITAMIN B_{12}, FOLATE, AND ALCOHOL	HEMOLYSIS AND AND GI BLEED
MCV < 80	MCV < 80	MCV > 80	MCV: normal
Retic index < 3	Retic index > 3		Retic index: > 3
Ferritin: Low	Ferritin: normal	Vitamin B_{12}: low	

MCV = mean corpuscular volume. Interventions are determined by the cause of the person's anemia.

20. Are there any current controversies about chemistry studies?

The most controversial issue in regard to laboratory chemistries involves the re-imbursement process from the insurance companies. Medicare depicts an exact diagnosis or International Classification of Disease (ICD) code for the clinician/laboratory to be reimbursed. It is highly recommended that the clinician become familiar with ICD codes. Patients may be responsible for the cost of studies that are not covered. Most importantly, however, the patient should be consulted in any decision-making process, regardless of their ability to afford the test. Tests that are indicated for the patient's health should be performed with the patient's consent. It is much less expensive to determine lipid status and treat undetected hyperlipidemia than it is to pay for a myocardial infarction and related disabilities.

BIBLIOGRAPHY

1. Cherneky C, Berger B: Laboratory Tests and Diagnostic Procedures, 2nd ed. Philadelphia, W.B. Saunders, 1997.
2. Eisenhauer L, Murphy M: Pharmacotherapeutics and Advanced Nursing Practice. New York, McGraw-Hill, 1998.
3. Ferri F: Clinical Advisor: Instant Diagnosis and Treatment. St. Louis, Mosby, 2000.
4. Hillis L, Firth B, Winniford M, Wilerson J: Manual of Clinical Problems in Cardiology, 5th ed. Boston, Little, Brown, 1995.
5. Mayo Clinic.com: Preventative Health Screening and Tests. Healthy Living Centers, 2001.
6. Nurse Practitioner Prescribing Reference: Spring 2001.
7. Tierney L, McPhee S, Papadakis M: Current Medical Diagnosis and Treatment, 37th ed. Stamford, CT, Appleton & Lange, 1998.

8. SPECIAL TECHNIQUES IN PELVIC EXAMS

Lori Settersten, PhD, RN, WHNP, C, FNP, BC

1. At what point during the physical examination is the pelvic exam performed?

Under the principle of progressing from less intimate to more intimate areas during the physical examination, most practitioners perform the majority of the examination before the pelvic exam. The practitioner can build rapport with the woman before conducting the pelvic exam. Some practitioners believe that women prefer to get the pelvic exam out of the way to decrease anxiety and do the pelvic exam first. Consider your rationale for why you do your physical examination in the order that you choose. Also consider asking female clients which order they prefer (i.e., pelvic exam first or last).

2. What are the options for pelvic examination position?

The position for a pelvic examination is usually dorsal lithotomy: the woman lies on her back with her knees bent and her heels fitted into the stirrups (foot rests). Most women are used to and prefer this position. Some women feel more in control in this position. They also have the opportunity to see what the practitioner is doing if they prefer. Women may prefer the semisitting position in combination with the dorsal lithotomy position: the head of the table is elevated to about 45–90°. In this position, the woman and the practitioner can make eye contact more easily.

Another option is the left lateral position: the woman lies on her left side with her right leg bent, her knee pointing upward at about a 90° angle from the table, and her foot placed on the table wherever comfortable. The stirrups are not usually used in this position, and the moveable foot end of the table is extended all of the way out. Some women feel less exposed in this position.

3. What concerns or fears do women commonly have before their first pelvic exam?

It is helpful to ask a woman what she has heard about the pelvic exam from others. Then you can address any myths or fears. Most often women have been told that it is going to be painful. Often they fear the unknown. You can explain the pelvic examination procedure and the sensations that the woman may feel (see the next question). You can clarify that she may feel some pressure sensations but that normally there should be no pain. You also can explain that most women, after having their first pelvic exam, say that it was not as bad as they thought.

Women may mention the "clamp thing" that they have heard about. You can explain that the speculum may look like a clamp but does not clamp onto anything. You can show her the speculum and how it works. You can explain that it helps to open the vagina gently and slowly so that you can see the cervix and collect any necessary tests (i.e., Pap smear and testing for sexually transmitted infections, as needed). Again, some pressure is usually felt, but normally the speculum exam should produce no pain.

4. What information should I provide before performing a woman's first pelvic exam?

It is important to explain what the pelvic examination consists of before conducting a woman's first pelvic exam. This explanation should include the steps of the pelvic exam as well as what the woman will feel during each step. It is also important to include the purpose for each of the components of the pelvic exam. The explanation may include the following:

1. "First, I will help you position yourself. You will need to slide down to the edge of the exam table. You can put your hands at the edge of the table so you can feel how far down you need to slide. Then I will help you place your heels on the foot rests."

2. "After I put on my gloves, I will ask you to let your legs fall back apart"; it is not recommended to say "spread your legs apart" because those words may have negative or sexual connotations. "Then I will examine around the outside of your vagina and the folds of tissue called the labia or lips. I will insert one finger into your vagina to check the glands (i.e., Bartholin's and Skene's) at the opening of your vagina."

3. "Next I will insert the speculum into your vagina to see the cervix and vagina. You might feel a little discomfort, sort of like a mild burning feeling, when the speculum slides into the vagina." When the speculum slides into the vagina, it may irritate the urethra, which is the tube that urine comes out of, located just above or in front of the vagina.

4. "This is what the speculum looks like (i.e., show the speculum). It is a little wider than a finger, but the worst part about it probably is the thought of something metal going into your vagina (if a metal speculum is used)." If a plastic speculum is used, you can say that the worst part about it probably is the thought of an instrument going into your vagina. If a plastic speculum is used, explain the clicking sounds that may be heard as the speculum is adjusted into place. Explain that only the blade of the speculum goes into the vagina. To help decrease any fear about the speculum, you can ask the woman to go ahead and touch the speculum after it has been warmed.

5. "Next I will do the Pap test as well as any testing for sexually transmitted diseases (if appropriate). You may feel a weird touching sensation during this testing." *Weird* is the most common word that women have used to describe the sensation while the Pap smear is collected. "Sometimes it may feel a little "pinchy" when the Pap test is done (depending on the type of specimen collection materials being used, such as a collection brush)." For the Pap test, explain that you will take a sample of cells from the cervix to be checked for abnormal cells. Inform her that the Pap test is done to screen for cervical cancer; however, point out that the Pap test is not diagnostic. If the Pap test is abnormal, other testing must be done to determine which type of abnormal cells are present and what method of treatment is necessary.

6. "After I have looked around in the vagina and on the cervix, I will remove the speculum."

7. "Finally, I will put two fingers into your vagina to make sure that the vagina, cervix, uterus, and ovaries feel normal. You will mostly feel pressure, sometimes deeper pressure, during this part of the pelvic exam." When the pelvic exam is completed, ask the woman to push back and sit up. Then ask her to take a deep breath, and congratulate her for making it through her first pelvic exam. Ask, "How was that experience for you?" Give her positive reinforcement for taking good care of herself.

5. When performing the first pelvic examination, particularly with a woman who is not sexually active, should I anticipate any findings that differ from the routine?

The hymen may or may not be intact even if a woman has never had sexual intercourse. Tampon use may have stretched the hymen open. If there has been limited or no previous sexual intercourse before the first pelvic exam and the hymen opening is narrow, a virginal speculum may be more comfortable for the pelvic exam. Advance the speculum slowly into the vagina according to the woman's comfort. You may need to delay the speculum exam until the hymen has been opened wider. The woman may use her finger at home to stretch the opening, or the hymen may be opened by future sexual intercourse or tampon use. You may be able to complete the bimanual exam even if you are unable to complete the speculum exam. Consider the woman's comfort level and risk for sexually transmitted infections, which is one of the main reasons to perform Pap smears on a regular basis. Human papilloma virus (HPV) has been associated with the majority of precancerous and cancerous lesions on the cervix.

Keep in mind that one finger inserted into the vagina may be more comfortable than two for the bimanual or internal exam. If you are not able to palpate the internal organs well enough with just one finger, you may keep your first finger in the vagina and insert your middle finger into the rectum. You should be able to feel the uterus, posterior cul-de-sac, and adnexal areas this way, if necessary.

6. Is there anything special that I should do with the speculum before using it for a pelvic exam?

The speculum should be warmed before use during a pelvic exam. Methods to warm the speculum include keeping speculums in a drawer of the exam table on top of a warming pad made especially for this use, running warm water over the speculum, or holding the speculum in your room hand (i.e., the hand that does not touch the client during the external genitalia and speculum exam) while you examine the external genitalia. The preferred method is the first.

7. How can a woman participate during her pelvic exam?

Be sure to give women explicit permission to ask questions. One way to do so is to ask specifically whether the woman has any questions about sexuality, orgasm, or sexual relations. By asking this specific question, you open the door for the woman to ask questions about sensitive topics and give her permission to ask other questions as well.

You may ask each woman if she would like to have someone with her during the pelvic examination to help allay anxiety or fear. This approach may be especially helpful for younger women or women having their first pelvic exams. Make sure that it is the woman's choice rather than coercion by the other person.

Each woman should have the opportunity to choose which position she prefers for the pelvic exam. She can choose whether she would like the head of the table flat or somewhat elevated. When elevating the head of the table, ask her after each adjustment if the position is comfortable for her or if she would like the head of the table elevated a little more.

It is important to help the woman remain in control of the situation as much as possible. Let the woman know that she may tell you to stop at any time if the pelvic exam becomes too uncomfortable. You must follow through and stop when requested to do so.

8. How can I help the woman who is particularly anxious about the examination?

It may be helpful to talk with her about the use of deep breathing techniques and mental imagery for relaxation as well as distraction. Breathing deeply and slowly helps the pelvic muscles to relax more and can decrease anxiety. In mental imagery, the woman can be asked to think about a place where she would like to be right now and to visualize being at that place in her mind. You can ask her questions about the place, such as, "What is it like to be in that place?", "How do you feel in that place?", and "What do you like about that place?" Distracting conversation may be just as helpful for relaxation and may be combined with informative explanations of the pelvic exam procedure. Humor is usually helpful for relieving tension and anxiety. Be careful, however, because humor may not be helpful for some women. You will need to use your instincts about people when considering which of the above techniques will be helpful for specific clients.

Although some women may prefer that you to do the exam without talking about it, most women want to hear about what you are doing. You can ask each woman if she would like you to tell her what you are doing as you go along. If a woman would like to hear about what you are doing and why, refer to question 4 for suggestions.

9. What else can I do to inform the woman who is particularly interested in learning about the examination and findings?

Ask each woman whether she would like to watch with a mirror while you perform the pelvic exam (i.e., the external genital inspection and speculum exam). Have the woman hold the mirror above and aimed at the external genitals. She can rest her forearm of the hand holding the mirror on her mid thigh on the side opposite to that from which you have the exam light focused. As you conduct the examination, explain with each step what you are looking at.

At the least, it is important to ask each woman if she would like to see her cervix and vagina. If she does, have her sit or lean up a little more on the table, resting on one elbow while her opposite hand holds the mirror. You will need to aim the exam light from below the speculum upward toward the upper blade of the speculum. The woman can hold the mirror a few inches immediately in front of and centered on the speculum to see her cervix and vagina. The cervix may be described either as a little bump with an opening in the middle or as doughnut-shaped bump.

Many women are interested in seeing their cervix and vagina. They can learn more about their bodies: what the cervix and vagina actually look like and what their functions are. On viewing their cervix and vagina, women often respond in a positive manner.

You may suggest to each woman, particularly one who has viewed her cervix and vagina, that she can feel her cervix at any time. Explain to her that it feels firm like the tip of her nose and that it is located about one finger length into her vagina.

10. In which situations is it especially important to ask a woman if she would like to see her external genitals, cervix, and/or vagina?

Women who are considering the use of a diaphragm for contraception or a pessary for urinary incontinence or uterine prolapse should be encouraged to see their cervix because they can see what they will be feeling for to ensure proper placement of these devices.

Women should be asked whether they would like to see abnormal examination findings, such as HPV lesions (i.e., venereal warts) on the external genitals, vagina, and/or cervix; molluscum contagiosum; folliculitis; and the erythema and excoriations associated with candidal vulvovaginal infections.

11. What else can I do to make the pelvic exam more comfortable for women?

When asking a woman to slide down to the edge of the table, you can ask her to feel for the edge of the table with her fingers so that she knows where it is located. You can let her know that sometimes if feels like her bottom is going to slide off the edge of the table, but this will not actually happen.

Remember to signal the woman before you start the pelvic exam. For example, let her know that you will be touching her on the thigh first, then on the labia or the lips, and so on. Always let her know what you will be doing before you do it. It is helpful to say the anatomic as well as the lay name of the body part that you are examining to help the woman learn more about her body and accurate descriptive terms.

Give the woman feedback after each part of the pelvic exam as well as a summary of your findings on completion of the exam. For example, when you finish examining the external genitalia, let her know that everything looks normal. When you finish with the speculum exam, let her know that her vagina and cervix look normal. Explain that the Pap smear will tell whether everything looks normal to the microscopic eye. Finally, when you are done with the bimanual exam, let her know that her uterus, tubes, and ovaries feel normal. Avoid using the phrase "feels good," which may be interpreted with sexual connotations.

12. How can I help to minimize the physical discomfort associated with the speculum examination?

One technique that is helpful for insertion of the speculum is to press down on the lower aspect of the vaginal introitus first with one finger; then add a second finger before inserting the speculum. This technique can help the pubococcygeus muscles to soften and relax in preparation for the insertion of the speculum. You also can explain to the woman that it makes the speculum exam more comfortable if she can soften or relax these muscles. Be specific in your feedback to women. For example, general "just relax" statements are usually not helpful and may lead to increased tenseness and anxiety about the speculum exam. Specific statements, such as "let these muscles soften or relax and sink down onto the table," are more helpful.

If a woman is having difficulty relaxing her vaginal muscles for a more comfortable insertion of the speculum, you can ask her first to tighten the muscles at the vaginal introitus and then relax them to help her know what it feels like to relax the muscles for the speculum exam. Also remember previous suggestions about the use of the relaxation and distraction techniques as well as humor.

13. What can I do if I have difficulty in locating a woman's cervix with the speculum?

If you have difficulty in finding a woman's cervix, first remove the speculum, and then insert your first finger into the vagina to locate the cervix with your finger. Then remove your finger and reinsert the speculum toward the direction in which you felt her cervix. Similarly, you may insert your finger further into a woman's vagina just after palpating the Skene's and Bartholin's glands to locate the cervix before you initially insert the speculum.

While you have the speculum open slightly, you also may look around and note where the smooth tissue of the cervix begins rather than where the rugated tissue of the vagina continues. Then close the speculum and reaim it toward the smooth tissue. You may need to move the speculum slightly from side to side or up and down while you open it slowly to coax the cervix into position at the end of the speculum.

It also may be helpful to have the woman slide down a little further toward you on the exam table so that her buttocks are slightly over the edge of the table. This positioning sometimes allows deeper insertion of the speculum.

Often women have a ridge of tissue in the posterior vagina. This ridge of tissue is usually located in the middle or anterior third of the posterior vagina. If you open the speculum and notice a ridge of tissue, close the speculum. Next, aim the speculum up and over that ridge of tissue; then continue in the usual downward and backward direction to locate the cervix.

14. Is there something I can do to visualize the cervix if the vaginal walls seem to fall inward, blocking the view?

Occasionally a woman's vaginal tissue may fold inward onto the speculum, making it difficult to view the cervix. In this setting, you should remove the speculum and slip either a cut glove or a cut condom over the speculum blades while the blades are closed. Then reinsert the speculum into the vagina with the cut glove or condom. The band of material around the speculum should help to keep the vaginal walls from closing around the speculum so that you can see the cervix better. However, because you cannot examine the vaginal walls with the cut glove or condom on the speculum, you need to examine the vaginal walls carefully while you are removing the speculum when you have finished your examination.

To prepare a cut glove, use a small or medium-sized glove. Cut off the finger portions so that a circular band remains. To prepare a cut condom, unroll a condom so that it is fully extended, then cut off the tip. Prepare a few of these cut gloves or condoms in advance and keep them handy, perhaps in one of the exam table drawers.

15. What can I do if I have difficulty in palpating a woman's cervix during the bimanual exam?

To locate a woman's cervix, you first need to place your own body in the most helpful position. You can place your foot (i.e., the foot on the same side of your body as the internal examining fingers) on the step of the examination table and brace the elbow of the internal examining hand on your ipsilateral hip to exert more pressure and push your fingers further into the vagina. While you are conducting the bimanual exam, be sure that your thumb and last two fingers stay off of the external genital area as much as possible. If you rest your thumb and last two fingers on the external genital area, they may block your first two fingers from reaching further into the vagina to palpate her cervix and uterus, or your thumb may accidentally press uncomfortably onto her clitoris. Instead, your thumb should be pointing away from the clitoris and toward the groin; your last two fingers should be folded over onto the palm of your hand. For practitioners with shorter fingers or for women who have longer vaginas, you can walk the two internal examining fingers along the anterior vaginal wall to bring the cervix closer to you while you put external pressure on the lower abdomen with the fingers of your other hand to press the uterus and cervix closer to your internal fingers.

16. What can I do if I have difficulty in palpating a woman's uterus during the bimanual exam?

To palpate a woman's uterus more easily, first locate her cervix. Then feel on either side of her cervix inward toward the uterus (i.e., into the lateral fornices) to palpate which direction her uterus is pointing. If her uterus seems to be pointing upward into the anteverted position, put two fingers on her cervix, and move her cervix upward and forward (i.e., in a forward C-shaped direction) to bring her uterus toward your internal fingers. Then put external pressure on her lower abdomen with your external fingers to push the uterus closer to your internal fingers. At this point, you will move your internal fingers into the anterior fornix, where you should now be able to feel the anterior aspect of the uterus, and determine whether there is some flexion in its position. If the uterus seems to be pointing downward (toward her back) into a retroverted position, put your two fingers on her cervix, and move her cervix downward and backward (i.e., in a backward C-shaped direction). This movement brings the uterus closer to where you will be moving your fingers next into the posterior fornix. Then put external pressure on her lower abdomen with your external fingers to push the uterus closer to your internal fingers, while you move your external fingers to her posterior fornix. With your fingers in the posterior fornix, you should be able to feel the posterior aspect of her uterus and determine whether there is some flexion in its position.

17. When should I perform a rectal exam on a woman?

A rectal exam should be performed for women ≥ 40 years old. For this part of the exam, explain to the woman that one finger will be inserted into the vagina and one finger into the rectum. Explain that the rectal walls, posterior cul-de-sac, uterine ligaments, and rectovaginal septum are assessed during this part of the exam—usually in that order. Also explain that the woman may feel like she is going to have a bowel movement, but reassure her that this will not actually occur.

A rectal exam may be performed on women who are younger than age 40 in certain circumstances. If a woman's vagina is very tight and it is difficult to insert more than one finger for the bimanual exam, you may find it easier to palpate the uterus and adnexal areas with one finger in the vagina and one finger in the rectum. Also, if you have difficulty palpating a woman's uterus and adnexal areas in any situation, or if there are any abnormal findings or symptoms, you may find it helpful to insert one finger into the vagina and one finger into the rectum to palpate the internal structures.

18. How do you perform a pelvic exam when the woman has significant physical limitations stemming from problems such as paralysis, spasticity, or acute pain?

It is helpful to have an electric examination table that can adjust from a table into the lithotomy position for women who have problems with paralysis or spasticity. Then their bodies are well supported during the transition into as well as in the lithotomy position. If you do not have access to one of these tables, you can try a number of alternative positions. In the side-lying position (usually on the left side), an assistant must be available to help hold the woman's upper leg comfortably elevated while you complete the pelvic examination. See the discussion in question 2 for a further description of this position.

Other position options include the obstetric stirrups position, the knee-chest position, the diamond-shaped position, the M-shaped position, and the V-shaped position. In the obstetric stirrups position, a woman lies on her back with her buttocks near the foot of the table; her legs are supported under the knee by the obstetric stirrups. In the knee-chest position, a woman lies on her side with both knees bent or with the lower leg extended. The top leg is usually brought closer to the chest. The handle of the speculum can be pointed toward either the abdomen or the back; remember to angle the speculum toward the small of the back, as usual, when you insert it.

For the diamond-shaped position, the woman lies on her back with her knees bent. Then ask her to move her heels so that they meet at the foot of the table and to let her legs fall back apart to form a diamond shape. In the M-shaped position, the woman lies on her back, her knees are bent and moved back apart, and her heels rest close to her buttocks on the examination table so that her legs form an "M" configuration. In the V-shaped position, the woman lies on her back on the examination table and keeps her legs straight but moves them wide apart in an upside-down "V" position. For this position, you need two assistants—one to support each leg at both the knee and the ankle. In each of these three positions, the speculum must be inserted with the handle pointing upward toward the woman's abdomen because the table will be extended and may interfere with the handle placement.

For women who are experiencing acute pain, try to complete the pelvic exam as gently and quickly as possible. Try a couple of different positions to find one in which she is most comfortable. Any of the positions described above may be used.

19. Are there any special techniques that I can use in performing a pelvic examination on an elderly woman?

Most elderly women do well in the semisitting lithotomy position. They may need help getting onto as well as off the exam table, depending on individual flexibility and strength. Alternative position options have been described previously.

20. What physical findings should I expect when performing a pelvic examination on an elderly woman?

The pelvic examination findings commonly seen in elderly women include a thinning of pubic hair, shrinkage of the labia minora, and flattening of the labia majora. The vagina mucosa looks paler with thinning of the epithelium and fewer rugae. Because of the thinning of the vaginal mucosa, an older woman's vagina may be narrower and shorter as well as less likely to distend. In addition, fewer secretions may be produced in the vagina. Because of the reduced secretions, you may need to use warm water on the speculum for added lubrication with insertion of the speculum. The vaginal pH changes from 3.5–4.5 to 6.0–8.0.

The cervix may protrude less into the vaginal canal because the surrounding fornices may be smaller. The squamocolumnar junction and transformation zone migrate high into the endocervical canal. In addition, the endocervical glandular tissue produces scant mucus. The uterus is smaller, and the ovaries are rarely palpable. Palpable ovaries should be considered suspicious, and an additional work-up may be required to rule out abnormalities.

BIBLIOGRAPHY

1. Boston Women's Health Book Collective: The New Our Bodies, Ourselves: A Book by and for Women. New York, Simon & Schuster, 1992.
2. Brown MS, Wheeler L, Malby P: Is there a right way? Acknowledging, respecting, and teaching different approaches to procedures. Midwifery Today Childbirth Educ 49:40–42, 1999.
3. Hubbard HS: Gynecologic examination of adolescents. Am J Nurs 101(3):24AAA–24DDD, 2001.
4. Kleinman DE, Hage ML, Hoole AJ, Kowlowitz V: Pelvic examination instruction and experience: A comparison of laywoman-trained and physician-trained students. Acad Med 71:1239–1243, 1996.
5. McCarthy V: Patient education review: The first pelvic examination. Pediatr Health Care 11:247–249, 1997.
6. Pokorny SF, Rome ES: Tips for the clinician: Pelvic examination of the virginal teenager. J Pediatr Adolesc Gynacol 12:37–38, 1999.
7. Scott JR, Di Saia PJ, Hammond CB, Spellacy WN: Danforth's Obstetrics and Gynecology, 8th ed. Philadelphia, Lippincott Williams & Wilkins, 1999.
8. Seidel HM, Ball JW, Dains JE, Benedict GW: Mosby's Guide to Physical Examination, 4th ed. St. Louis, Mosby, 1999.

9. SCREENING FOR PROSTATE CANCER

Mary Jo Goolsby, EdD, MSN, APRN, ANP-C

1. Describe the incidence and significance of prostate cancer.
Prostate cancer is a significant health problem and was responsible for over 30,000 deaths among U.S. men in 1999. It is the most common form of cancer among U.S. men when skin cancers are excluded.

2. What are the most efficient means of screening for prostate cancer?
The most effective way to screen for prostate cancer is the combination of a digital rectal examination (DRE) with a prostate-specific antigen (PSA) level. By combining the two tests, a greater number of prostate cancers are detected. In one treatment center, up to 35% of men treated for prostate cancer had a normal PSA, but disease was detected through an abnormal DRE exam; 60% of men treated for prostate cancer had a normal DRE exam, but disease was detected through an abnormal PSA.

3. Should all men be screened for prostate cancer?
This issue is controversial. Most recommendations suggest leaving the determination to the individual patient once he has been given information on which to base his decision. Every man should be informed of the availability of prostate cancer screening and the risks and benefits associated with screening and detection and allowed to participate in screening, if interested. Some men may leave the decision to be tested up to the provider, in which case the American Cancer Society recommends that they be tested.

4. When should screening begin?
Most guidelines recommend screening for men who are at least 50 years of age. It is also suggested that men who are at increased risk for prostate cancer should be offered screening at an earlier age (40–45). Some authorities suggest that screenings should stop once a man no longer has a 10-year life expectancy. The rationale for this recommendation is that older men with undiagnosed prostate cancer most likely have a form that will not shorten life expectancy and would not be treated aggressively, if identified. This principle, of course, is not universally true; you and your patients must decide when screening is no longer warranted.

5. Which men are at highest risk for developing prostate cancer?
The incidence of prostate cancer rises with age. However, men who have first-degree relatives with prostate cancer and/or who are African American are at higher risk than others. Research is under way to establish the significance of other potential risk factors, including history of vasectomy, high intake of dietary fat, occupational exposures, and tobacco use. Overall, however, the greatest risk factors remain family history and race.

6. What type of information should men consider before electing to be screened?
Men should be provided information about the PSA test and DRE examination as well as prostate cancer. By briefly addressing each of the following issues, the man is given the opportunity to ask questions.
- Importance of prostate cancer as a significant health problem
- Procedures for testing (PSA and DRE)
- Risk for false-negative or false-positive results
- Potential for early detection in relation to screening
- Benefits of early detection, including potential for lifetime cure

• Significance of prostate cancer if undetected
• Potential benefits and risks associated with prostate cancer treatments, including potential affects on quality of life
• Individual risk factors for prostate cancer

7. What types of benefits are associated with prostate cancer screenings?

The most important benefit is early detection of prostate cancer at a curable stage. Aggressive forms of prostate cancer are associated with great morbidity and significant mortality risk; disease detected early (while it remains in the prostate capsule) usually responds well to available treatments. If advanced cancer is detected, a benefit may be selection of a therapy to halt or minimize advancement of the disease.

8. What types of risks are associated with prostate cancer screenings?

One often mentioned risk is the potential anxiety associated with screening and a real or false diagnosis. The treatments for prostate cancer also bear some risks.

9. How often should prostate cancer screenings be performed?

Annual screening is generally recommended. In fact, an important aspect of evaluating PSA results involves looking at serial results to detect a significant increase from one year to another.

10. What are the important techniques to remember in performing a DRE?

Although the prostate is a multidimensional organ, you can palpate only the posterior- and inferior-most aspects. In addition to determining the superficial surface characteristics, by moving the finger over the palpable surface, you also should strive to determine tissue consistency beneath the surface and to judge symmetry and size. An assymetrical, nodular, hard, indurated, or otherwise abnormal prostate should trigger evaluation by a urologist. When assessing the prostate, remember to include detection of rectal lesions as well.

11. What is the norm for PSA?

The usually accepted norm for PSA level is 4.0 ng/ml. However, when this level is chosen as the cut-off for normal across all age groups, there is a greater risk that malignancy will be missed in younger men and that an older man with no significant form of prostate cancer will be subjected to needless anxiety and testing.

12. What is the risk of a false negative with the PSA test?

The sensitivity or likelihood that PSA will detect a malignancy is 67–80%; conversely 20–33% of malignancies may be missed.

13. Is there any way to improve the sensitivity for my patients?

One way to improve PSA sensitivity is to use age-specific norms. A younger man's PSA norm is lower than that of an older man. Another method involves monitoring serial PSA levels. The rate at which PSA doubles is a hundred times faster in prostate cancer, and an increase > 0.75–0.8 ng/ml in one year is significant. Using this method, the provider may obtain a PSA level as often as 3 times/year to detect an increase.

Age-Specific PSA Norms

40–49 yr	< 2.5 ng/ml
50–59 yr	< 3.5 ng/ml
60–69 yr	< 4.5 ng/ml
70–79 yr	< 6.5 ng/ml

14. Can prostate cancer be present despite a normal PSA and a normal DRE?

Yes. Although using methods to improve sensitivity helps eliminate this problem, prostate cancer does not always cause PSA elevation. A patient with a normal DRE may still have cancer. Although no one test or combination of tests identifies all malignancies, the combination is more successful than any test alone.

15. What is the risk that a PSA will result in a false-positive finding?

The risk of a false positive is 30–40%; up to 40% of abnormal PSA levels may not be associated with prostate cancer. Thus the specificity of PSA is 60–70%.

16. How can I improve the specificity of PSA tests?

One way is through the use of the age-specific norms, which also lower the incidence of false positives in older men. Another method involves considering the ratio of free to total PSA, which is lower with malignancy than with benign disease. The PSA norm also can be adjusted, based on prostate size; a larger prostate is more likely to produce a greater amount of PSA. The best way to determine prostate size, however, is through ultrasound; a urologist usually makes this distinction. It is important to remember that by improving specificity, you sometimes decrease sensitivity so that more malignancies may be missed.

17. What nonmalignant factors can increase PSA levels?

Prostate massage (not DRE), prostatitis, prostatic hyperplasia, and even physical activity. If a PSA is elevated, you must consider whether any nonmalignant cause may explain the elevation. In this case, you may treat the cause and then obtain another PSA. Prostate biopsies significantly increase the PSA level, and a PSA level should not be done for 4 weeks after a biopsy.

18. Does the DRE increase the PSA level?

A DRE may cause a slight elevation in PSA, but it is not significant. You need not wait to obtain a PSA level after DRE.

19. What factors can decrease PSA levels?

Finesteride decreases PSA by 50% once it has been taken for 6 months. Treatment for prostate cancer, if successful, decreases PSA. In fact, PSA is used to monitor response to treatment.

20. If a patient is taking finesteride, how can I interpret the PSA reading?

You should double the PSA result in a man who has taken finesteride for an extended time before comparing it to the norms. Failure to do so may result in missed detection of a malignancy.

21. What nonmalignant factors cause an abnormal DRE?

Some of the same nonmalignant prostate diseases that increase PSA also alter DRE findings, including prostatitis and prosatic hyperplasia. However, with any questionable DRE findings and no definite nonmalignant disease (such as acute prostatitis), you should be suspicious of malignancy. Of course, malignancies can coexist with other disease processes.

22. What should I do if I find an elevated PSA or abnormal DRE?

With any elevation of PSA or an abnormal DRE finding, you should arrange for the patient to be seen by a urologist.

23. If I must refer a patient to a urologist for an abnormal PSA or DRE, what can I tell him to expect?

The urologist probably will review or obtain a medical history and perform a physical examination, both focused on assessment of the prostate. The DRE and possibly the PSA will be repeated. The patient probably will be scheduled for a transrectal ultrasound (TRUS) with prostate biopsy. All of the information will be considered in the determination and staging of any malignancy or other disorder. If cancer is detected, the urologist will discuss with the patient the likely stage of the cancer and treatment options.

24. Once a patient has been treated for prostate cancer, how often should he be monitored for recurrence with PSA?

The urologist or oncologist determines the schedule for monitoring. One common regimen includes PSA and DRE assessment quarterly for at least 1 year, then twice a year for the next 4 years. After 5 years, the PSA and DRE may be performed annually. This schedule, of course, is also highly individualized.

25. What controversies surround prostate cancer screening?

Whether all men over a given age (usually 50 years) should be screened is still debated, although the most common recommendation is that screening should be offered and discussed individually and completed after men choose to participate. Other controversies involve whether to use a single, standardized norm for PSA levels or whether age-specific norms, free-to-total ratios, or other means of improving detection is warranted. Some authorities continue to believe that early detection is not warranted because historically the outcomes after treatment were not optimal. In the past, the high number of men diagnosed with advanced cancer did not fare well, and a high number experienced adverse effects associated with the treatments, including incontinence and erectile dysfunction. However, PSA has been available for over a decade and has allowed early detection so that most prostate cancers are now identified while they are still localized. Ongoing studies show favorable outcomes, resulting from earlier detection. At the same time, surgical techniques have been improved so that the incidences of incontinence and erectile dysfunction are lower after radical prostatectomy. In addition, new treatments, including implanted radioactive seeds, or brachytherapy, are showing favorable outcomes. The good news is that currently several substantial clinical trials are seeking answers to the many questions surrounding the cause, detection, treatment, and outcome of prostate cancer. For now, practitioners should consider the potential risk and benefit associated with screening and help the patient to make the decision that is right for him.

BIBLIOGRAPHY

1. Coley CM, Barry MJ, Mulley A: Screening for prostate cancer. Ann Intern Med 126:468–484, 1997.
2. Ferrini K, Woolf S: Screening for prostate cancer in American men: American College of Preventive Medicine policy statement, 1998. Available on-line: URL: http://www.acpm.org/prostate.htm (accessed March 2001).
3. Gunby P: Prostate cancer's complexities of causation, detection, and treatment challenges researchers. JAMA 277:1580–1582, 1997.
4. Smith R, et al: American Cancer Society guidelines for the early detection of cancer: Update of early detection guidelines for prostate, colorectal, and endometrial cancers and update 2001: Testing for early lung cancer detection. Cancer J Clin 51:38–75, 2001. (also available on-line: URL: http://www.cancer.org).
5. Thompson I, et al: Prostate-specific antigen (PSA) best practice policy. Oncology 14:267–286, 2000 (also available on-line: URL: http://www.cancernetwork.com/journals/oncology/o0002e.htm).

10. SEXUAL ABUSE AND ASSAULT

Vicki Ellison Burns, PhD(c), RN, FNP-BC

1. What is the difference between sexual abuse and sexual assault?

Generally speaking, sexual abuse is defined as the involvement of immature children or adolescents in sexual activities that they do not fully comprehend, to which they are unable to give informed consent, or that violate taboos or family relationships. Sexual assault, which is used when the victim is an adult, is defined as any sexual act performed by one person on another without consent.

2. What is the usual setting in which sexual abuse/sexual assault victims are seen by health care professionals?

Adult victims of sexual assault usually are seen in hospital emergency departments, although they may choose to be seen by their primary care physician. Children and adolescents, however, are often frightened and intimidated by the bright lights, clinical atmosphere, and crowded conditions of an emergency department. Whenever possible, children and adolescents should be seen in an alternative setting such as a designated child advocacy center. In addition, providers in all health care settings should be alert for signs of possible sexual abuse and assault and make appropriate reports and referrals.

3. How does a child advocacy center function?

A child advocacy center is an institution established for the specific purpose of evidentiary collection in cases of suspected child sexual abuse. Children are referred to advocacy centers after a report of sexual abuse has been made to either the Division of Family Services or law enforcement. Most advocacy centers are not connected to hospitals or clinics and are set up in residential locations with a home-like atmosphere. Staff members usually include a director, forensic examiner, one or more case managers, registered nurse who assists the examiner, one or more professionals who conduct forensic interviews, and support staff.

4. Can any health care professional perform an evidentiary examination on a victim of sexual abuse or assault?

The person performing the evidentiary examination should have specialized training in sexual abuse/assault forensic exams.

5. How does one train to perform sexual abuse/assault forensic exams?

Training programs and opportunities vary from state to state, as do educational requirements for examiners. Many nurse examiners are trained at the advanced practice level, although some are not. Trained examiners adopt various titles, depending on where and how they were trained. Common titles include SAFE (sexual abuse forensic exam) provider, SANE (sexual assault nurse examiner), SANC (sexual assault nurse clinician), and FNE (forensic nurse examiner). Many examiners also are physicians. Scope of practice and specific duties vary from state to state and program to program. For more information about the specifics of training, interested parties can log on to the U.S. Department of Justice Office for Victims of Crime website at http://www.ojp.usdoj.gov/ovc/.

6. Should a licensed physician performing an evidentiary exam on a victim of sexual abuse or assault also have had specialized training in forensic exams?

Absolutely. The field of forensics is a specialty unto itself, and no health care degree qualifies a person to collect forensic evidence unless additional specialty training has been obtained. Evidence of specialty training also lends credibility to examination findings and legal testimony.

7. What are the specific priorities in evidentiary collection for victims of sexual abuse or assault?
- To provide efficient, thorough, and professional forensic evidence collection, documentation, and preservation of evidence
- To protect the victim from further harm
- To test for and provide treatment for sexually transmitted diseases
- To make appropriate referrals for follow-up medical care and counseling
- To assist law enforcement agencies to obtain meaningful evidence and successfully prosecute sexual abuse/assault cases

8. Do persons who perform evidentiary exams on victims of sexual abuse or assault have to testify in court about their findings?
An examiner can be subpoenaed as an expert witness to testify about an examination that he or she performed on a victim. The possibility of subpoena is only one of many reasons why clear, precise, and accurate documentation of findings is absolutely essential.

9. What are the specific components of a typical forensic examination for an adult victim of sexual assault?
- Written consent from the victim to perform the exam
- History of the assault in the victim's own words, including orifices where violence was used or penetration occurred
- Pertinent medical information, including allergies, pregnancy status, and menstrual history
- General physical assessment for trauma
- Assessment of designated orifices for trauma
- Sperm and seminal fluid swabs of involved orifices
- Fingernail clippings or scrapings
- Pubic hair combings
- Blood for typing and DNA studies
- Urine specimen, especially if rape drug use is suspected
- Collection of stained or torn clothing

10. What are the primary purposes for the evidence collected during such an examination?
- To confirm recent sexual contact
- To show that coercion and/or force were used
- To help identify the perpetrator
- To corroborate the story told by the victim

11. Is any special equipment used to perform an examination on a sexual assault victim?
Most hospital emergency departments are equipped with rape kits, which contain swabs, bags for clothing, tweezers, slides and envelopes for storage of specimens, and detailed instructions about how to collect evidence. A Woods lamp, an ultraviolet light source that illuminates the presence of sperm on clothing and tissue, also is commonly used during an examination on a sexual assault victim.

Some facilities have access to a colposcope, which provides high magnification and a powerful light source to better visualize the anogenital tissue and assess for trauma. Many colposcopes have photographic capability as well, both still and video, so that the examination can be videotaped and the video entered into evidence. Staining preparations such as gentian violet and toluidine blue are sometimes used to enhance visualization of genital injuries.

12. Within what time frame should a sexual assault victim be seen by health care professionals to collect the best evidence?

A sexual assault victim should be seen as soon as possible after the incident—definitely within 72 hours. The longer a victim waits to be seen, the more likely it is that healing of traumatic injuries and compromise of forensic evidence will occur.

13. Is the absence of anogenital trauma on a sexual assault examination an indication that the victim is not telling the truth about the incident?

No. The presence or absence of anogenital injury is a poor indicator of sexual assault. Most rape victims do not experience anogenital trauma. One recent study found that only 22 of 83 adult rape victims (27%) exhibited genital injuries. Anogenital tissue is resilient and heals rapidly, and the absence of injuries should not influence an examiner's testimony about the validity of a sexual assault.

14. If anogenital injury does occur, where it most likely to be found?

The most common sites for anogenital trauma are the outer or inner labia, the hymenal ring, the vaginal tissue, the posterior fourchette, the fossa navicularis, and/or the anal tissue in females and the penis, scrotum, and/or anal tissue in males.

15. Does the examiner take a formal statement from the sexual assault victim about exactly what happened during the assault?

The examiner takes a history of the assault for the purposes of focusing the exam, but the victim's formal statement is taken by law enforcement officials.

16. What is the final step in the sexual assault examination after the physical assessment is complete?

The final (and critical) step is to make appropriate referrals for follow-up care and counseling. If injuries require further treatment or need to be re-checked, arrangements should be made before the victim leaves the treatment facility. In addition, lists of rape crisis, violence, and victim centers that offer specialized counseling for victims of sexual assault should be provided.

17. What is the biggest challenge for health care professionals in performing examinations of sexually abused children?

The biggest challenge for health professionals is coming to terms with the idea that adults use children for sexual gratification. Willingness to consider a diagnosis of child molestation seems to be directly related to level of training and education in the field, which is another argument for focused, specialized training.

18. What important behavioral indicators of possible sexual abuse may be picked up by a parent or a health care professional before the abuse is disclosed?

- Acute traumatic response (newly manifested clinging behaviors and irritability in young children)
- Regressive behaviors (loss of bowel and bladder control, withdrawal, renewed use of a security blanket, thumb sucking)
- Sleep disturbances (nightmares, fear of sleeping alone, bedwetting, sleepwalking)
- Problems at school (change in academic achievement, distractibility, inability to concentrate)
- Social problems (depression, anger, fighting, hyperactivity, poor relationships, sexualized behavior inappropriate for age and development)
- Long-term sequelae (guilt, low self-esteem, suicidal ideation, psychosomatic illness, promiscuity, legal trouble, substance abuse, eating disorders)

19. How do I decide whether to report suspected abuse?

All health care professionals are mandated reporters. You are bound by law to report any case of suspected child abuse or neglect that comes to your attention.

20. Are female children more likely to be sexually abused than males?

Recent statistics indicate that approximately 1 in every 4 female children and 1 in every 6 male children experience some form of sexual abuse by the time they reach their eighteenth birthday. It is unknown, however, whether the lower incidence in males is a result of reduced reporting.

21. Since children are typically examined at child advocacy centers, can anyone, including a parent or a health care professional, call a center and make an appointment for a child?

No. Child advocacy centers typically take referrals only from the Division of Family Services or law enforcement officials. In other words, a case of suspected child sexual abuse must be reported to the proper authorities before an advocacy center can become involved.

22. What is the forensic medical examiner's role at a child advocacy center?

The forensic medical examiner at a child advocacy center typically takes the child's medical history and history of the alleged incident from whoever has brought the child to the appointment (parent, legal guardian, social worker, or law enforcement officer). The medical examiner also performs the forensic examination of the child.

23. What does the medical examination of a pediatric sexual abuse victim involve?

Typically, the medical examination involves (1) a physical assessment of eyes, ears, nose, throat, heart, lungs, abdomen, and reflexes, and (2) an intensive examination of the anogenital area, most often under video colposcopy. Testing for pregnancy and/or sexually transmitted diseases is performed as indicated.

24. Is it more likely that genital trauma will be found in pediatric victims of sexual assault than in adult victims?

No. Physical evidence of sexual abuse is found in only about 20% of children who have been molested. As in adults, anogenital tissue in children is highly resilient and, even when injured, heals quite rapidly. A perfectly normal exam is possible in a child only a few days after an incident involving full intercourse. In addition, many forms of sexual abuse in children, such as fondling and oral sex, create no physical injury and therefore leave no physical sign. Generally speaking, some type of penetrating genital trauma, either with a finger, penis, or foreign object, has to occur for physical evidence to be present. Again, however, it is important to remember that *even when penetrating trauma has occurred, physical evidence is present in only around 20% of cases.*

25. If an injury is evident, where will it most likely have occurred?

The most common sites for anogenital injury in children are the same as those for adults: the inner or outer labia, the hymenal ring, the vaginal tissue, the posterior fourchette, the fossa navicularis, and/or the anal tissue in females, and the penis, scrotum, and/or anal tissue in males.

26. What kinds of injuries may an examiner see when they do occur?

An examiner may see any number of changes in the anogenital tissue, including bruising, lacerations, severe inflammation and friability of the tissue, evidence of sexually transmitted disease, and/or interruptions in the integrity of the inner edge of the hymen (e.g., tears, notches, thinning of the hymenal tissue).

27. Can any of the tissue changes mentioned in question 26 be attributable to factors other than sexual abuse in children?

Certain factors can cause changes in anogenital tissues in children that are similar to changes seen in cases of sexual abuse. Examples include congenital anomalies, straddle injuries, and certain skin conditions. In adolescents, prior sexual activity, use of tampons, and previous speculum exams also can contribute to anogenital findings. In general, however, whenever changes and abnormalities are found in anogenital tissue, sexual abuse cannot be ruled out as the cause at the time of the forensic examination. If an alternative medical explanation is suspected, the child should be referred to an appropriate specialist for follow-up evaluation as indicated.

28. What happens if a child refuses the anogenital portion of an examination?

If a child refuses to undergo the anogenital portion of the examination, his or her wishes are respected. Force and physical restraint are not used on children to obtain a forensic exam. Children who already may have been victimized should not be made to feel like victims again as a result of being examined.

29. Can a child's parent or guardian be present during the examination?

Absolutely. Parents are encouraged to be with their children to promote feelings of safety and comfort. The only instance in which a parent or guardian is not allowed in the examination room is when the child requests that they remain outside.

30. Are rape kits used for children at advocacy centers just as they are for adults in emergency departments?

They can be but usually are not. If a child alleges rape and the center keeps kits on hand, they may be used. In general, however, advocacy centers do not stock rape kits. Instead, they rely on evidence compiled from the forensic interview and examination.

31. In addition to the physical examination, what else can a child expect to happen at an advocacy center?

Generally speaking, a child undergoes a forensic interview and physical examination in the course of an appointment at a child advocacy center. The forensic interview is conducted by an employee of the center who has specialty training in forensic techniques. The interview is done with the child only, and a social worker and law enforcement official typically observe from behind a two-way mirror. Interviews are most often videotaped. Whether the child receives both an interview and an examination is up to the person who made the advocacy center referral. In some cases, children may receive only an interview or only an examination.

32. What is the final step in the forensic process for suspected sexual abuse of a child?

Just as in adult sexual assault cases, the final step in the forensic process for children is appropriate referral for follow-up treatment and counseling as indicated. Parents or guardians of the child are provided with a packet of information before they leave the facility, which contains lists of crisis and victim centers where counselors who specialize in working with children and adolescents are available. One of the primary goals of the advocacy center team is to do everything possible to prevent the long-term sequelae of child sexual abuse, as outlined in question 2.

BIBLIOGRAPHY

1. Adams JA, Knudson S: Genital findings in adolescent girls referred for suspected sexual abuse. Arch Pediatr Adolesc Med 150:850–857, 1996.
2. Boyer D, Fine D: Sexual abuse as a factor in adolescent pregnancy and child maltreatment. Fam Plann Perspect 24:4–11, 19, 1992.
3. Farber E, Showers J, Johnson C: The sexual abuse of children: A comparison of male and female victims. Clin Child Psychol 13:294–297, 1984.
4. Heger A, Emans SJ: Evaluation of the Sexually Abused Child. New York, Oxford University Press, 1992.
5. Herman J: Trauma and Recovery. New York, Basic Books, 1997.
6. Ledray LE: Sexual Assault Nurse Examiner (SANE): Development and Operation Guide. Minneapolis, Sexual Assault Resource Service, 1998.
7. Monteleone JA: Child Maltreatment: A Clinical Guide and Reference, 2nd ed. St. Louis, G. W. Medical Publishing, 1998.

III. Clinical Challenges

11. IMPAIRED VISION

Mary Jo Goolsby, EdD, MSN, APRN, ANP-C

1. Should patients who complain of a change in vision or other visual impairment be routinely referred to an ophthalmologist?
No. First, you should determine the nature of the patient's complaint and whether it is likely to be purely an ophthalmologic problem or to stem from another, more systemic cause. You also should determine the urgency of the complaint. Patients who presents with a problem that may be sight-threatening or an otherwise urgent risk should be immediately referred.

2. What types of complaints are covered by the umbrella term "visual impairment"?
Patients complaining of impaired vision may be referring to any one of several types of problems. Examples include hazy or diminished vision, dim color perception, color blindness, visual halos, double vision, blurred vision or difficulty in focusing, scotomas, total blindness, and intermittent visual loss or alterations.

3. What "red flag" indicates that the problem is urgent?
When a patient complains of sudden onset of visual impairment, you should be concerned about the potential for permanent, irreversible visual loss. Sudden onset of altered vision, whether painless or painful, is a common finding of many of the causes of irreversible vision loss and requires urgent evaluation and intervention.

4. List some of the urgent causes of vision impairment.
Temporal arteritis, retinal detachment, retinal occlusion, acute open angle glaucoma, amaurosis fugax, and cerebrovascular accident (CVA).

5. What major characteristics help NPs to recognize the problems listed above?
- Temporal arteritis causes partial or total, sudden, monocular visual loss and is commonly associated with pain of the head, scalp, or temporal area. It generally occurs in older patients.
- Retinal detachment causes floaters, scotomas, blurring, or complete monocular visual loss with sudden onset and often follows some trauma.
- Retinal artery occlusion causes sudden, painless, persistent (or slowly resolving) monocular visual loss.
- Acute open-angle glaucoma is characterized by sudden onset of monocular blurring, halos, or vision loss, often triggered by a dark environment and commonly associated with severe head pain, nausea, and/or vomiting.
- Amaurosis fugax causes full or partial transient loss of vision in one eye, often described as if a curtain were drawn across the visual field.
- CVAs cause a variety of visual disturbances, including sudden onset of visual loss of specific fields as well as impairments due to neuromuscular deficits, such as double vision or color discrimination problems.

6. List common causes of nonemergent visual impairment.
Many of the causes of visual impairment require timely but not immediate response. Examples include cataracts, open-angle glaucoma, diabetic retinopathy, macular degeneration,

and migraines as well as changes due to chronic disorders such as thyroid disease, hypertension, and diabetes.

7. **What are the common presentations of the above problems?**
   - Cataracts commonly present as a gradual onset of monocular or binocular impaired vision, which may be noticed initially as dimming of vision, halos around lights, or altered color perception.
   - Open-angle glaucoma is often accompanied by the gradual onset of peripheral vision loss.
   - Diabetic retinopathy can cause either monocular or binocular gradual loss of selected fields or full fields.
   - Macular degeneration causes the gradual loss of central vision, with preserved peripheral vision.
   - Migraine episodes may involve transient scotomas or other visual disturbances, often followed by unilateral headache. The visual disturbance is detected in both eyes, a finding that helps to differentiate between migraine and amaurosis fugax.

8. **When a patient complains of altered vision, what are the key components of the history?**
   When a patient complains of visual impairment, the history must be sufficient not only to rule out urgent causes but also to discriminate among the other potential causes, including systemic diseases. The following questions are helpful:
   - What makes the symptoms better? Worse?
   - Under what, if any, circumstances are the symptoms most likely to occur?
   - What do you mean by impaired vision (or other term)?
   - How much, or to what percentage, would you estimate your vision is altered?
   - What, if any, specific portion of vision is most affected?
   - Are both eyes equally affected?
   - Using this paper to represent your visual field, mark the areas where your vision is affected.
   - How, if at all, has the vision change affected your ability to perform usual activities?
   - Have you noticed any associated symptoms? Pain, nausea or vomiting, dizziness, weakness?
   - Describe the onset of your symptoms. Was it sudden or gradual?
   - Have the symptoms been constant or intermittent?
   - Do you have any major health problems? Hypertension, diabetes, kidney disease, heart disease, stroke?
   - Have you had any prior eye problems? Any surgeries?
   - How much, if any, tobacco do you use?
   - What, if any, prescription or over-the-counter medications do you take?
   - It is also wise to do a brief review of system, particularly of the systems that are most often implicated in visual impairment: neurologic, cardiologic, and endocrine.

9. **What physical examination is suggested for visual impairment?**
   Of course, a thorough examination of the eyes is always indicated when a patient presents with altered vision. Further examination of the cardiovascular, neurologic, endocrine, or other symptoms should be performed based on the history and physical findings.

10. **What specific components of the eye examination are essential?**
    You should check close and far visual acuity, central and peripheral vision, color vision, ocular movement and alignment, and external eye structures and complete a thorough funduscopic examination.

11. **How do you test close and far vision?**
    - **Distant vision** is assessed most accurately with the Snellen chart. The patient should stand exactly 20 feet from the chart in a well-lighted room.

• **Close vision** is assessed most accurately using a standardized tool such as a Rosenbaum or Jaeger chart, both of which should be held within 14 inches. Scoring systems are similar to that of the Snellen chart. When these tools are not available, ask the patient to read standard newsprint.

12. Can visual acuity be tested if the patient is unable to read the largest print on a standardized chart?

When the patient cannot read the largest print, you may move the patient closer to the chart and document the distance at which the largest print can be read. For instance, using the Snellen chart, visual acuity should be recorded as "15/200" if the patient can read the 200-ft line at a distance of 15 feet or 5/200 if read at 5 feet from the chart. If the patient cannot read the largest print despite moving progressively closer, document whether the patient can count fingers or detect hand motion at a distance of 2 feet or perceive light.

13. How do you test central and peripheral vision?

• **Central vision** is tested when the near and distant vision are assessed, as described above. If visual acuity is not tested with a standardized chart, you can also assess central vision by asking the patient to identify a common object held directly in front of the visual field.

• **Peripheral vision** is assessed by tests of confrontation.

14. If a patient wears glasses or contact lenses, should the vision be assessed with or without correction?

You can check both corrected and noncorrected vision. However, the corrected vision gives you the most accurate assessment of any alteration in vision.

15. What is "legal blindness"?

Legal blindness is defined as visual acuity of 20/200 or less in the better eye.

16. How can color vision be tested?

The Snellen eye chart includes red and green color strips to test color perception. Ishihara plates, actually designed for color blindness screening, can be used to assess color discrimination. If you do not have access to Ishihara plates or a Snellen chart, you can ask the patient to identify the color of various objects.

17. What ocular movement deficits should be observed in evaluating altered vision?

When visual disturbance is due to thyroid disease, the patient may have limited ocular motion, particularly looking upward. Lid lag with gaze downward is a strong indication of thyroid eye disease. If the problem is related to myasthenia gravis, the examination may be normal initially, but fatigue may be evident after the patient is asked to hold an upward gaze for at least 1 minute. The full test of cardinal fields of vision detects isolated or combined deficits related to specific cranial nerves or muscle weakness/paralysis.

18. Are any particular pupillary changes common to specific vision disorders?

Most eye disorders described above usually present with normal round, reactive, and equal pupils. Sometimes an afferent defect is present with retinal artery occlusion, chronic open-angle glaucoma, or retinal detachment. The pupil may be fixed and mid-dilated during an acute attack of open-angle glaucoma.

19. Is it necessary to examine the cornea when a patient presents with impaired vision but no injury?

Yes. Corneal deposits, which can alter vision, may be associated with medications such as gold or other heavy metals and can be detected on close examination. In acute open-angle glaucoma, the cornea may have an edematous, "steamy" appearance. In examining the cornea, tangential lighting should be used to detect any "shadowing," which is found with a narrowed anterior chamber, another sign of acute closed-angle glaucoma.

20. Is eye redness an important finding in association with impaired vision?

Yes. Although most causes of visual disturbance present without redness, a reddened eye can indicate acute closed-angle glaucoma, uveitis, or corneal injury.

21. How can the appearance of the optic disc be used to determine the cause of altered vision?

A pale disc with no visible vessels is associated with atrophy of the optic nerve, which may occur with transient or persistent retinal artery occlusion. With ischemic optic neuropathy related to temporal arteritis, the optic disc is pale white and edematous. An enlarged cup is associated with increased intraocular pressure and glaucoma. A hyperemic disc with blurred margins and no visible cup is associated with papilledema, which can cause visual disturbances when persistent.

22. What funduscopic vessel changes are important to the differentiation of visual change?

- Amaurosis fugax: emboli may be visible within the arteries, or the examination may appear normal.
- Retinal artery occlusion: obstructions may be visible in the artery.
- Hypertensive eye disease: crossing variants and engorged vessels may be seen.

23. What funduscopic background changes are important to the differentiation of a visual disturbance?

- Amaurosis fugax: areas of the retina may be pale or white, and the fovea may appear "cherry red" if the occlusion has persisted long enough for infarction.
- Retinal artery occlusion: patchy or consistent milky white retina, with "cherry red" fovea.
- Retinal detachment: wrinkled appearance; a flap or tear may be visible.
- Macular degeneration: drusen bodies and/or exudates may be visible; neovascularization.
- Hypertensive eye disease: background hemorrhages and/or exudates.
- Diabetic eye disease: background hemorrhages, exudates, and/or neovascular changes as well as any changes from related macular degeneration, vitreous hemorrhages, glaucoma, or retinal detachment.

24. What medications are associated with vision changes?

Several medications can affect the vision. Review the patient's medication profile and investigate specific medications if you are unsure of their potential visual effects. Common examples include the following:

- Digitalis: altered color perception, "yellowing" of vision.
- Ethambutol: altered color perception, "greening" of vision, optic neuropathy.
- Antihistamines: blurred vision.
- Antimalarials: retinopathy, corneal deposits, visual field defects.
- Phenothiazines: retinopathy, corneal deposits, lens deposits/cataracts, oculomotor dysfunction.
- Heavy metals: corneal deposits.
- Steroids: cataracts, glaucoma, optic neuropathy.

25. If the patient's complaint is diplopia, what are the possible causes?

Myasthenia gravis, thyroid ophthalmoplegia, and oculomotor nerve disorders are among the problems associated with diplopia.

26. If an urgent cause of visual disturbance is suspected, to whom should the patient be referred?

When in doubt, you can either refer the patient to an ophthalmologist for an immediate and more detailed assessment or obtain a phone consultation with the ophthalmologist. The ophthalmologist performs a dilated examination (unless contraindicated, as in acute-angle closure glaucoma) and use much more sophisticated and accurate techniques of assessment. The ophthalmologist determines whether the patient also should be seen by a cardiologist, neurologist, or other specialist and can provide more detailed findings.

However, when nonophthalmic emergencies are suspected, the appropriate service should be consulted immediately, because referral to an ophthalmologist only delays the appropriate treatment of an urgent problem, such as an evolving CVA. If a patient presents with visual complaints and physical findings consistent with a CVA, prompt referral to a neurologist or stroke center is indicated. Similarly, if the history is consistent with amaurosis fugax and the medical history includes risk factors for this disorder (e.g., hyperlipidemia, hypertension, peripheral vascular disease), you may order carotid studies, but refer the patient immediately to a neurologist.

BIBLIOGRAPHY

1. Anderson P, Knoben J: Handbook of Clinical Drug Data. New York, McGraw-Hill, 1998.
2. Andreoli TE, Bennett JC, Carpenter CC, Plum F: Cecil's Essentials of Medicine. Philadelphia, W.B. Saunders, 1998.
3. Caplan L, Hinchey J: Visual loss. In Hurst JW (ed): Medicine for the Practicing Physician. Stamford, CT, Appleton & Lange, 1998, pp 1783–1794.
4. Chang D: Ophthalmologic examination. In Baughan D, Asbury T, Eva-Riordan P (eds): General Ophthalmology. Stamford, CT, Appleton & Lange, 1999, pp 27–56.
5. Eagle R: Eye Pathology: An Atlas and Basic Text. Philadelphia, W.B. Saunders, 1999.
6. Eisenbauer L, Murphy M: Pharmacotherapeutics and Advanced Nursing Practice. New York, McGraw-Hill, 1998.
7. Gans L: Ocular emergencies. In Stine R, Chudnofsky C (eds): A Practical Approach to Emergency Medicine. Boston, Little, Brown, 1994, pp 911–933.
8. Horton J: Disorders of the eye. In Fauci AS, Braunwald E, Isselbacher KJ, et al (eds): Harrison's Principles of Internal Medicine, 14th ed. New York, McGraw-Hill, 1998, pp 159–172.
9. Kanski J: Clinical Ophthalmology. Woburn, MA, Butterworth-Heinemann, 1999.
10. Newell F: Ophthalmology: Principles and Concepts. St. Louis, Mosby, 1996.
11. Swartz M: Textbook of Physical Diagnosis. Philadelphia, W.B. Saunders, 1998.

12. FORGETFULNESS

Valerie T. Cotter, MSN, CRNP

1. How do I recognize when forgetfulness is a symptom of an underlying medical condition?

It is important to differentiate cognitive changes that result from "normal aging" and changes that are signs of a disease. Cognitive changes, such as slight declines in memory and the ability to manage multiple tasks simultaneously and a slowing in the speed of thought processing are thought to be part of the normal aging process. Age-associated memory impairment (AAMI) or age-related cognitive decline is not significant enough to interfere with daily functioning: instrumental activities of daily living (IADLs; driving, shopping, housekeeping, cooking, using the telephone, managing finances and medications) or activities of daily living (ADLs; bathing, dressing, ambulating, using the toilet, feeding). Increasing memory complaints with age are common, but the course of cognitive function in normal aging has not been well defined.

2. What is the difference between AAMI and mild cognitive impairment (MCI)?

Patients with MCI meet the following criteria:
- Memory complaint by the patient or a knowledgeable informant
- No change in the ability to perform IADLs and ADLs
- Normal cognitive function, except for abnormal memory for age (1.5 SD below age- and education-matched scores)
- No dementia

3. Why is it important to identify patients with MCI?

Patients with MCI are at an increased risk of developing Alzheimer's disease at the rate of 10–12% per year compared with rates of 1–3% in controls. Studies are under way to assess the benefits of cholinesterase inhibitors and other pharmacologic interventions to delay progression. No adequate and well-controlled clinical trials demonstrate that pharmacologic interventions slow the progression from MCI to AD. Patients with MCI should be followed more closely to identify cognitive and functional declines suggesting dementia and treated appropriately.

4. How do you make the diagnosis of dementia?

Dementia is a clinical syndrome characterized by deficits in at least two cognitive domains that interfere with daily functioning in an alert patient. Diagnosis requires memory impairment and deficits in one or more other cognitive domains (language, attention, apraxia (inability to carry out motor activities despite intact motor function), agnosia (inability to recognize or identify objects despite intact sensory function), and deficits in executive function (planning, organizing, sequencing, abstracting). The extent of deficits in each cognitive domain helps to establish the particular clinical diagnosis of the dementia. This principle is most prominent in frontotemporal dementia; patients have little-to-no memory impairment in the early stages of the disease, but as the dementia progresses memory is affected.

5. What diseases are the most common causes of dementia?
- Alzheimer's disease (AD) (60–80%)
- Frontotemporal dementia (FTD) (10–20%)
- Dementia with Lewy bodies (DLB) (10–20%)
- Vascular dementia (VaD) (5%)

6. What other conditions are associated with cognitive impairment and may be confused with dementia?

Cognitive complaints and decline may be a secondary symptom of depression. Depression is often a prodromal or early sign of dementia. In fact, patients who experience a first episode of depression late in life are at high risk to develop dementia, notably AD, within a few years. Depression frequently coexists with dementia and contributes to cognitive impairment and functional disability in older adults with AD. Depression should be treated aggressively and cognitive function measured at appropriate intervals to identify and treat coexisting dementia.

Cognitive impairment is a core feature of delirium, but is differentiated from dementia by abrupt onset and relatively shorter duration and usually is associated with an underlying acute medical condition. Persons with dementia are at higher risk for developing delirium.

Hypothyroidism, vitamin B_{12} deficiency, drug toxicity, neurosyphilis and other medical conditions may cause cognitive impairment. Medications such as anxiolytics and sedatives are notorious causes of cognitive impairment.

7. What is the most efficient and effective method of evaluating a patient who complains of forgetfulness?

A detailed history focusing on functional, cognitive, mood, and behavioral changes is the most sensitive method of evaluating forgetfulness. In assessing functional changes, it is important to focus on changes caused by cognitive rather than physical impairments. A thorough description of the initial symptoms is most important to help differentiate the cause; behavioral or language symptoms in FTD, visual hallucinations with a fluctuating course in DLB, insidious memory loss in AD, and focal neurologic symptoms in VaD. Many patients with dementia lack insight and awareness about their functional and cognitive declines; therefore, a careful history should be obtained from a knowledgeable informant, such as a spouse, partner, adult child, or friend, in addition to the patient. The physical examination identifies neurologic or other medical abnormalities that may cause or contribute to forgetfulness.

8. How do I assess cognitive function?

Standardized cognitive tests, such as the Mini-Mental State Examination (MMSE), assist in the diagnosis and staging of dementia and are helpful measurements of cognitive function against which to compare future testing. The Brief Cognitive Screen (BCS) is another efficient way to measure cognitive function and takes less than 10 minutes to complete. A score of 0–4 indicates no cognitive impairment; 5–8 indicates mild cognitive impairment; and a score > 8 indicates probable dementia. (See Figure 1, page 66.)

In addition to short mental status tests, structured assessments of functional performance also should be included. The Functional Assessment Screen (FAS) is a screening version of the Dementia Severity Rating Scale (DSRS). A screening score > 4 indicates meaningful cognitive impairment, and further comprehensive evaluation is recommended. (See Figure 2, page 67.)

9. When should screening for cognitive impairment be done?

There are insufficient data to recommend cognitive screening of asymptomatic people. Those who have self-reported or knowledgeable informant-reported memory complaints or cognitive decline should undergo further comprehensive assessment.

10. What is included in a comprehensive assessment of dementia?

A more thorough mental status evaluation, including mood, affect, and presence of psychotic symptoms, should be done. Laboratory evaluation with blood chemistry, electrolytes, liver function, complete blood count, thyroid function, vitamin B_{12}, and, when appropriate, a screen for neurosyphilis is done to rule out potentially reversible causes of dementia or to identify medical illness that can contribute to cognitive impairment. Brain imaging with either noncontrast computed tomography (CT) or magnetic resonance (MR) scan rules out conditions such as subdural hematoma, brain tumor, or stroke. Atrophy suggests a neurodegenerative dementia.

Name: _____   Date: _____

Orientation *(These 3 questions are not necessary for assessment but may be useful to build confidence)*
                One Point for Each Incorrect Item   Error score   Max. score

Date: Day of week:_____   _____   ____1_

                Day of month:_____   _____   ____1_

                Month:_____   _____   ____1_

                Year:_____   _____   ____1_

Address: Street & number:_____   _____   ____1_

                Town/City:_____   _____   ___1_

                ZIP:_____   _____   ____1_

Phone: Area code:_____   _____   ____1_

                Seven digit number:_____   _____   ___1_

Memory   Ask to repeat and remember three words (apple, table, penny)

Serial subtractions   (appropriate if education > 12 years) Give first example $(100 - 3 = 97)$
                Reset to correct # if subject errors. Score one point for each **incorrect** number

        100   97   94   91   88   85   _____   ___4_

Clock draw to indicate the time of 8:20
                (See examples on back for scoring guidelines)   _____   ___3_
                0 = normal | 2 = moderately impaired
                1 = mildly impaired | 3 = severely impaired

Verbal Fluency

                Number of unique animals in 60 seconds: _____   _____   ___3_
                0 = > 12 animals | 2 = 5-8 animals
                1 = 9-12 animals | 3 = < 5 animals

Delayed recall   (score number not recalled)

                apple   table   penny   _____   ___3_

---

        no cognitive impairment   0 - 4
        mild cognitive impairment   5 - 8   **Total errors**   [   ]
        probable dementia   >8

FIGURE 1.   Brief cognitive screen (to be completed by provider). (From Clark CM, Arnold SE, Karlawish JHT, Horowitz D. Brief Cognitive Screen. From Dementia Disease Management Program, University of Pennsylvania Health System, 1999. Retrieved April 26, 2001 from the UPHS Intranet; http://uphsnet.med.upenn.edu/dm/dementia.)

11. What is the most useful way to stage patients with dementia?

Patients are generally staged as mild, moderate, severe, profound, or terminal. (See table, page 68.) Of the numerous dementia-staging systems in the literature, some are better suited for patients in the early-to-moderate stage and others for late-stage patients. The Clinical Dementia Rating Scale (CDR) is useful to stage patients with early AD, and the Functional Assessment Staging (FAST) is more advantageous for assessing functional change in the severe, end-stage immobile patient with AD.

Current staging systems were developed in groups of patients with AD and follow the progression of AD (memory loss and IADL impairments in the early stage and ADL impairments in the later stages). Patients with other dementia diagnoses may not fit well into the various stages. For example, a patient in mild-stage FTD typically has early ADL impairments, such as incontinence and personal hygiene neglect, but less memory and IADL impairment.

PERSON COMPLETING FORM: _____   RELATIONSHIP TO PATIENT: _____
In each section, please circle **one number** that **most closely applies** to the patient. This is a general form, so no one description may be exactly right -- please circle the answer that seems most appropriate at this time.
Please circle only one number per section.

MEMORY

0   Normal memory.

1   Occasionally forgets things that they were told recently. Does not cause many problems.

2   Mild consistent forgetfulness. Remembers recent events but often forgets parts.

3   Moderate memory loss. Worse for recent events. May not remember something you just told them. Causes problems with everyday activities.

4   Substantial memory loss. Quickly forgets recent or newly learned things. Can only remember things that they have known for a long time.

SPEECH AND LANGUAGE

0   Normal ability to talk and understand others.

1   Sometimes cannot find a word, but able to carry on conversations.

2   Often forgets words. May use the wrong word in its place. Some trouble expressing thoughts and giving answers.

3   Usually answers questions using sentences but rarely starts a conversation.

DATE AND TIME

0   Normal awareness of the time and which day of the week it is

1   Some confusion about what time it is or what day of the week it is, but the problem is not severe enough to interfere with everyday activities.

2   Frequently confused about the date and/or time.

ABILITY TO MAKE DECISIONS

0   Normal - as able to make decisions as before.

1   Only some difficulty making decisions that arise in day-to-day life.

2   Moderate difficulty. Gets confused when things get complicated or plans change.

ABILITY TO GET FROM PLACE TO PLACE

0   Normal, able to get around on their own (May have physical problems that require a cane or walker).

1   Sometimes gets confused when driving or taking public transportation, especially in new places. Able to walk places alone.

2   Cannot drive or take public transportation alone, even in familiar places. Can walk alone outside for short distances. Might get lost if walking too far from home.

FIGURE 2.   Functional assessment screen (to be completed by knowledgeable informant). (From Clark CM, Arnold SE, Karlawish JHT, Horowitz D. Functional Assessment. From Dementia Disease Management Program, University of Pennsylvania Health System, 1999. Retrieved April 26, 2001 from the UPHS Intranet; http://uphsnet.med.upenn.edu/dm/dementia.)

12. Describe the behavioral and mood symptoms common in dementia.

Up to 50% of patients experience depression, especially mild depression, at some point in the illness. Verbal or physical agitation, delusions, hallucinations, sleep disturbance, and aggressiveness are common in the moderate stage and peak in the severe stage. Assessment can be difficult because of overlap of symptoms of depression and dementia. In particular, psychomotor agitation or slowing, appetite and sleep changes, social withdrawal, and psychotic symptoms are present in both. Behavioral and mood symptom assessment should be incorporated into every patient encounter.

13. What causes behavioral symptoms?

The environment influences behavior in dementia and should be evaluated. Fatigue, boredom, overstimulation, and change in routine or caregiver are common precipitants of behavioral symptoms. Medication, such as beta blockers, alpha blockers, sedatives, steroids, or anticholinergic agents and acute medical illness, constipation, or dehydration may cause or contribute to symptoms.

14. Describe the consequences of behavioral symptoms for patient and caregiver.

Early accurate diagnosis of symptoms is important to improve function, quality of life, and disability in both patient and caregiver. Depression leads to greater functional impairment

Stages of Dementia

	MILD	MODERATE	SEVERE	PROFOUND	TERMINAL
Function	IADL-independent or decreased ability with complex tasks ADL-independent	IADL-dependent or assistance needed ADL-independent or reminders, assistance needed	IADL-dependent ADL-dependent (incontinent, able to feed self, still ambulatory)	IADL-dependent ADL-dependent (loss of ambulation, feeds with assistance)	Inability to walk or sit up without assistance Inability to smile or hold head up > 10% body weight loss, pressure ulcers > stage 2 urinary tract infection, aspiration pneumonia
Cognition	Difficulty in learning new information, memory loss interferes with everyday functions Difficulty with time relationships Mild word finding difficulty Able to carry on social conversation Mild judgment impairment	Substantial memory loss, disoriented in time, often to place Conversation disorganized, rambling Judgment impaired Decreased attention span	Oriented to person only Only fragments of memory remain Severe language impairment Inconsistent recognition of familiar people Very short attention span	Speaks < 6 words Consistent difficulty in recognizing familiar people	Few words spoken
Behavior	Mild personality changes Less engaged in relationships Appears normal	May have psychotic, wandering, elopement, agitated verbal or physical symptoms Sleep disturbance Appears well enough to be taken to functions outside of home	Emotional lability Restlessness Inability to focus on tasks Appears to ill to be taken to functions outside the home	Repetitive vocalizations, calling out More passive	Passive
Cognitive scores	MMSE ≥ 19	MMSE 12–19	MMSE 6–11	MMSE < 6	Not testable

and decreased quality of life for the patient. Caregiver education and support, emphasizing problem-solving and coping with behavioral symptoms, delay nursing home placement by about 1 year.

15. What are the current goals for the management of dementia?

Focus interventions not only on the patient with dementia but also on the caregiver. The overarching goal of all dementia care is to enhance function and quality of life and prevent excessive disability.

16. Describe current pharmacologic treatments in dementia.

Pharmacologic therapies to improve cognitive symptoms and slow progression are the standard of care for patients with dementia. Cholinesterase inhibitors, such as donepezil (Aricept), rivastigmine (Exelon), and galantamine (Reminyl), are prescribed for improvement in symptoms in mild-to-moderate AD. Gastrointestinal side effects, such as loose stools, nausea, and stomach upset, are usually mild and dose-related and abate over time. Clinician, patient, and caregiver impressions of change in cognition, function, and behavior measure success. Doses usually are increased at 4-week intervals. Treatment can be continued indefinitely, although evidence is insufficient to recommend it in the later stages. No data support the benefits of one cholinesterase inhibitor over another, but if the patient does not respond, consider a trial of a different agent.

Alpha-tocopherol (vitamin E), an antioxidant, slows progression in AD. At a dose of 1000 IU twice daily, it has been shown to delay functional deterioration and time to institutionalization or death. It is well tolerated, but the dose is decreased with concomitant anticoagulation therapy.

Clinical trials have failed to show clinically meaningful benefit of gingko biloba, estrogen, or nonsteroidal anti-inflammatory drugs to treat symptoms or slow decline in AD.

17. What pharmacologic interventions should you recommend in depression or agitated behaviors?

Selective serotonergic reuptake inhibitors (SSRIs), trazodone, and anticonvulsants (valproic acid, carbemazepine) are useful treatments. Atypical antipsychotics (risperidone, olanzapine, quetiapine) are reserved for patients with psychotic symptoms that are distressing to the patient or lead to aggressive behavior toward others.

18. What behavioral interventions support the person with dementia?

Communication should validate and respect the person's reality and needs. Recommend meaningful social interventions and individualized activities through adult day care or similar recreation programs in long-term care facilities. Special care units in long-term care may improve quality of life but have not been shown to slow functional decline.

19. What recommendations should be given to caregivers?

Caregivers need education about the disease process and what to expect in the future. Emotional support, problem-solving, and management of behavioral symptoms enable caregivers to withstand the stresses of caregiving and defer institutionalization. The Alzheimer's Association (1-800-272-3900 or http://www.alz.org) and local agencies of aging are useful referrals for information and support.

BIBLIOGRAPHY

1. American Psychiatric Association: Diagnostic and Statistical Manual of Mental Disorders, 4th ed. Washington, DC, American Psychiatric Association, 1994.
2. Clark CM, Arnold S, Karlawish HT, Horowitz D: Brief cognitive screen. From Dementia Disease Management Program, University of Pennsylvania Health System, 1999. Accessed April 2001 from the UPHS Intranet: http://uphsnet.med.upenn.edu/dm/dementia.

3. Clark CM, Arnold S, Karlawish HT, Horowitz D: Functional assessment screen. From Dementia Disease Management Program, University of Pennsylvania Health System, 1999. Accessed April 2001 from the UPHS Intranet: http://uphsnet.med.upenn.edu/dm/dementia.

4. Devanand DP, Sano M, Tang MX, et al: Depressed mood and the incidence of Alzheimer's disease in the elderly living in the community. Arch Gen Psychiatry 53:175–182, 1996.

5. Folstein MF, Folstein SE, McHugh PR: "Mini-Mental State": A practical method for grading the cognitive state of patients for the clinician. J Psychol Res 12:189–198, 1975.

6. Logsdon RG, Teri L: The pleasant events schedule—AD: Psychometric properties and relationship to depression and cognition in Alzheimer's disease patients. Gerontologist 37:40–45, 1997.

7. Mittelman MS, Ferris SH, Shulman E, et al: A family intervention to delay nursing home placement of patients with Alzheimer disease. JAMA 276:1725–1731, 1996.

8. Petersen RC, Smith GE, Waring SC, et al: Apolipoprotein E status as a predictor of the development of Alzheimer' disease in memory-impaired individuals. JAMA 273:1274–1278, 1995.

9. Petersen RC, Smith GE, Waring SC, et al: Mild cognitive impairment: Clinical characterization and outcome. Arch Neurol 56:303–308, 1999.

10. Phillips CD, Sloane PD, Hawes C, et al: Effects of residence in Alzheimer disease special care units on functional outcomes. JAMA 278:1340–1344, 1997.

11. Reisberg B: Functional assessment staging (FAST). Psychopharmacol Bull 24:653–659, 1988.

12. Rovner B, Broadhead J, Spencer M: Depression in Alzheimer' disease. Am J Psychiatry. 146:350–353, 1989.

13. Sano M, Ernesto C, Thomas RG, et al: A controlled trial of selegiline, alpha-tocopherol, or both as treatment for Alzheimer's disease. N Engl J Med 336:1216–1222, 1997.

14. Washington University ADRC Clinical Dementia Rating Scale. Accessed May 2001 from the world-wide web: http://www.adrc.wustl.edu/adrc/cdrScale.html.

13. ANXIETY AND GRIEF REACTIONS

Valerie A. Hart, EdD, APRN, BC

1. Patients often present to a primary care setting with either anxiety or depression. What questions should I first ask patients with either or both problems?

In assessing psychosocial behavioral symptoms, ask for a precipitating event. "When did this first occur, and what was happening in your life?" Then assess level of functioningby asking questions such as, "Has this affected your ability to work?" "How are you sleeping?" "Any changes in appetite or weight loss?" "Tell me about your home life and relationships." A useful tool is the BATHE technique. **BATHE** is an acronym for the important components of an interview and fits easily into a 15-minute format. Assessment is made of the **b**ackground situation, the patient's **a**ffect, the problem that is most **t**roubling for the patient, and the method the patient is using to **h**andle the problem. The interview concludes with **e**mpathy.

2. What potential diagnoses do I look for if the main presenting complaint is anxiety?

Anxiety disorders are common (10% of visits) and often undiagnosed in primary care. Examples include panic disorder, generalized anxiety disorder (GAD), posttraumatic stress disorder (PTSD), social phobia, and obsessive-compulsive disorder (OCD). Patients often present with somatic complaints rather than complaints of pure anxiety or nervousness.

3. What interview techniques are most useful in detecting anxiety disorders?

Open-ended questions that cannot be answered by "yes" or "no" are paramount. Other techniques are active listening and observation. The nurse practitioner (NP) needs to inquire about the relationship of stress to the presenting symptoms.

4. What are the common complaints in patients with panic disorder?

In primary care settings patients may describe chest discomfort, dizziness or shortness of breath, choking sensation or "lump in the throat," excessive sweating, hot flashes, nausea, or abdominal distress in the absence of a detectable medical pathology. Peak age of onset is 15–20 years; after age 40 an underlying medical condition or depression is suspected. Other symptoms include fear of dying, sudden feeling of fright for no apparent reason, fear of losing control or going crazy, feeling detached from part of one's body, experiencing trembling or shaking, and rubbery legs. Patients also may have a preoccupation with health concerns and make frequent appointments.

5. What questions should I ask to elicit information that relates to panic disorder?

"Have you ever had a sudden attack of anxiety, with rapid heartbeat, sweating, and feeling of dread?" and "Are you aware of any specific trigger?" Panic attacks are untriggered; if a specific trigger can be identified, specific phobia, PTSD, or social phobia may be the primary diagnosis.

6. What symptoms are associated with GAD?

Three areas hold clusters of symptoms: motor tension, autonomic hyperactivity, and vigilance and scanning. Complaints of easy fatigue, muscle soreness, and trembling, shaking, or twitching are associated with motor tension. Dizziness, dry mouth, palpitations, shortness of breath, trouble with swallowing, hot flashes and chills, sweating or clammy hands, frequent urination, and nausea or diarrhea are related to autonomic hyperactivity. Irritability, difficulty in concentrating, trouble with falling or staying asleep, and exaggerated startle response are related to vigilance of the environment.

7. What symptoms are common in patients with social phobia?

Patients report a fear of social or performance situations and the judgment of others. Symptoms usually occur during adolescence and rarely have onset after age 30. The patient experiences excruciating distress and begins making life adjustments that create a disability. A common story is trying to avoid social situations, which cause extreme anxiety. Patients fear humiliation or embarrassment and, to deal with the demands of ordinary school life, may report the use and abuse of drugs or alcohol. Most patients have a comorbid psychiatric or substance-use diagnosis such as depression. Patients with a specific social phobia, such as performance anxiety, need to be differentiated from a more generalized social phobia, in which a myriad of situations are feared.

8. Does the treatment differ for specific social phobia and generalized social phobia?

Yes. Patients with specific social phobia benefit from beta blockers, and patients with generalized social phobia should try selective serotonin reuptake inhibitors (SSRIs) as first-line agents in a primary care setting. Psychotherapy is also indicated in both types of phobias, along with pharmacotherapy and patient education.

9. What symptom are most prominent in patients with PTSD?

PTSD is precipitated by exposure to a traumatic event that evokes an initial reaction of shock, fear, and a sense of helplessness. When a combination of re-experiencing the trauma in the form of nightmares or flashbacks and the experience of avoidance/numbing and hyper-arousal is present for at least 1 month, the diagnosis is made. Comorbidity with depression and substance abuse is high; the incidence of medical illness also is increased.

10. What treatment is recommended for PTSD?

Psychotherapy remains the treatment of choice. Medication may play a supportive role.

11. Is OCD commonly seen in primary care? What are the symptoms to look for?

OCD is frequently missed because of the patient's profound sense of shame and embarrassment. Although patients may be highly functioning in their career or personal life, they must go to great lengths to conceal certain behaviors. Most do not seek treatment directly unless their functioning becomes significantly impaired. Peak ages of onsets are adolescence and mid-30s. **Obsessions** are intrusive thoughts, and **compulsions** are rituals or repetitive behaviors; both tend to be chronic. Common obsessions involve contamination, harming others, performing routine tasks, and sexual behaviors. Compulsions involve rituals of cleaning, checking, or doing tasks over and over again. An awareness of the thoughts or behaviors and a realization that they are extreme must be present at some point for the diagnosis to be made.

12. What sort of treatment and referral are required if OCD is diagnosed?

Cognitive-behavioral therapy is the treatment of choice. If symptoms are severe, the addition of medications is indicated. SSRIs are the most effective category of medications.

13. When is a referral for psychotherapy a wise decision in dealing with anxiety disorders?

- Suspicion of substance abuse
- Failure of pharmacologic treatment to relieve symptoms
- Distress due to interpersonal issues in the patient's life
- More than one relapse
- Comorbid depression
- PTSD
- Social phobia
- Specific phobia

14. What is the general prognosis for anxiety disorders?

Anxiety disorders tend to be chronic. Although medications and therapy may help to alleviate incapacitating symptoms, patients experience periods of both symptom reduction and recurrence.

15. Who is at increased risk for developing an anxiety disorder?

Children of parents with anxiety disorders, children with an anxious temperament and behavioral inhibition, and victims of trauma.

16. When do symptoms of anxiety indicate a reaction to an external event or inner psychological conflict rather than an anxiety disorder?

Mild and moderate anxiety presents with an increase in physiologic functions, whereas more severe anxiety is accompanied by a slowing of functions. Normal anxiety results from a realistic perception of danger and can be motivating and useful. In abnormal anxiety the perception of danger is distorted, unrealistic, and out of proportion. Counseling the anxious patient about relaxation techniques, regular exercise, and avoidance of stimulants such as caffeine, diet pills, and decongestants is recommended.

17. What is the appropriate treatment of acute situational anxiety that may be a precursor of GAD?

A referral for traditional psychotherapy or supportive psychotherapy is indicated.

18. What are the symptoms of a normal grief reaction? Are there differences in different populations?

Somatic complaints such as gastrointestinal, cardiovascular, respiratory, and sleep disturbances; anxious and depressed mood; suicidal wishes (not ideation or intention); anger and guilt; and preoccupation with an image of the deceased are within the parameters of a normal grieving process. Grieving is a process with phases of shock, disbelief, avoidance, acute mourning (when most symptoms appear), and resolution and reorganization. Because grief is a dynamic and adaptive process, symptoms and corresponding phases wax, wane, and overlap. Although normal grief process applies to children and adolescents, age-specific responses to death must be considered. Bereaved children may evidence guilt, anger, and apathy but also may display somatic distress, insomnia, and appetite disturbances rather than sadness and grief. Adolescents' response to a significant death may be especially acute because of their limited view of the future. Parents grieving the death of a child generally experience more intense and prolonged symptoms. Cultural differences affect the grief response. Gender differences also exist: widowers suffer more depression, mental illness, and morbidity than widows and the general male population. In the second year after bereavement widows and mothers are at a higher risk for depression.

19. What are the risk factors and health consequences of bereavement?

Prior mental illness, preexisting medical conditions, sudden and unexpected death, survivors of homicides or accidents, and lack of social support are risk factors. PTSD may retard normal grieving. Low socioeconomic status and concurrent life stresses may affect overall health status and create compromised coping resources.

20. In dealing with a grieving patient, what are the differential diagnoses to consider?

Depressive disorder, anxiety disorders, PTSD, and adjustment disorder are the differential diagnoses. Assessment of normal depressive mood changes and normal apprehensions are required. Because these disorders are debilitating and indicate a need for both psychotherapy and pharmacotherapy, diagnosis must be accurate. In children and adolescents, adjustment disorder is associated with morbidity, overanxious disorder, oppositional disorder, avoidant disorder, and attention-deficit disorder with hyperactivity and poor outcome. Major depression occurs in 10% of grieving patients and needs to be considered in patients with marked psychomotor retardation, suicidal ideation, obsessional guilt, disturbed self-esteem, and feelings of worthlessness.

21. What type of somatic and behavioral complaints suggest a possible grief response?

Somatic complaints include appetite and subacute gastrointestinal disturbances and fatigue. Sleep disturbances and depression may be the presenting complaints. Behavioral problems include substance abuse and social, school, or work difficulties.

22. What primary care interventions are appropriate for grieving patients?

Empathetic affirming of reality, normalizing, education about the grief process, and referral to support groups are appropriate interventions in primary care. Follow-up for a grieving patient should include a 1- to 2-year plan. Accepting the reality of the loss, experiencing the pain of grief, adjusting to life without the deceased, and reinvesting in new activities and relationships constitute the goals for the grieving patient. By monitoring these tasks, the clinician can ensure that the process is proceeding and that adjustment is occurring over time.

23. How is pathologic grief defined? How common are conditions in this category?

The various types of responses include delayed grief, inhibited grief, absent grief, and chronic grief. Twenty-five (25%) of bereaved adults experience complications of some kind. Delayed grief occurs in 10–15% of pathologic responses and is hallmarked by an onset delayed more than 2 weeks after the loss. Inhibited grief occurs in 5% of pathologic responses when the patient continues to have exaggerated symptoms and is associated most often with an anniversary of the event. When no symptoms of grief are present for 6 months or more after the loss, absent grief is the diagnosis. Chronic grief represents 75% of pathologic responses and is diagnosed when acute symptoms continue past the first year or when symptoms of loss worsen. Chronic grief may be the aftermath of delayed, absent, or inhibited grief. In summary, if the NP does not see progress over time through the phases of grieving, the patient may be "stuck" in one of the phases. Remaining excessively sad or angry indicates that the patient may be struggling with the stage of resolution and would benefit from referral for psychotherapy. Delayed grief reactions can occur years after the death or loss and may not be part of the patient's consciousness when they present as somatic complaints. Anniversary reactions to a death or loss also may be at an unconscious level.

24. What should one consider when patients exhibit both depressive and anxiety symptoms?

With the exception of panic disorder, mixed anxiety and depressive disorders are the rule. In GAD, social phobia, and PTSD, many patients also suffer from a depressive disorder. Although the anxiety symptoms are usually chronic, the depressive symptoms tend to be episodic. Comorbid patients are likely to have a more severe illness, with greater risk for hospitalization and suicide attempts and a poorer long-term outcome.

25. Do any controversies surround evaluation or treatment of either anxiety disorders or grief reactions?

Most patient with anxiety disorders are treated in nonmental health settings—that is, primary care settings. Yet research continues to focus on patients who visit mental health providers and are not treated in primary care settings. Recognition and treatment of anxious patients in primary care settings must be a priority to bring research findings into proper realistic perspective. This problem presents an interesting turf issue among primary care providers, mental health clinicians, and researchers.

A movement is still brewing to create a separate diagnostic category for complicated grief reaction, which is defined by three sets of symptoms: intrusions, avoidances, and failures to adapt to the specific loss event.

When the *Diagnostic and Statistical Manual of Mental Disorders*, 4th edition, was revised in the early 90s, the subcommittee on PTSD recommended a separate category of diagnoses for stress response syndromes. The subcommittee wished to combine several diagnoses in which stress or events precipitate symptom formation. Examples include pathologic or complicated grief, acute stress disorder, PTSD, dissociative amnesia, and adjustment disorder. This suggestion was rejected, but the debate will continue when the next edition is developed.

BIBLIOGRAPHY

1. Barlow D, Wincze J: DSM-IV and beyond: What is generalized anxiety disorder? Acta Psychiatr Scan 98:23–29, 1998.
2. Barbee J: Mixed symptoms and syndromes of anxiety and depression. Ann Clin Psychol 10:15–29, 1998.
3. Feldman M: Managing psychiatric disorders in primary care: Anxiety. Hosp Pract 7:77–84, 2000.
4. Horowitz M, Siegel B, Holen A, et al: Diagnostic criteria for complicated grief disorder. Am J Psychiatry 154:904–910, 1997.
5. Newman M, Borkovek T, Hope D, et al: Future directions in the treatment of anxiety disorders: An examination of theory, basic science, public policy, psychotherapy research, clinical training and practice. J Clin Psychol 55:1325–1345, 1999.
6. Norton P, Gordon J, Asmundson G, et al: Future directions in anxiety disorders. J Anxiety Disord 14:69–94, 2000.
7. Price D, Beck A, Nimmer C, Benson S: The treatment of anxiety disorders in a primary care HMO setting. Psychol Q 71:31–45, 2000.
8. Sanders C: Risk factors in bereavement outcome. In Strobe M (ed): Handbook of Bereavement: Theory, Research and Intervention. Cambridge, Cambridge University Press, 1993.
9. Sansone R, Sansone L, Righter E: Panic disorder: The ultimate anxiety. J Womens Health 7:983–989, 1998.
10. Steen K: A comprehensive approach to bereavement. Nurse Practit 23:54–64, 66–68, 1998.

14. EARACHES AND EAR DRAINAGE

Ann Marie Ramsey, RN, MSN, CPNP

1. What are the diagnostic criteria for acute otitis media (AOTM)?

1. Fluid must be present in the middle ear space but can be accurately assessed only by pneumatic otoscopy or tympanometry. The usual landmark of the long arm of the malleous may be obscured by bulging of the tympanic membrane.

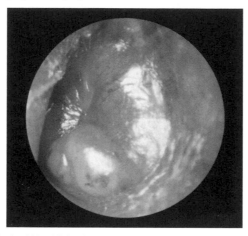

Acute otitis media. Note lack of identifiable landmarks due to bulging of tympanic membrane. (From A Guide to the Use of Diagnostic Instruments and Ear Examinations [educational pamphlet]. Skaneateles Falls, NY, Welch Allen, Inc, 1996, with permission.)

2. The fluid in the middle ear must be infected. Infection frequently is manifested by a yellow cast to the tympanic membrane, indicating the presence of purulence in the middle ear space.

3. The child must be symptomatic. Symptoms include fever, irritability, change in sleep patterns, and change in feeding patterns.

2. What organisms are most commonly associated with AOTM?

1. The three most commonly cultured organisms in AOTM are:
   - *Streptococcus pneumoniae* (cultured in 40–50% of all isolates)
   - *Haemophilus influenzae* (cultured in 20–30% of all isolates)
   - *Moraxella catarrhalis* (cultured in 10–15% of all isolates)

2. Viral organisms coexist with bacterial organisms in 95% of isolates and are the sole organism in 5% of isolates. Commonly found viruses include influenza A, respiratory syncytial virus, coxsackie virus, adenovirus, and parainfluenza.

3. How is AOTM treated?

The Centers for Disease Control and the American Academy of Pediatrics have developed principles for judicious use of antimicrobial agents for AOTM:
   - There must be an accurate diagnosis of AOTM.
   - Only AOTM is treated with antimicrobials. Sterile fluid in the middle ear, known as otitis media with effusion (OME), is not routinely treated with antimicrobials.
   - The diagnosis of AOTM requires documentation of infected middle ear fluid *and* clinical symptoms.

- Children younger than 2 years of age should be treated with a 10-day course of antibiotics.
- Children older than 2 with uncomplicated AOTM may be treated with a 5- to 7-day course.
- Persistent middle ear effusion after resolution of AOTM should not be treated.
- Prophylactic antibiotics should be used rarely and selectively.

4. What are the best antibiotics to use to treat AOTM?

Amoxicillin is universally recognized as the most effective agent for AOTM in nonallergic patients. The child with AOTM who is not in day care and has not had antibiotics in the past month should receive low-dose amoxicillin for the length of time specified above. Children who have had antibiotics in the past month or are in group day care may receive high-dose amoxicillin, amoxicillin-clavulanate, or cefuroxime axetil. Children who are allergic to penicillin may receive azithromycin. In the past, cefaclor and trimethoprim/sulfamethoxazole were utilized for penicillin-allergic patients. In recent years, increasing numbers of resistant organisms and potential side effects associated with these agents have resulted in their declining use. A complete list of all antimicrobial agents approved by the Food and Drug Administration (FDA) for acute otitis media, their dose ranges, advantages and disadvantages is summarized in the table on pages 78 and 79.

5. The child has not clinically improved in 48–72 hours. What are the next steps?

1. Reexamination of the child is recommended to ensure that physical findings are consistent with persistent AOTM.
2. Pharmacologic options depend on first-line treatment.
   - If first-line treatment was low-dose amoxicillin, a second-line option is to increase the dose of amoxicillin to 90 mg/kg.
   - If first-line treatment was either low- or high-dose amoxicillin, another second-line option is amoxicillin-clavulanate or cefuroxime axetil.
   - If either amoxicillin-clavulanate or cefuroxime axetil was used as a first-line treatment, the alternative agent may be used.
3. Ceftriaxone may be used as a second-line choice in patients with severe infection or patients in whom compliance or ability to tolerate oral antibiotics is believed to be an issue.

6. What is recommended follow-up for a child with AOTM?

1. Children should be reexamined if they do not show clinical improvement within 48–72 hours of beginning antimicrobial therapy.
2. 60% of children recovering from AOTM have middle ear fluid 4 weeks after resolution of the infection; 10% of children have fluid 12 weeks after infection.
3. Routine follow up should be scheduled at 6–10 weeks after diagnosis.

7. What is the role of the new 7-valent pneumococcal vaccine in the prevention of AOTM?

The American Academy of Pediatrics recommends that all children under the age of 2 be vaccinated with the 7-valent pneumoccocal vaccine, which is directed at the 7 serotypes identified by epidemiologic data as the primary pathogens in 86% of cases of bacteremia and 83% of cases of meningitis. Thus, the vaccine was directed at the most invasive disease entities and not at otitis-specific serotypes.

In a Finnish study, the 7-valent vaccine was found to be 34% efficacious in preventing pneumoccocal otitis of all serotypes and 57% effective in preventing pneumoccocal otitis from the vaccine-specific serotypes. A study at Kaiser reported a 7% decrease in all episodes of AOTM and 23% reduction in repeat episodes. Therefore, although this vaccine is not specifically indicated for the prevention of AOTM, clinical evidence suggests that AOTM prevention may be an added benefit.

Antimicrobial Agents Approved for the Treatment of Acute Otitis Media

DRUG NAME	TRADE NAME	DOSE	STRENGTH	WEAKNESS	COMMENTS
Amoxicillin	Amoxil, and others	40–90 mg/kg twice daily	Broad reliable coverage	Ineffective against penicillin-resistant S. pneumoniae and beta-lactamase producers	First-choice agent for non-allergic patients. Use high dose for patients with risk factors.
Amoxicillin-clavulanate	Augmentin	40–90 mg/kg/day based on amoxicillin in 2 or 3 doses	Excellent broad-spectrum coverage, including beta-lactamase producers	GI complaints, expensive	Recommended second-line choice for amoxicillin failures or first-line choice for patients with risk factors.
Trimethoprim-sulfamethoxazole	Bactrim/Septra	8 mg/kg/day based on trimethoprim twice daily	Broad-coverage capabilities	High allergic profile, potential for fatal side effects	S. pneumoniae resistance patterns have rendered it a drug with moderate-to-poor efficacy; generally not used.
Erythromycin with sulfisoxazole	Pediazole	30–50 mg/kg/day based on erythromycin in 3 doses	Broad coverage	High allergic profile High incidence of resistant strains	Emerging resistant strains have caused this drug to fall out of favor as a first-line choice for penicillin-allergic children.
Azithromycin	Zithromax	10 mg/kg day 1 5 mg/kg days 2–5	Broad coverage, including beta-lactamase producers	Emerging strains of resistant S. pneumoniae	First-choice therapy for patients allergic to penicillins and cephalosporins.
Clarithromycin	Biaxin	15 mg/kg/day in 2 doses	Broad coverage, including beta-lactamase producers	Emerging strains of resistant S. pneumoniae Very bad, grainy taste	No clinical advantage over azithromycin.
Cefixime	Suprax	8 mg/kg/day	Excellent gram-negative coverage	Poor S. pneumoniae coverage	Not recommended because of effect on gut flora
Ceftibuten	Cedax	9 mg/kg/day	Excellent gram-negative coverage	Poor S. pneumoniae coverage	Not recommended because of effect on gut flora.
Cefdinir	Omnicef	14 mg/kg/day in 1 or 2 doses	Broad spectrum	Poor S. pneumoniae coverage	Some authors cite similar efficacy rates as Augmentin at lower cost.

(Table continued on next page.)

Antimicrobial Agents Approved for the Treatment of Acute Otitis Media (cont'd)

DRUG NAME	TRADE NAME	DOSE	STRENGTH	WEAKNESS	COMMENTS
Ceftriaxone	Rocephin	50–75 mg/kg/day IM for 1–3 days	Broad and reliable coverage	IM injection, requires office visit, expensive	Recommended as second-line therapy for severe infections or in cases of questionable compliance or intolerance of oral antibiotics.
Loracarbef	Lorabid	30 mg/kg/day in 2 doses	Broad coverage, tastes great	Somewhat beta-lactamse–sensitive, expensive	Fair second-line choice.
Cefprozil	Cefzil	30 mg/kg/day in 2 doses	Broad coverage	Somewhat beta-lactamse–sensitive	No clinical advantage to this agent.
Cefpodoxime	Vantin	10 mg/kg/day in 2 doses	Broad, reliable coverage	Tastes very bad, bitter after-taste, poorly tolerated	Poor tolerability have made this a fair second-line choice.
Trimethoprim	Primsol	8 mg/kg/day in 2 doses	Intermediate coverage	*S. pneumoniae* and *M. catarrhalis* resistant	Covers only one of 3 major organisms of AOTM; therefore, generally not used. Adverse effects include rash.
Cefuroxime axetil	Ceftin	30 mg/kg/day in 2 doses	Excellent broad-spectrum coverage, including beta-lactamase producers	Suspension has gritty, bitter taste	Recommended second-line choice for amoxicillin failures or first-line choice for patients with risk factors; first-line choice for patients with penicillin allergy (not anaphylasis or other severe allergy).
Cefaclor	Ceclor	40 mg/kg/day in 2 doses	Broad coverage	Increasing incidence of resistance; associated with serum sickness	Increasing patterns of resistance and high potential for significant side effects make this a poor choice. Generally not utilized for AOTM any more.

8. What is otitis media with effusion (OME)?

OME is defined as fluid in the middle ear space that is not infected. The fluid may be thin (commonly termed serous effusion) or be very thick (termed a mucoid effusion or "glue ear").

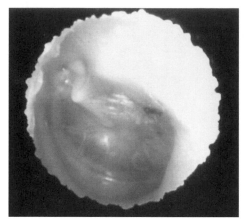

Otitis media with effusion. Note air-fluid level and visible landmarks. This condition is *not* treated with antibiotics. (Photo: ©Ann Marie Ramsey, RN, MSN, CPNP.)

9. What causes OME?

The most common cause of OME is eustachian tube dysfunction. The eustachian tube does not properly drain and ventilate the middle ear space. Factors believed to place a child at risk for development of OME include:

1. Exposure to second-hand smoke in the home environment.
2. Attendance at group day care
3. Family history of ear disease

10. What are the symptoms of OME?

Most patients are asymptomatic. Complaints of ear pain are rare. Affected children are identified most frequently by hearing loss. Many are referred when they fail school hearing screens or when the family has concerns about hearing loss. Some children present with speech delay or significant decline in speech.

11. How is OME treated?

The Agency for Healthcare Research and Quality (formerly Agency for Health Care Policy and Research) convened a group of otolaryngologists, pediatricians, and family practice health care providers to develop guidelines for the treatment of OME. These guidelines apply to otherwise healthy children.

Initial identification of bilateral OME with hearing loss

1. Observation (highest recommendation)
2. Control of risk factors listed in question 9 (highest recommendation)
3. One course of antibiotics (lower recommendation) is estimated to improve outcomes in approximately 14% of cases.
4. Bilateral myringotomy and tubes are *not* recommended at this time.

Persistent OME for 3 or more months with hearing loss

1. Control of risk factors listed in question 8
2. Bilateral myringotomy and tube placement
3. If the child is over 4 years of age, adenoidectomy may be performed concurrently with tube placement.

12. What are ear tubes?

Ear tubes, also called pressure-equalizing tubes (PETs), are placed in the tympanic membrane through a small incision called a myringotomy. This procedure is usually done while the child is under general anesthesia. The ear tube functions just like the eustachian tube to allow fluid in the middle ear to drain and to keep the middle ear ventilated.

13. What are the criteria for consideration of PET placement?

The following are general indications for referral to an otolaryngologist for evaluation:

1. Recurrent AOTM. Children who have 4–6 episodes of AOTM within 4–6 months. Children with significant drug allergies may be referred sooner because of the limited antimicrobial options.

2. OME. Children who have bilateral OME that has persisted longer than 3 months and is associated with hearing loss.

14. Do PETs prevent ear infections?

No. PETs drain and ventilate the middle ear space. Fluid in the middle ear space can serve as a medium for bacterial growth and a subsequent AOTM. Children can still get infections in the middle ear space while the tube is in place. Instead of building up behind the tympanic membrane, pus drains out through the tube. Children typically do not present with the fever, irritability, and ear pain common to AOTM.

15. What are the possible complications of PETs?

Generally PETs are well tolerated and provide predictable relief from recurrent AOTM and OME. Most children have no complications. Possible complications include:

- Ear drainage, which may be episodic or chronic.
- Formation of granulation tissue around the tube, resulting in bleeding from the ear (episodic or chronic).
- Chronic drainage or granulation tissue formation, which may require surgical removal of the tubes.
- Extrusion of the tube into the middle ear space
- Hearing loss

16. How do I treat a child with PETs and ear drainage?

In 2000 the American Academy of Otolaryngology convened a consensus panel of practicing otolaryngologists and infectious disease experts to recommend treatment for three common otologic problems. For drainage through a PET, *the panel recommends topical antibiotics alone as first-line treatment, finding no evidence that oral antibiotics alone or in conjunction with topical antibiotics result in improved outcomes.* There has been extensive research on the safety of ototopical antibiotics. The fluroquinolone antibiotics, which include ciprofloxicin and ofloxicin have been found to be safe and non-ototoxic. They have excellent antimicrobial activity, low systemic absorption, and a low allergic profile. Ofloxacin, the antibiotic found in Floxin (Diachii Pharmaceuticals), has received FDA approval for use in the presence of an open tympanic membrane.

17. How can antibiotic drops be used if the child has ear drainage?

The pus and cellular debris must be removed from the external auditory canal to allow antibiotic drops to penetrate to the level of the tympanic membrane. There are several ways to accomplish this goal:

1. The child may be referred to an otolaryngologist for aural hygiene in the office, using suction under direct visualization with an otological microscope.

2. The ear my be irrigated with a solution of half white vinegar and half warm tap water, using a 10-ml syringe with a butterfly set connected to the end. The needle and all but 1 cm of

the butterfly set is cut off, thereby leaving only the tip, which directs the irrigating solution into the ear canal.

3. The drainage may be wicked out of the ear with a cotton swab.

18. How do I treat a child with a PET and bleeding ear?

Bleeding from the ear of a child with tubes usually results from the formation of granulation tissue around the tube. Granulation tissue is polypoid-appearing tissue with a rich vascular supply that is an end-product of the inflammatory cascade. Granulation tissue may form spontaneously or in response to an episode of drainage. Treatment involves cleaning the ear to allow visualization of the tympanic membrane and tube and identification of the granulation tissue. Many primary care providers find debridement of the bloody ear difficult and often refer the patient to an otolaryngologist. Treatment of ear granuloma involves application of topical steroid drops. In cases of severe granuloma, surgical removal may be necessary.

19. What is laser-assisted myringotomy? How do I know if it is right for my patient?

Laser-assisted myringotomy is a new technology used as an alternative to placement of tubes. A laser is used to make a hole in the tympanic membrane. This hole typically heals in approximately 6 weeks. Topical local anesthesia is applied to the tympanic membrane via an otowick device. The procedure is performed with the child awake and in the parent's arms. Advantages include avoidance of general anesthetic, parental separation, and a foreign body (PET) in the ear. The main disadvantage is the short-term duration of ventilation of the middle ear space. In young children who have a significant amount of time before the eustachian tube is expected to mature, symptoms tend to recur when the hole closes. Many such children eventually require placement of tubes.

At present, the technology is too new to have a firm set of indications (i.e., children for whom the procedure is most recommended). Preliminary practice experience has revealed that school-aged children with unilateral effusion seem to have the most favorable outcomes, defined as long-term resolution of the effusion and low incidence of the need for tube placement. To avoid disappointment by parents if their child is not a candidate for this procedure, it is probably best not to refer a child specifically for this purpose; instead, inform the parent that several therapeutic options are available and that the provider to whom you are referring the child will help them to select the best option.

20. When should a child with ear pain or ear drainage be referred to an otolaryngologist?

1. Emergent referral for ear pain or infection if intracranial or intratemporal complication is suspected, such as acute mastoiditis (cardinal sign: unilateral facial paralysis)

2. Urgent referral for refractory otitis media in a significantly symptomatic child for the purpose of tympanocentesis

3. Routine referrals
   • Child who meets criteria listed above for consideration of PET placement
   • Child with chronic drainage (lasting for 6 weeks or longer) from the ear(s) despite appropriate treatment

21. What controversies are associated with otitis media?

Two current controversies involve whether children with tubes should protect their ears from water and whether tympanocentesis should be recommended as a primary care option for cases of refractory AOTM.

22. Should children with tubes protect their ears from water with plugs?

The rationale for use of ear plugs is based on the fact that the natural protection of the middle ear space by an intact tympanic membrane is lost when a tube is placed. Water may carry bacteria, which may seed in the middle ear space and result in drainage from the ear. Current research, however, suggests otherwise. Lee performed a meta-analysis of 64 studies examining the relationship between otorrhea in children with PETs and water exposure and found that children who swam without ear protection have the same or fewer episodes of otor-rhea than children who swam with ear protection. Herber put a head model through a series of water exposure scenarios. Results showed no water entry with showering, hair rinsing, or sub-mersion of the head less than 2 feet in clean water. Water entry was associated with head sub-mersion in more than two feet of water and when soap was introduced into the water. Salata used an experimental design to determine whether ear plugs and/or prophylactic drops de-creased swim-related otorrhea in children with tubes. He found no statistical difference in rates of swim-related otorrhea between children who wore ear plugs or used antibiotic drops after swimming and children with no ear protection at all.

When counseling families about the use of plugs and/or drops during exposure to water, it is important to be consistent with the operating otolaryngologist's recommendations. In the absence of recommendations, current research suggests that the potential for water entry into the middle ear space during routine showering, hair rinsing, and swimming is relatively low; hence, no protection is required. Because exposure to soapy water (as occurs in a bathtub) in-creases the potential for water penetration to the middle ear, children should not lay or put the head under the water in the bath. Submersion of the head under more than 2 feet of water and diving also should be discouraged.

23. Should tympanocentesis be recommended as a primary care option for cases of re-fractory AOTM?

Proponents' rationale

1. Before the antibiotic era, primary care physicians routinely performed tympanocente-sis. The technique is described by experts as "relatively simple," easily learned, and easily carried out in all children with the exception of small infants.

2. It allows treatment based on culture, thereby taking the "guess work" out of treatment for refractory cases. This evidence-based approach may decrease the use of multiple courses of antibiotics and the likelihood of resistant organisms.

Opponents' rationale

1. Tympanocentesis is not routinely taught in pediatric or family practice residency programs. Of all board-certified pediatricians in the United States, only 100 know how to perform tympa-nocentesis and only about 50 perform the procedure on a routine basis, according to Pichichero.

2. Cases of true refractory AOTM are not common; therefore, there is no opportunity to practice and refine this skill in the primary care setting.

3. Some experts recommend providing conscious sedation before the procedure, which requires monitoring of the child's airway and availability of emergency equipment and trained personnel in the event of airway emergency. This requirement, along with cost and time, pre-clude many busy primary care offices from routinely performing the procedure.

4. Generally patients with refractory AOTM can be referred, if necessary, to an otolaryn-gologist trained and expert in the procedure.

Bottom line: Tympanocentesis is unlikely to make a grand reemergence in the primary care arena. The procedure is costly and time-intensive and frequently requires resources outside the scope of a primary care office. A better alternative plan is to establish a relationship with a local otolaryngologist to whom children with refractory acute otitis media can be referred for care.

ACKNOWLEDGMENT

The author acknowledges the assistance of Heather VandenBussche, Pharm.D., Pediatric Clinical Pharmacist at the University of Michigan, in ensuring the accuracy of the drug information presented in the antibiotic table.

BIBLIOGRAPHY

1. Blumer JL: Fundamental basis for rational therapeutics in acute otitis media. Pediatr Infect Dis J 18:1130–1140, 1999.

2. Dowell SF, et al: Acute otitis media: Management and surveillance in an era of pneumococcal resistance: A report from the drug-resistant *Streptococcus pneumoniae* therapeutic working group. Pediatr Infect Dis J 18:1–9, 1999.
3. Dowell SF: Otitis media: Principles of judicious use of antimicrobial agents. Pediatrics (Suppl Pt 2):165–171, 1998.
4. Hannley MT, Denneny JC, Holzer SS: Use of topical antibiotics in treating three common ear diseases. Arch Otolaryngol Head Neck Surg 122(6):934–940.
5. Herbert RL, et al: Tympanostomy tubes and water exposure: A practical model. Arch Otolaryngol Head Neck Surg 124:1118–1121, 1998.
6. Klein JO: Review of consensus reports on management of acute otitis media. Pediatr Infect Dis J 18:1152–1155, 1999.
7. Lee D, Youk A, Goldstein NA: A meta-analysis of swimming and water precautions. Laryngoscope 109:536–540, 1999.
8. McCracken GH: Prescribing antimicrobial agents for treatment of aute otitis media. Pediatr Infect Dis J 18:1141–1146, 1999.
9. Pichichero ME: Controversies in the medical management of persistent and recurrent acute otitis media: Recommendations of a clinical advisory committee. Ann Otol Rhinol Laryngol 102(Suppl Pt 2):1–12, 2000.
10. Ramilo O: Role of respiratory viruses in acute otitis media: Implications for management. Pediatr Infect Dis J 18:1125–1129, 1999.
11. Salata JA: Water precautions in children with tympanostomy tubes. Arch Otolaryngol Head Neck Surg 122:276–280, 1996.

15. SYNCOPE

Tina Hackney, MSN, RN, CS, FNP

1. Define presyncope.

Presyncope may be defined primarily as dizziness without true vertigo and may be an early warning sign of an impending seizure. Presyncope may or may not lead to an actual syncopal episode. The following findings are present:
- Sensation of dizziness
- Lightheadedness/faintness
- Impending loss of consciousness

Other symptoms include visual blurring, diaphoresis, and heaviness in the lower limbs, leading to postural sway.

2. What is syncope?

Syncope is classically defined as a *sudden* transient loss of consciousness, caused by an acute drop in blood flow to the brain. Syncope accounts for 5–10% of emergency department visits and hospitalizations. It usually occurs while the patient is standing and may be preceded by a presyncopal episode or occur suddenly. A syncopal episode has no definite seizure activity. The following variables are present in a true syncopal episode:
- Loss of motor function with postural collapse
- Transient, reversible decrease in cerebral blood flow
- Spontaneous recovery

Other symptoms include weak, thready pulse; pallor; and diaphoresis.

3. List common causes of syncope.

CIRCULATORY	CEREBRAL	RESPIRATORY	OTHER
Arrhythmia	Stroke	Hypoventilation	Hypoglycemia
Carotid sinus sensitivity	Transient ischemic attack	Hypoxia Hyperventilation	Psychogenic (anxiety, panic)
Valsalva maneuver/ vasovagal	Seizure (more likely related to a pre-		Situational (coughing, eating, defecation may in-
Myocardial infarction	syncopal event)		duce vasovagal response)
Aortic/pulmonic stenosis			Drug induced
Pulmonary embolism			
Orthostatic hypotension			

4. Which questions are most important to include in the key history-taking?
- What time of day did the event occur?
- Was the event related to meals?
- What happened in the preceding 24 hours?
- Did the event occur in association with bladder/bowel habits?
- Was the patient taking any new medications? (Review all medications, prescription and over the counter)
- Was there a witness to describe any preceding symptoms?
- How long did the episode last?
- Were there any precipatating or aggravating circumstances?
- In what position was the patient at the time of the episode?

- Is this the first episode?
- Was the person exposed to intense pain or the sight of blood before the episode?

5. Describe the pertinent physical findings.

1. You should always assess orthostatic vital signs. Take the left and right blood pressure and pulse with the patient in the supine position; repeat each immediately after the patient moves to a sitting position. Next, have the patient stand, as you repeat left and right blood pressure and pulse measurements at baseline, 30 seconds, and 60 seconds. A normal response is to notice a slight decrease in blood pressure and increase in heart rate immediately on standing, but values should normalize at the 30- and 60-second intervals. Have a second person assist, taking the pulse and blood pressure on one side, as you do the same on the opposite side. The presence of a second person to assist is important in case the patient begins to sway. Failure of blood pressure and pulse to normalize as expected may indicate vasovagal response, dehydration, blood loss, or medication response.

2. Cardiac exam is imperative. Carotid bruits may indicate significant stenosis interrupting blood flow to the brain. Have the patient hold his or her breath, and listen with the bell of the stethoscope for a high-pitched sound. Listen on the right and left sides. Make sure that the patient is told to resume breathing. Auscultation of the heart is important for detecting murmurs (aortic/mitral stenosis), extra heart sounds (cardiomyopathy), and tachycardias/bradycardias. Be attentive for both diastolic and systolic murmurs as well as an S_3, S_4, click, or snap.

3. Neurologic exam is essential to identify any deficits indicative of stroke, tumor, or seizure. Assess the cranial nerves as well as coordination, strength, and sensation. The pattern of any neurologic deficits may help to differentiate among potential neurologic causes. If the patient is seen soon after a seizure, he or she may still be groggy or confused and/or smell of urine (if incontinent during the episode). When considering potential neurologic causes, also look for signs of physical injury. In contrast to episodes of true syncope, patients with a neurologic deficit are less likely to have an awareness of the need to break their fall; thus, they are more likely to sustain injury.

6. What diagnostic studies are used in diagnosing the causes of syncope?

The first episode of syncope may not need any diagnostic testing. However, any suggestion of a cardiac arrhythmia requires a more aggressive work-up.

- Electrocardiogram: gives a "snapshot" of actual heart rate and rhythm; may be useful in detecting bradycardia/tachycardia or irregular rhythm and measuring QRS interval.
- Laboratory tests: blood glucose (hypoglycemia), hematocrit/hemoglobin (anemia), serum chemistry (electrolyte imbalances), and drug screen.
- Holter monitor: needs to be worn for at least 48–72 hours to detect a cardiac arrhythmia, especially if the events are infrequent. Patients may need to wear the monitor for an even longer period.
- Exercise stress test: may be useful in trying to detect arrhythmia or bradycardia.
- Echocardiogram (if indicated by physical exam): detects aortic, mitral, and tricuspid valve stenosis; left ventricle hypertrophy; and left atrial enlargement; measures ejection fraction.
- Computerized tomography (CT) or magnetic resonance imaging (MRI): useful if any neurologic deficits are noted to rule out a brain tumor.
- Electroencephalogram (EEG): useful if seizure disorder is suspected.
- Tilt-table test (performed by specialist): may induce severe bradycardia, hypotension, presyncope, or syncope. Because of the severity of these induced symptoms, most patients cannot or will not tolerate this test, which may be extremely frightening, especially to elderly patients.
- Worth mentioning, although not recommended, is a carotid sinus massage. If syncope is truly related to the carotid sinus, it is most noticed when the patient turns the head

quickly from side to side or wears tight clothing around the neck. If carotid massage is done on both carotids and the patient has unknown stenosis, the massage may lead to cerebral ischemia.

7. Describe the treatment for orthostatic hypotenstion.
- Caution patients to change positions slowly, especially when moving from a supine position to a standing or sitting position. Patients should sit up for a few seconds to make sure that they are not feeling dizzy or lightheaded before standing up.
- Sleep with the head of the bed elevated.
- Stretch/exercise the legs before getting out of bed.
- Wear elastic stockings to help prevent pooling of blood flow to the lower extremities.
- Eat frequent smaller meals.
- Avoid alcohol.
- Avoid overheating (e.g., hot showers and baths, hot weather).

8. What do you do when someone faints?
1. Elevate the patient's feet and legs (this position permits maximal blood flow to the brain).
2. Loosen all tight articles of clothing.
3. Maintain a good airway.
4. Drizzling (not splashing) cold water on the face may help.
5. If, however, the person faints in cold weather, covering the person with blankets may be more beneficial.
6. When the person regains consciousness, do not allow him or her to get up until all symptoms of lightheadedness or dizziness have passed. The patient then should be monitored for a few more minutes to make sure that no further symptoms have occurred.

9. How is the treatment of vasovagal syncope handled?
Elastic stockings may help. Beta blockers (atenolol, 25–50 mg/day) can be used as first-line drug therapy. They are the most common pharmacologic approach to managing vasovagal syncope. Beta blockers reduce the severity of catecholamine stimulation of the cardiac receptors. Anticholinergic agents, such as a scopolamine patch applied every 2–3 days, also can be tried.

If these medications do not work, fluorocortisone acetate (Florinef), 0.1–0.3 mg/day, or fluoxetine (Prozac), 10 mg/day, can be tried. Fludrocortisone, however, should *not* be used in patients with congestive heart failure. Increased sodium intake helps to increase volume. Again, this method should *not* be used in patients with congestive heart failure.

10. If carotid sinus syncope is suspected, how should it be treated?
1. Loose clothing is of paramount importance. People should be taught to turn the entire body when looking to the side as opposed to turning only the head.
2. Potential fall hazards also should be reduced. Rubber mats may be placed in the bathtub and on the bathroom floor. Soft surfaces are preferrable to hard surfaces for walking.
3. Reducing potential falls is important because trauma from a fall related to a syncopal episode can be a bigger hazard for elderly people than the syncopal episode itself.

11. Whom do you admit to the hospital for a work-up as opposed to an outpatient work-up?
- Anyone who has a syncopal episode with known cardiovascular disease, angina, or significant electrocardiographic changes.
- Anyone who sustains an injury due to abrupt loss of consciousness should be admitted and evaluated.
- Anyone with exertional syncope requires an aggressive work-up to determine how much exertion induces syncope.
- In people older than 70 years, syncope may signal an arrhythmia or heart block. Severe arrhythmias or heart block may signal a need for a permanent pacemaker.

12. When do you refer to a specialist (cardiologist or neurologist)?
• Physical examination suggests carotid artery obstruction (bruits).
• History suggests cardiac origin of syncopal episode.
• Seizure disorder is suspected.
• New cardiac murmurs indicating valvular disease or cardiomyopathy.
• Holter monitor provides proof of heart block, tachyarrhythmia, or bradycardia.

13. What are the major differential diagnoses of syncope?
1. **Hypoglycemia**: Severe hypoglycemia usually points to a serious disease (tumor), advanced adrenal/hepatic disease, or an excess of insulin administration. Mild hypoglycemia usually occurs 2–5 hours after eating and is not associated with actual syncope.

2. **Anxiety (panic attack)**: Usually described as a feeling of dizziness without actual loss of consciousness. Symptoms are *not* relieved by elevating the legs above the head. The attack usually can be reproduced by hyperventilating, which results in decreased blood flow to the brain. Epinephrine release during an anxiety attack also contributes to the feeling of dizziness/faintness.

3. **Acute hemorrhage**: Usually in the gastrointestinal tract. This diagnosis may remain a mystery until the person passes a black, tarry stool or has hematemesis or abdominal pain.

4. **Cerebral transient ischemic attack**: Usually occurs in people with artherosclerotic stenosis or emboli to the major arteries in the brain. Isolated loss of consciousness in this setting is uncommon.

5. **Seizure activity**: Usually some other symptom occurs at the time of the event, such as extremity shaking, loss of bowel/bladder control, or drooling.

BIBLIOGRAPHY

1. Blatt CM, Graboys TB: Evaluation of the patient with syncope. In Alpert JS (ed): Cardiology for the Primary Care Physcian, 2nd ed. Philadephia, Current Medicine, 2001, pp 73–78.
2. Bloomfield DM: A symposium: A common faint: Tailoring treatment for targeted groups of patients with vasovagal syncope. Am J Cardiol 8A:1Q–2Q, 1999.
3. Darooff RB, Martin JB: Faintness, syncope, dizziness, and vertigo. In Fauci AS, et al (eds): Harrison's Principles of Internal Medicine, 14th ed. New York, McGraw-Hill, 1998, pp 100–104.
4. Futterman LG, Lemberg L: A novel device in evaluating syncope. Am J Crit Care, 9:288–293, 2000.
5. Hoole AJ, Pickard CG, Ouimette R, et al: Disorders of the nervous system. In Brogan JE (ed): Patient Care Guidelines for Nurse Practitioners, 5th ed. Philadelphia, J.B. Lippincott, 1999, pp 411–413.
6. Hughes R, Disrud BJ: Dizziness and syncope. In Mladenovic J (ed): Primary Care Secrets, 2nd ed. Philadelphia, Hanley & Belfus, 1999, pp 360–363.
7. Linzer M, Yang EH, Estes NA III, et al: Diagnosing syncope. Part 2: Unexplained syncope. Clinical Efficacy Assessment Project of the American College of Physcians. Ann Intern Med 127:76–86, 1997.
8. Luria DM, Shen WK: Syncope in the elderly: New trends in diagnostic approach and nonpharmacologic management. Am J Geriatr Cardiol 10:91–96, 2001.
9. Massie BM: Heart. In Tierney LM, et al (eds): Current Medical Diagnosis and Treatment, 35th ed. Stamford, CT, Appleton & Lange, 1996, pp 358–359.
10. Seller RH: Dizziness/lightheadedness and vertigo. In Seller RH (ed): Differential Diagnosis of Common Complaints, 3rd ed. Philadelphia, W.B. Saunders, 1996, pp 109–119.
11. Uphold CR, Graham MV: Presyncope/syncope. In Uphold CR, Graham MV (eds): Clinical Guidelines in Adult Health, 2nd ed. Gainesville, FL, Barmarre Books, 1999, pp 394–399.

16. ASTHMA

Deborah M. Judd, MSN, RN-C, FNP

1. What impact does asthma have on morbidity and mortality in the United States?

Asthma is the sixth most common chronic disease in the United States. It affects blacks more frequently than whites and females more often than males. More than 17 million people today are affected by this chronic lung condition. Asthma accounts for over 450,000 hospitalizations, 2 million emergency department (ED) visits, and about 5,000 deaths annually. It is estimated that asthma accounts for more than 10 million missed school days and over $3 million lost from work each year. Asthma continues to be the most common chronic condition treated in primary care settings.

2. Does the incidence of asthma differ by age?

Until recent years, there was an equal distribution of asthma between pediatric and adult populations. The general prevalence of asthma has almost doubled in the past 20 years, whereas the incidence among young children and infants has tripled during the same period. Morbidity and mortality related to asthma affect primarily the very young, the elderly, and people of lower socioeconomic status.

3. Why is the prevalence of asthma increasing?

Reasons for the dramatic increases in both prevalence and associated costs of asthma are somewhat controversial. Several theories have been proposed:

Reasons for Asthma Prevalence Increase

Too clean theory	Childhood infections provide protection against allergy or asthma development; increased use of cleaners, sanitizers, and antibiotics decreases exposure to infectious and/or environmental organisms.
Pollution theory	"Dirty air" damages lung tissue and increases airway reactivity. There is a significant increase in asthma in inner city and large city environments; premature and low birth weight infants are especially affected.
Videogame or computer use theory	People are spending more time indoors and thus are overexposed to indoor allergens (cockroach excreta, dust, rodent droppings, molds).
Greater awareness theory	Medical providers are much more aware of the diagnosis of asthma. Increased awareness leads to more correct diagnosis.
Less healthy lifestyle	Increased sedentary activities, prepackaged items, and processed foods allow more exposure to chemicals, preservatives, and man-made goods.
Consumer knowledge	Increased consumer knowledge of medical care encourages patients to seek care for treatment and improvement of lung disease.
Better access to care	This is not a universal situation, but there are many opportunities for people to seek care paid for by insurance or other health care programs.

4. Are there different types of asthma?

Asthma can be classified in different ways. The most commonly accepted system, developed by the National Institutes of Health (NIH), classifies asthma by disease severity (see question 14). Asthma can be classified by etiology, presentation pattern, and/or trigger pattern. This information allows the nurse practitioner (NP) to initiate appropriate treatment.

ETIOLOGY	PRESENTATION	TRIGGER PATTERNS
Allergic: triggered by allergens, common family/personal history of atopic diseases	Perennial vs. seasonal Episodic vs. continuous Diurnal vs. nocturnal Home setting vs. work setting	Allergy-induced: exposures to environmental stimuli triggers symptoms, often with rhinitis
Nonallergic: triggered by exposure to pollutants, medications, stress, upper respiratory infection (URI)	Healthy vs. sick	Exercise-induced: cough or dyspnea triggered by exercise; preexercise metered-dose inhaler response
Mixed: any combination of factors		Nocturnal: frequent cough and sleep disturbances; worse in early morning (associated with gastroesophageal reflux disease) Temperature-induced: symptoms occur with exposure to cold air, humidity, and/or dry heat URI-induced: colds or flu trigger asthmatic bronchitis

5. What is reactive airway disease?

Certain people experience asthma symptoms only when they are ill. They generally are diagnosed with reactive airway disease (RAD) and may or may not later develop true asthma.

6. What happens during an asthma attack?

An asthma attack is commonly characterized by two phases:

Early phase. Onset begins within 20 minutes of trigger exposure. Chemical mediators are released without actual airway inflammation. Symptoms spontaneously resolve in 1–2 hours.

Late phase. Onset begins 5–6 hours after the early phase, lasting from days to weeks. It is characterized by airway hyperresponsiveness, airway inflammation, and mucus hypersecretion.

7. What are the classic symptoms of asthma?

The three most common complaints are dyspnea, wheezes, and cough. Less frequent complaints include chest pain (usually described as tightness), sleep disturbances, choking sensation, exercise intolerance, and shortness of breath associated with upper respiratory infections.

DYSPNEA	WHEEZE	COUGH
Most commonly reported symptom	Often felt as well as heard	May be the only sign of asthma
Highly subjective complaint	Associated with chest discomfort	Usually dry and nonproductive
Not usually correlated to disease severity	Wheezing is expiratory in asthma	Often described as "irritating"
PFTs validate disease severity	With inspiratory wheezes, alternate diagnoses should be explored	During exacerbation, cough may become productive
PEF rate most useful indicator	Many asthmatics have COPD (inspiratory/expiratory wheezes)	Generally worse at night

COPD = chronic obstructive pulmonary disease, PEF = peak expiratory flow, PFTs = pulmonary function tests.

8. What factors should be used to diagnose asthma?
- Subjective history of recurrent cough, wheeze, or dyspnea
- Reversibility of airflow obstruction demonstrated by spirometry (PFTs), with or without broncodilator therapy
- Airway reactivity demonstrated during cold air or exercise testing
- Positive methacholine challenge even with normal spirometry (PFTs) results
- Exclusion of any other diagnoses

9. How can you differentiate asthma from chronic obstructive pulmonary disease (COPD)?

Differentiation is important because appropriate treatment depends on appropriate diagnosis.

DIAGNOSIS CHARACTERISTICS	COPD	ASTHMA
Age	Usually over 40 yr	Can be seen at any age
Smoking history	Current smoker or past smoker for > 10 yr	Not correlated to smoking history; may be trigger
Dyspnea	Occurs with exertion generally	Episodic attacks, often associated with trigger
Wheezes	Can be both inspiratory and expiratory	Generally expiratory
Cough	Productive; most productive in morning	Cough more frequent at night
Spirometry	FEV_1 low, ratio of FEV_1/FVC < 70%	Variable during exacerbations: FEV_1/FVC ratio low until ill
Peak flow	Little variation, generally low; often low values well tolerated	Morning values low; values vary with triggers/attacks
Inhaled corticosteroid (IC) response	Variable—only 20–30% improve with IC use	Improvement: continued IC use decreases symptoms
Chest x-ray	Overinflation demonstrated	Normal except in exacerbation; may show overinflation

FEV_1 = forced expiratory volume in 1 minute, FVC = forced vital capacity.

10. What diagnostic tests validate the diagnosis of asthma?
- Pulmonary function tests (PFTs): 20% posttreatment change in FEV_1 from baseline.
- Peak flow meter monitoring: monitor diurnal pattern for 2 weeks; morning values tend to be lower than early afternoon values. Measure before and after beta$_2$ agonist administration during the same period.
- Chest x-ray: helpful in distinguishing other lung diseases by demonstrating hyperinflation vs. chronic changes; generally excludes other diseases.
- Upper gastrointestinal studies: to rule out gastroesophageal reflux disease or esophageal problems.

11. What other diagnoses should be considered in diagnosing asthma?
- **Chronic obstructive pulmonary disease (COPD):** commonly misdiagnosed as asthma. Pure COPD is not responsive to aggressive asthma therapy, because the airway obstruction is generally irreversible.
- **Congestive heart failure (CHF):** prevalent in the elderly. CHF presents with wheezes, but no history of respiratory disease and concurrent symptoms of edema and orthopnea.
- **Esophageal spasm:** despite frequent dyspnea and cough, there is no response to asthma treatments. PFTs are normal. Diagnosis confirmed by esophageal manometry.

- **Vocal cord dysfunction**: no response to inhaled corticosteroids (ICs) or bronchodilators. Often a voice change is present. Endoscopy reveals abnormal function or lesion.
- **Gastroesophageal reflux disease (GERD)**: may present as "nocturnal asthma" (frequent night-time cough). Patients may or may not have heartburn, eructation, or other symptoms typical of GERD. There should be a high degree of suspicion for GERD in patients with poorly controlled asthma and/or frequent nocturnal symptoms.

In addition, upper airway obstruction, Churg-Strauss syndrome, and bronchiectasis should be considered.

12. What specific triggers can initiate an asthmatic process?

A thorough history can elicit specific triggers. The following triggers should be considered in gathering information. A diary completed by the patient once he or she is aware of potential triggers can guide the NP in a specific treatment plan and strategies for trigger avoidance.

Potential Triggers

Upper respiratory infections (viral or bacteria)	Weather changes	Seasonal plant/tree allergens
Humidity	Tobacco smoke	Fire smoke/wood burner smoke
Aspirin/NSAIDs	Food preservatives (sulfites)	Fragrances (i.e., perfumes)
Pet dander	Cockroach excreta	Molds/spores
Occupational exposures	Dust—any kind	Food allergies
Exercise	Temperature changes	Emotions
Illness	Stress	Chemicals/fibers

NSAIDs = nonsteroidal anti-inflammatory drugs.

13. Is it important to know the actual severity of a specific patient's asthma?

To treat asthma, the severity of the disease must be assessed. Current asthma management focuses on (1) recognition of the disease as an inflammatory process, (2) treatment of the severity of symptoms, and (3) involvement of the patient in managing the symptoms to prevent exacerbations and disease progression.

14. How is asthma severity classified?

Asthma Classification

CATEGORY	SYMPTOMS SEVERITY/FREQUENCY	NOCTURNAL SYMPTOMS	PULMONARY FUNCTION VALUES
Step 1: mild intermittent	Symptoms 2 times wk or less Brief exacerbations (last only hours) Exacerbation intensity varies	Not more than twice monthly	FEV_1/PEF rate: at least 80% of predicted PFTs may be normal
Step 2: mild persistent	Symptoms more than twice weekly but not daily Exacerbations last longer, affect activities	More than twice monthly but not weekly	FEV_1/PEF rate: 80% or less of predicted PEF rate variability: 20–30%

(Table continued on next page.)

Asthma Classification (cont.)

CATEGORY	SYMPTOMS SEVERITY/FREQUENCY	NOCTURNAL SYMPTOMS	PULMONARY FUNCTION VALUES
Step 3: moderate persistent	Daily symptoms Daily use of beta$_2$ agonist for rescue Exacerbations affect activities Exacerbations last more than 1 day	More than once each week	FEV$_1$/PEF rate: 60–80% of predicted PEF rate variability > 30%
Step 4: severe persistent	Continuous daily symptoms Frequent exacerbations Limited physical activities due to SOB	Frequent symptoms, often every night Symptoms may be worse at nighr rather than during the day	FEV$_1$/PEF rate: at least 60% of predicted PEF rate variability > 30%

FEV$_1$ = forced expiratory volume in 1 minute, PEF = peak expiratory flow, PFTs = pulmonary function tests, SOB = shortness of breath. Adapted from the National Institutes of Health Guidelines for the Diagnosis and Management of Asthma.

15. If symptoms fluctuate, how is the category determined?

Assess by the most severe symptoms experienced before treatment. This classification should be maintained as the patient's asthma type, even when symptoms improve to be consistent with a lower classification with treatment. Once the severity is determined, the most appropriate treatment can be initiated.

16. What management is recommended for asthmatics according to NIH step classification?

Step Therapy Treatment Plan for Asthma

STEP CATEGORY	TREATMENT RECOMMENDATIONS
Mild intermittent (step1)	Inhaled short-acting beta$_2$ agonists as needed Treat triggers, infections, and exacerbations appropriately
Mild persistent (step 2)	Treatment as for step 1 *plus* Daily inhaled corticosteroids (ICs) (lowest dose) to prevent frequent symptoms
Moderate persistent (step 3)	Treatment as for step 2, except use medium dose of IC *plus* Trial of long-acting beta$_2$ agonist Trial of antileukotrienes Treat nocturnal symptoms with H$_2$ blocker
Severe persistent (step 4)	Treatment as for step 3, except use high dose IC *plus* Trial of oral steroids (lowest effective dose) Consider oral beta$_2$ agonists Consider inhaled mast-cell stabilizer (e.g., cromolyn) Monitor closely and reduce oral steroid use when possible

Adapted from National Institutes of Health Guidelines for the Diagnosis and Management of Asthma.

17. What is meant by the terms *controller medications* and *rescue medications*?

Controller medications are routinely used to prevent exacerbations/symptom onset (example: inhaled corticosteroid or beta$_2$ agonist).

Rescue medications are used to treat a symptomatic episode (example: short acting beta$_2$ agonist).

18. Is there a simple way to know when to use a controller medication?

One way to know when a controller medication is indicated is the "rule of two's." Any patient who meets *any* of the following criteria should be prescribed a controller medication:
- 2 beta$_2$ agonist cannisters/year ($\geq$ 400 puffs)
- 2 doses beta$_2$ agonists/week
- 2 symptom-related nocturnal awakenings/month
- 2 unscheduled asthma-related visits/year
- 2 prednisone bursts/year

19. What should be done to manage a patient with chronic daily symptoms?

Management of chronic asthma is a process of individualized trial and response to treatment, based on the recommended stepwise plan. When severity levels change during certain periods of the patient's life, treatments change accordingly.

20. How are peak flow meters (PFM) used in asthma management?

PFMs provide a simple, reliable measure of the severity of airway obstruction, identifying airway changes hours to days before asthma symptoms are actually manifested. The results are reproducible and objective. Accurate measurement is technique-dependent and is used to determine personal best and perhaps worst values. PFM demonstrates exacerbation severity, guides therapeutic measures and decisions for both NP and patient, confirms effectiveness of a treatment plan, determines medication use according to "zone values," and allows disease self-management.

21. How are PFM personal best values determined?

A patient's personal best should be determined by values collected over 1 month while the patient is well. The best measures are obtained while the patient is standing (the lungs fill completely). The PFM should be checked at different times of the day and both before and after any prescribed beta$_2$ agonist administration. Usually, the best values occur between 12 noon and 2 PM, and the lower values occur on awakening.

22. How does PFM guide self-management?

The patient should be informed of what self-care activities are indicated by PFM readings and when to call for further guidance. The following zone system works well for most people, but others may have to be given an actual number (i.e., call when your PFM is below 250).

Green zone ($\geq$ 80% personal best): usual medications; IC and short acting beta$_2$ agonist as needed.

Yellow zone (50–80% personal best): IC medications; start regular use of an inhaled beta$_2$ agonist; monitor PFM readings; check with provider for other suggestions.

Red zone ($\leq$ 50% personal best): rescue beta$_2$ agonist; seek medical care or go to emergency department.

23. When should patients use a spacer?

All patients who use inhalers should be provided a spacer and instructions in its use. A spacer more effectively delivers inhaled medications to the lung, decreasing the amount deposited in the oral cavity. A spacer is most beneficial for children and older adults who have difficulty with coordinating "the puff" and "inhalation." *They should not be used with diskus delivery systems.*

24. How do you ensure proper use of a spacer?

Patients should be instructed in proper technique and asked to demonstrate use of the spacer before leaving the clinic. Have patients demonstrate how they use their inhalers and spacers at each visit.

25. When should nebulized medications be prescribed?

Nebulized medications are better delivered to the lung tissues and should be used when they give greater benefit than metered-dose inhalers (MDIs). Nebulized medications are often used during periods of exacerbation or when patients cannot use a spacer or coordinate the use of an MDI canister (e.g., very young children, elderly patients, and patients with significant shortness of breath). Use of a nebulizer requires less coordination than an MDI canister but is more time-consuming and expensive than a MDI. The results often justify the use of a nebulizer despite added time or cost.

26. Is the response to nebulized medications different from the response to an MDI?

Because a nebulizer delivers medications more efficiently, patients may experience more apparent side effects than with an MDI. It is also not uncommon for patients who have been significantly short of breath and/or who are sleep deprived to become relaxed and even sleepy during the nebulized treatment.

27. What role do short-acting beta$_2$ agonists play in managing asthma?

• Small, frequent dosing available
• Can be used up to 4–6 times/day (see question 39)
• Provide safe, immediate relief as airways dilate
• Used as an adjunctive therapy with ICs
• Usually inhaled (tablets are available as well as a liquid form for pediatric patients)

28. Why use a long-acting beta$_2$ agonist?

Long-acting beta$_2$ agonists keep the airways open for 12 hours but should not be used for relief of acute symptoms. They should be used in combination with ICs. They help to prevent nocturnal asthma episodes. Currently only one long-acting beta$_2$ MDI is available, but several long-acting tablets are on the market. Although some patients prefer an oral medication to another inhaler, inhaled medications provide direct relief and have fewer systemic side effects.

29. What are the benefits of inhaled corticosteroids?

ICs are recommended as the most effective means of preventing inflammatory changes within the airways and are considered the cornerstone of asthma therapy. The many benefits of ICs include:

• Decreased mortality and morbidity
• Decreased hospitalizations and emergency department visits
• Decreased exacerbation frequency
• Improved asthma control on a daily basis
• Reduced airway inflammation
• Improved lung function/PFT measures
• Suppressed chronic persistent symptoms
• Prevention of irreversible airway damage (remodeling)

30. How are ICs dosed?

The lowest dose of any IC that controls symptoms should be used. Some ICs offer different dosage strengths, whereas others are adjusted by changing the frequency of dosing and the number of puffs prescribed. For example, Azmacort has a single dose strength but can be dosed 2–4 times/day, whereas three different doses of Flovent are available. The dose may be increased during an exacerbation and decreased during remission (see question 39).

31. When should a methylxanthine be used to treat asthma?

Theophylline is a controller medication used to dilate the airways for up to 12 hours. It is more commonly used to treat COPD but has some efficacy for asthma, particularly during prolonged exacerbations or hospitalization. It does not provide immediate relief, as do other medications. Theophylline is also thought to boost the effect of concurrently used ICs. The wide range of available doses allows titration, which helps to prevent airway restriction.

32. With long action and flexible dosing, why is theophylline not considered a first-line therapy?

Theophylline has more reported side effects and potential drug interactions than many of the newer medications. A patient taking theophylline also requires periodic blood tests to monitor drug level and toxicity, adding to the cost and associated risk.

33. Should the anticholinergic drug ipratropium (Atrovent) be used for asthma?

Ipratropium is used to treat COPD more commonly than asthma, but it is a good alternate "quick-fix" medication for patients who cannot use or tolerate a beta$_2$ agonist. It does not act quite as quickly as beta$_2$ agonists but is still highly effective. It may be used as an adjunct to a beta$_2$ agonist during exacerbation for more effective rescue relief.

34. What role do antileukotriene drugs play in the treatment of asthma?

Leukotrienes are responsible for both acute and chronic symptoms in asthmatic patients. Antileukotrienes target important inflammatory pathways, blocking symptom development and decreasing the possibility for an exacerbation. They also can augment the effects of ICs, inhaled nasal steroids, and oral antihistamines in an allergic asthmatic patient.

Pulmonary effects of antileukotrienes
- Broncodilatation (improved FEV$_1$ in persistent asthma)
- Bronchoprotection (prevents airways from narrowing even in the presence of triggers)
- Reduces overall airway inflammation
- Decreases eosinophil levels, reducing sputum production

Nonpulmonary effects of antileukotrienes
- Blocks inflammation in allergic rhinitis
- Improves night-time rhinitis symptoms
- Reduces ocular effects

35. Do all antileukotriene drugs have the same actions and considerations?

No. They are classified as either a leukotriene modifier or a leukotriene inhibitor.

LEUKOTRIENE MODIFIERS (Montelukast and Zafirlukast)	LEUKOTRIENE INHIBITORS (Zilueton)
Block leukotriene receptor sites	Block synthesis of leukotrienes
Prevent leukotriene mediated symptoms	Decrease airway inflammation
Decrease nocturnal awakenings	Decrease number of sick days during an exacerbation
Decrease inhaled beta$_2$ agonists use	Require liver enzyme monitoring
Dosed at bedtime or in the morning	Dosed 4 times/day

36. When should oral corticosteroids be used?

Oral steroids are used to treat mild-to-severe asthma exacerbations, to prevent further exacerbation development, and to diminish morbidity and mortality associated with an asthma flare. With significant decreases in PFM readings and/or increased shortness of breath, use of oral steroids should be considered. Patients who are reliable with a plan of self-care can be given a prednisone asthma rescue prescription to be initiated when an exacerbation occurs.

37. How are oral steroids dosed?

A typical oral steroid treatment involves a taper over 3–12 days. There are many variations, but the typical adult regimen starts with 60 mg, using multiple 20-mg tablets, and is tapered over many days. A child's rescue taper uses prednisolone (Prelone), 1–2 mg/kg (maximum of 4 mg/kg/day) in 2 or 3 doses/day for 3–5 days.

38. Why are antihistamines and intranasal steroids often prescribed to treat asthma?

The upper and lower airways are part of the same mucosal system. Allergic rhinitis affects a large percentage of asthmatics and is the most common cause of chronic cough. Thus antihistamines and intranasal steroids are used to control the symptoms of chronic rhinitis. Intranasal steroids, like ICs, are a topical treatment resulting in little, if any, adverse reactions. They make a significant difference in the process of chronic rhinitis.

Antihistamines are useful in treating allergic rhinitis, but most are systemic and have more adverse reactions than intranasal steroids. They are most effective when used before the release of histamine and apparent allergy symptoms.

39. What are the most common therapeutic drugs used to treat asthma? What are the typical doses and potential adverse reaction(s) for each?

Please refer to the table on page 98 and 99.

40. What is the goal in treating a more significant acute asthma attack?

During an acute attack, management is aimed at keeping adequate oxygen saturation (> 93%). In addition, rapid reversal of airway obstruction is attempted to prevent further airway restriction and to avoid respiratory arrest. Unfortunately, asthma can progress to death if not appropriately treated. Early treatment is the best therapy to manage exacerbations.

41. What is the accepted treatment regimen for an acute exacerbation?

Management of an acute attack not responsive to the suggested stepwise plan includes:
1. Nebulized albuterol treatments every 30 minutes (maximum of 3 treatments)
2. Intramuscular (IM) or intravenous (IV) corticosteroids
3. Treatment of infection: appropriate antibiotic class for suspected organisms
4. Close monitoring of patient response/improvement

42. What should be done if the patient does not respond to treatment for an acute exacerbation?

If the patient responds poorly to the above treatments, aggressive therapy should be delivered by a certified provider of advanced cardiac life support in an emergency-equipped setting (e.g., acute care clinic with an observation unit, emergency department, or hospital unit). Treatment then may include:
- Subcutaneous epinepherine or terbutaline to improve poor respiratory effort
- Aggressive nebulizer treatments (albuterol with either ipratropium or atropine)
- IV aminophylline bolus followed by continuous IV infusion
- Intubation, sedation, and mechanical ventilation

43. What factors indicate that a patient may be at risk of death from asthma?
- History of sudden onset of exacerbations
- Two or more hospitalizations during the past year
- Three or more emergency department visits within the past year
- Use of more than two inhaled beta$_2$ agonist MDI canisters per month
- Recent withdrawal from oral corticosteroids
- Comorbidity (e.g., COPD or coronary artery disease)
- Low socioeconomic status with urban residence
- Prior intubation for shortness of breath or asthma

44. When and to whom should you refer a patient with asthma?
Refer to pulmonologist (adult patients)
- No improvement with recommended stepwise treatments
- Diagnosis of asthma in question (atypical or no response)
- Patients with COPD/asthma mix

CLASS	BRAND NAME	GENERIC NAME*	DOSAGE RANGE	IMPORTANT NOTES
Beta₂ agonists Short-acting	Alupent Brethine Maxair Proventil Ventolin	Metaproterenol Terbutaline Pirbuterol Albuterol Albuterol	2–4 puffs every 4–6 hr prn 2.5 mg tid (12–15 yr) or 5 mg tid (> 15 yr) 1–2 puffs every 4–6 hr prn MDI, 2 puffs every 4–6 hr prn (oral form also) MDI, 2 puffs every 4–6 hr prn (oral form also)	Side effects: tachycardia, nervousness, palpitations, nausea, vomiting, dry mouth, hypertension, hypokalemia, hypotension
Long-acting	Serevent	Salmeterol	2 puffs bid or 2 puffs 30 min before exercise qd	Do not use for acute attack or more than twice daily
Anticholinergics	Atrovent	Ipratropium	MDI, 2 puffs qid prn or 500 μg jet neb tid/qid Do not use under age 12 yr	Side effects: dizziness, insomnia, elevated liver enzymes
Inhaled corticosteroids (a dose range and/or no. of puffs to determine potency range from low to high)	Aerobid Azmacort Beclovent, Vanceril Flovent	Flunisolide Triamcinolone Beclomethasone Fluticasone	2 puffs bid 2–4 puffs bid–qid (> 12 yr) (children: 4–12 puffs/day divided bid to qid) Preferred pediatric drug 2 puffs tid–qid (> 12 yr) (children: 4–12 puffs/day divided tid/qid) 44 μg MDI, 2 puffs bid (> 12 yr) (4–12 yr often dosed 1 puff bid) 110 μg MDI, 2 puffs bid (> 12 yr) (4–12 yr often dosed 1 puff bid) 220 μg MDI, 2 puffs bid (> 12 yr)	Side effects: candidiasis, anxiety, weight gain, cough, extrapyramidal symptoms, tachycardia, nervousness, palpitations, nausea, vomiting, dry mouth, hypotension, hypertension, hypokalemia
	Pulmicort	Budesonide	1–2 puffs bid	
Combination inhalers	Combivent Advair	Albuterol/ipratropium Fluticasone/salmeterol diskus	2 puffs qid, maximum of 12 puffs/day IC/beta₂ ratio: 3 dose strengths by μg 100/50, 250/50, 500/50	See individual drugs above.
Leukotriene modifiers	Accolate Singulair	Zafirlukast Montelukast	20 mg bid, taken 1 hr ac or 2 hr pc 10 mg qd (> 12 yr) 5 mg qd (6–12 yr)	Use with caution in hepatic disease. Increases levels of warfarin. Macrolides and theophylline decrease drug activity.

(Table continued on next page.)

CLASS	BRAND NAME	GENERIC NAME*	DOSAGE RANGE	IMPORTANT NOTES
Leukotriene inhibitors	Zyflo	Zileuton	600 mg qid (adult use only)	Possible liver enzyme changes. Frequent dosing required. Side effects as above.
Methylxanthines (Dose per serum level: target range: 10–20 µg/ml)	Elixophyllin	Theophylline elixir	80 mg/15 ml, initial dose: 3–5 mg/kg	Side effects: nausea, vomiting, epigastric pain, palpitations, tachycardia, insomnia
	Respbid	Theophylline	250 mg and 500 mg bid or tid	Interactions: lithium, OCP, macrolide antibiotics, propranolol, rifampin, phenobarbital, amiodarone, fluoroquinolone
	Slo-bid	Theophylline	100 mg, 200 mg, and 300 mg	
	Theo-24	Theophylline	100 mg, 200 mg, 300 mg, and 400 mg	
	Theo-Dur	Theophylline	100 mg, 200 mg, 300 mg, and 450 mg	
	Uniphyl	Theophylline	300 mg and 600 mg	
		Aminophylline	12–18 mg/kg/day age 1–9 yr	
			13 mg/kg/day age 9–12 yr	
			10 mg/kg/day age > 12 yr	
Anti-inflammatory	Solu-Medrol	Methylprednisolone	IV or IM every 4–6 hr for acute exacerbation; check protocols for dose range	Side effects: insomnia, mood swings, increased appetite, skin changes, acne, edema, osteoporosis, ulcer disease, cushingoid habitus
	Medrol, Prednisone	Methylprednisolone	PO taper over 10–12 days (see question 35) Medrol pack: prepackaged per label for 6 days	
Antihistamines Sedating (first generation)	Atarax	Hydroxyzine	25 mg tid or qid	Side effects: drowsiness, dizziness, headache, hypotension, dry mouth, fatigue, confusion
	Benadryl	Diphenhydramine	25 mg every 4–6 hr OTC or 50 mg only by prescription	
	Chlortrimeton	Chlorpheniramine	4 mg qid OTC or 8 mg bid only by prescription	
	Deconamine SR	Chlorpheniramine/ pseudoephedrine	8/120 mg tablet bid	
	Phenergan	Promethazine	12.5–25 mg every 6–8 hr: for nausea and allergy	
Nonsedating (second generation)	Allegra	Fexofenadine	60 mg bid or 180 mg qd (extended release)	Side effects: drowsiness (~ 2%), nausea, dyspepsia, dysmenorrhea, headache
	Claritin	Loratadine	10 mg qd (children use for ages > 6 yr common)	
	Zyrtec	Cetirizine	5–10 mg qd (children use 5 mg dose)	

prm = as needed, bid = 2 times/day, tid = 3 times/day, qid = 4 times/day, qd = each day, neb = nebulizer, MDI = metered-dose inhaler, IC = inhaled corticosteroid, ac = before meals, pc = after meals.
* Active ingredient.

- Patients with severe persistent asthma (level 4)
- Patients with multiple exacerbations

Refer to pulmonologist (pediatric patients)
- Unusual findings (e.g., barrel chest, clubbing, reflux)
- Severe symptoms not responsive to treatment
- Hospitalization within the past year for asthma
- Frequent emergency department visits for shortness of breath
- Exercise-induced asthma associated with syncope
- Severe persistent asthma (level 4)

Refer to allergist
- Allergies and asthma not controlled with usual medications
- Frequent asthma exacerbations with no obvious cause
- For allergy desensitization

Refer to asthma care manager (NP, physician's assistant, physician)
- Moderate-to-persistent asthma (all level 3 and 4 patients)
- New asthmatics (education and equipment)
- Frequent emergency department visits for shortness of breath
- Evaluation of PFTs

45. What are the special considerations for pediatric patients with asthma?

Pediatric patients are treated much the same as adult patients, using the step-level severity system and appropriate dosing. In the youngest pediatric patients, inhaled medications are generally delivered via a jet nebulizer.

Oral beta$_2$ agonists often are used and are available as a syrup (2 mg/5 ml). For patients under 6 years of age, a 0.1mg/kg/dose is prescribed 3 times/day. For patients 6–12 years of age, a 2-mg/kg dose is used 3 times/day.

ICs are now used more routinely in children. Patients as young as 4–5 years of age can use ICs delivered via an aerochamber. Despite some concern over possible growth retardation, ICs are generally believed to be safe. Adequate control of asthma is believed to outweigh any risks associated with long-term IC use. The lowest effective IC dose should be used. Oral steroids also may be prescribed for an asthmatic child but should be used sparingly to avoid systemic side effects (possibility of cushingoid syndrome and growth retardation).

Cromolyn is frequently used to treat chronic pediatric asthma, but the initial response may not be observable for 1–4 weeks. It is effective as a pre-exercise or pre-allergen contact controller therapy. The preventative effects last about 4 hours. It is used for infants and small children because it is a safe medication.

46. What gender differences are involved in the management of asthmatic patients?

Treatment for males and females is generally the same. However, asthma exacerbations may occur more frequently at menarche in adolescent girls or in relation to menses in women.

After menopause, many women experience decreased asthma symptoms. Women who use hormone replacement therapy (HRT) seem to experience an increased number of asthma exacerbations. Of interest, women on HRT show improved PFTs.

47. What are the special considerations in managing asthma during pregnancy?

Asthma management during pregnancy is based on the stepwise treatment approach. The mother's oxygenation is essential to fetal health. Although asthma symptoms are highly individualized, woman who experience significant asthma before pregnancy typically have more exacerbations during pregnancy. There is generally a consistent pattern from one pregnancy to the next in the same woman. If a woman with asthma uses tobacco, she should be strongly encouraged to abstain during pregnancy.

48. What is known about the role of specific asthma medications and their effect on the fetus?

Pregnancy Treatments

MEDICATION	FETAL EFFECTS	SAFETY	INDICATIONS	OTHER INFO
Salmeterol	Unsure of fetal risks; minimal fetal effects in animals	May be used any time, try albuterol first (category C)	Moderate to severe asthma, not responsive to beta$_2$ agonists	Useful if previous response known
Ipratropium	No fetal defects noted in animal study	Use if good response before pregnancy (category B)	Acute asthma not responsive to inhaled beta$_2$ agonists	Inhaled; hence immediate bronchodilation
Nedocromil	Nonteratogenic	May continue use during pregnancy: (category B)	Mild-to-moderate asthma	Less effective than ICs or cromolyn
Leukotriene modifiers	Unknown; fewer fetal (animal) changes with montelukast and zafirlukast	Not recommended as first line therapy (category C)	Mild-to-severe asthma already responding to this class of medications	Zileuton is not recommended; do not initiate leukotriene modifiers during pregnancy, if patient is not current user
Oral steroids	Oral cleft changes documented with use; restrict use during first trimester	Benefits of medication outweigh fetal risks (category B)	Asthma exacerbation or recalcitrant asthma, nonresponsive to other treatments	May predispose mother to preeclampsia last trimester
Inhaled steroids	Litle data on inhaled steroids (nasal or pulmonary)	Considered safe in patient with good response to ICs (category C)	Use to prevent asthma exacerbations and maintain degree of wellness	Efficacy suggests use if warranted Budesonide and beclomethasone are ICs of choice
Antihistamines first generation (sedating)	Considered safe	Safe, but avoid any medication not needed during pregnancy (category B/C)	Allergic rhinitis trigger for asthma exacerbations	Use diphenhydramine or chlorpheniramine as first choice
Antihistamines second generation (nonsedating)	Use controversial; animal studies show some defects	Avoid use during first trimester (category C)	Use if need nonsedating effects and no response to topical or other therapy	May use loratadine or cetirizine if no other antihistamine response

49. What effect does smoking have on asthma and asthma exacerbations?

Smoking is a trigger for asthma, especially among children. A higher percentage of children exposed to second-hand smoke develop asthma. Tobacco smoke exposure is associated with decreased PFTs, increased medication requirements, and altered school and work attendance.

50. What methods should be used to encourage smoking cessation?

Smoking cessation should be a priority of asthma management. Intensive interventions are more effective than brief reminders. Successful smoking cessation strategies include medication therapy, behavioral modification, and a support system consisting of family, friends, and providers.

51. What should the educational plan for a patient with asthma include?

In addition to initiating and managing appropriate therapy, NPs should provide education about:

- Daily/regular IC use as a controller therapy for best results
- Appropriate rescue medications
- Overused beta$_2$ agonist and/or other rescue medications
- Importance of spacer use and rationale
- Rationale for PFM monitoring, when to check and when to seek care
- Trigger identification: develop strategies for avoidance and treatment
- Treatment of asthma: not treated only when symptoms are present
- Asthma symptoms: result from preventable airway inflammation and bronchospasm
- Asthma basics: disease process, chronicity, and variability
- Discussion of how medications work, adverse effects, and rationale
- Emphasize that exacerbations are usually preventable if self-care plan is followed
- Emphasize need for regular clinic follow-up to maintain health
- Avoidance of aspirin and nonsteroidal anti-inflammatory medications (potential triggers)

52. What factors influence treatment outcomes and self-management in asthmatic patients?

Developing a successful and positive relationship with the patient is of utmost importance and is best achieved through long-term association. This type of relationship is not always possible because of time constraints and changes in medical care delivery. Open communication is essential in the relationship, and the NP must have an adequate understanding of each patient's personality, interests, life situation, financial resources, and support system. An adequate explanation that allows an understanding of the disease process, treatment options, and medication rationale at the patient's educational level is necessary. Each patient has certain cultural experiences, knowledge level, treatment expectations, and life experiences. Optimal self-management requires each patient to be treated with these factors in mind.

53. What are the major barriers to self-management?

- General lack of understanding, ignorance
- Difficulty in obtaining medications
- Improper use or administration of medications
- Lack of knowledge about self-care measures (e.g., PFM and safety zones, spacers)
- Nonsupportive family and friends
- Low socioeconomic status
- Denial of illness

54. What alternative therapies are used in asthma management today?

The use of alternative or complementary medical approaches to disease management is common. Herbal remedies, homeopathy, yoga and meditation, hypnotherapy, biofeedback, acupuncture, therapeutic massage, and chiropractic manipulation are used to treat asthma. There is a lack of research to support many of these modalities. With increased use of alternative therapies, more research is under way to assess response and rationale for action.

55. What herbal/nutrient remedies are used to treat asthma?

AGENT	RATIONALE FOR AGENT	DOCUMENTED ACTIONS
Omega-3 fatty acids	Inhibits formation of prosta-glandins and leukotrienes	No observed FEV_1 changes in studies
Ascorbic acid	Believed to be low in asthmatics	Improved FEV_1 and decreased asthma symptoms
Zinc	Low zinc levels identified in asthmatics and those with allergic rhinitis	Positive association between low zinc and increased bronchial hyperactive noted
Magnesium	Believed to have bronchodilating effects	No data about PFT changes
Ma huang	Contains ephedrine which acts on $beta_2$ receptors	Causes bronchial relaxation
Ginkgo	Old Chinese medicine—uncertain action that changes PFTs	FEV_1 improves after 8–10 weeks
Saiboku-to	Combination of herbal product containing 10 different ingred-ients—multiple actions	Effective in decreasing steroid use in steroid dependent bronchial asthma
Tylophora	An Indian medicine—action uncertain	15% improvement of FEV_1 and decreased asthma symptom frequency

There is a need for research to validate actions of these substances in asthma management (see chapter 29).

56. What other alternative or complementary therapies are used for asthmatics?

COMPLEMENTARY THERAPY	COMMENTS ABOUT THERAPY
Homeopathy: the use of dilute substances that cause disease can actually cure it	Dilute primary allergen(s) used for 4 weeks or longer. Significant symptom reduction reported. FEV_1 and FVC are shown to improve.
Yoga and meditation: the use of a variety of body positions and breathing techniques	Yoga alone may be of benefit due to stress reduction. Breathing practices are responsible for improved FEV_1, whereas yoga postures and breathing increase exercise tolerance and fitness. Breathing exercises should be done slow and deep for 15 minutes twice daily
Hypnotherapy: a state that allows suggestion to institute physiologic changes	Do not use if patient has any psychosis. Limited studies show decreased hypersensitivity and bronchodilator MDI use. Some improvement in PFTs documented.
Biofeedback: learning conscious control of bodily functions normally controlled by unconscious mechanisms	Useful in decreasing stress and effects on body function. Reported decrease in symptoms, yet no significant changes in PFTs. May decrease respiratory resistance.
Acupuncture: insertion of stain-less steel needles at trigger or specific body points	Considered a safe practice. Not enough data to assess effectiveness, results contradictory.
Therapeutic massage: touch ther-apy and massage to body surfaces	Improvement in subjective symptoms and decreased anxiety documented. No significant improvements seen in PFTs.
Chiropractic manipulation: uses spinal manipulation to relieve symptoms and treat chronic disease	No significant changes seen in FEV_1 or FVC. Slight decrease in bronchodilator MDI use in some patients.

BIBLIOGRAPHY

1. Asthma in America: Asthma Statistics, Background on Asthma, and Managing Asthma: http://www.asthmainamerica.com (accessed February 2001).
2. Byrd RP Jr, Krishnaswamy G, Thomas R: Difficult-to-manage: How to pinpoint the exacerbating factors. http://www.postgradmed.com/issues/2000/11_00/byrd.htm.
3. Di Gregorio GJ, Barbieri EJ: Commonly Prescribed Drugs [handout]. 15th ed. Nutley, NJ, Roche Laboratories, Medical Surveillance Inc., 2000.
4. Mitchell I, Ford G: Recognizing and treating asthma in women. Women Health Primary Care 3:507–519, 2000.
5. National Institutes of Health: Advances in Allergic Diseases. An Update for the New Millennium. Bethesda, MD, NIH, 2001.
6. National Institutes of Health Guidelines for the Diagnosis and Management of Asthma: Expert Panel Report. NIH publication no. 98-4051. Bethesda, MD, NIH, 1999.
7. Nogueras D: Asthma management: Focus on children. Adv Nurses Feb:13–16, 2001.
8. Perlman A, Serbin JS: Complementary and alternative medicine: Does it have a role in treating asthma. Women Health Primary Care 4:282–288, 2001.
9. Perlman A, Serbin JS: Nontraditional approaches to asthma: Homeopathy, yoga, hypnosis, biofeedback, acupuncture, chiropractic, massage: A review of the evidence. Women Health Primary Care 4:405–410, 2001.
10. Sandrini A, Chapman KR: Asthma therapy: Will your patient benefit from leukotriene receptor antagonists? Consultant Feb:205–216, 2001.
11. Suissa S, Ernst P, Benayoun S: Low-dose inhaled corticosteroids and the prevention of death from asthma. N Engl J Med 343:332–336, 2000.

17. CHEST PAIN

Leslie L. Davis, MSN, RN, CS, ANP

1. When a patient presents with chest pain, what are the immediate goals?

Of course, the most immediate goals are to assess airway, breathing, and circulation (ABCs) and to establish the patient's stability and needs. Obviously, if the patient complains of chest pain, establish that the airway is open and the patient is breathing. Next, do a brief assessment of vital signs and perform a general survey to determine the need to obtain an immediate electrocardiogram (EKG) or arrange transport to an urgent care center.

Once the immediate stability of the patient has been established, the most important goal for evaluation of nontraumatic chest pain in adults is risk stratification—in other words, what is the likelihood of coronary artery disease (CAD)? Essential components needed for risk stratification include a detailed symptom assessment (history), a focused physical exam, and a directed risk factor assessment. The levels of risks fall into three categories:

1. High risk: patients with known CAD, men ≥ 60 years old, women ≥ 70 years old, patients with significant EKG changes indicative of ischemia.

2. Intermediate risk: classic symptoms of CAD in men < 60 years old or women < 70 years old; atypical symptoms in diabetics or patients with ≥ 2 risk factors, or less specific EKG changes suggestive of ischemia.

3. Low risk: symptoms probably not angina, with ≤ 1 risk factor, normal EKG.

2. What pearls are useful in the evaluation of chest pain?

- Maintain a high index of suspicion for ischemia as a cause for chest pain. Treat all chest pain, including patients with atypical symptoms, as myocardial ischemia until the diagnosis is sorted out.
- There is little relationship between severity of chest pain and gravity of cause.
- A careful history is augmented by a focused physical exam and simple diagnostic testing.
- Know which pain characteristics and associated symptoms are most likely to be predictive of ischemia. However, a single nonischemic feature should not cancel the ischemic features because chest pain symptoms are complex.
- Risk factors are cumulative: the more factors, the greater risk of cardiac disease.
- If the chest pain has subsided, spend more time obtaining a history of the present illness, past medical history, risk factors, family/social history, and physical exam; otherwise keep the history and physical exam focused for rapid evaluation and triage of the likely cause of chest pain.

3. What are the essential questions to ask the patient with nontraumatic chest pain?

- Presence or absence of chest pain at the time of assessment
- Character and severity of pain (crushing, burning, stabbing, tearing)
- Location and radiation of pain (substernal, epigastric; radiation to left arm, shoulder, jaw, neck, throat, back)
- Precipitating factors (abrupt or gradual onset)
- Duration of symptoms (seconds, minutes, hours, days)
- Aggravating and relieving factors (exercise, rest, emotional stress, eating, deep breaths/coughing, changing positions)
- Associated symptoms (nausea, vomiting, diaphoresis, dyspnea, palpitations, syncope)
- Does this pain represent a change from the patient's "baseline"?

• Risk factors (hypertension, diabetes, tobacco use, hyperlipidemia, male gender or post-menopausal women, age, family history, obesity)
• Underlying disorders to assist with the differential diagnosis

4. What unique features associated with ischemic chest pain are not found with other causes?

Although many patients with ischemic chest pain may present with atypical symptoms (i.e., elderly patients and women) most have typical symptoms.

ISCHEMIC CHEST PAIN	TYPICAL FEATURES
Stable angina	Substernal; predictable pattern of frequency; brought on by exertion or meals; brief duration; prompt relief with nitrates or rest
Unstable angina (USA)	Less predictable pattern; new onset or change in pattern of angina (more frequent/lasts longer); pain may be more intense, occur at rest, or awaken patient with pain; more associated symptoms; may or may not be relieved by nitrates or rest
Acute myocardial infarction (AMI)	Prodromal symptoms common; pain lasting ≥ 1 hour; more instability; more associated symptoms; not relieved by nitrates

5. How do I quickly determine whether the chest pain is most likely associated with ischemic cardiac changes?

Risk stratification, assessment of the symptoms, patient's risks and likelihood of CAD, other possible diagnoses, and the 12-Lead EKG. Symptoms most predictive of AMI include the following:
• Chief complaint of chest pain with radiation to the left arm
• Wider extension of pain
• History of myocardial infarction (MI)
• Associated symptoms such as nausea, vomiting, diaphoresis
• Physical exam predictors: hypotension, third heart sound, crackles
• Most predictive EKG changes: new ST-segment elevation, new Q waves, new conduction defects, ST-segment depression, T-wave peaking or inversion.
Symptoms less predictive of an AMI include the following:
• Pleuritic, sharp, stabbing, positional, or reproducible chest pain
• Normal EKG

6. What are common nonischemic causes of acute chest pain?
• Gastrointestinal disease (gastroesophageal reflux, esophageal spasm)
• Musculoskeletal disorder (costrochondritis)
• Respiratory disease (pneumonia, pleurisy)
• Anxiety
• Mitral valve prolapse
• Acute pericarditis

7. What other nonischemic causes of chest pain are life-threatening?
• Acute aortic dissection
• Pulmonary embolism
• Pneumothorax

8. How do the complaints and findings in such patients differ from those in patients with ischemia?

CAUSES OF CHEST PAIN	UNIQUE SYMPTOMS	UNIQUE SIGNS	DIAGNOSTIC TESTS FOR CONFIRMATION
GERD and esophageal spasm	Chest pain most mimics MI pain; burning, constricting, squeezing pain; may have radiation; worse when supine, bending over, or with certain foods (spicy, caffeine, alcohol); associated symptom: bitter taste	Partial relief when sitting upright, food/fluids, or when given antacids or nitroglycerin; may have epigastric tenderness	After CAD ruled out, GI studies (barium swallow, esophageal manometry, or 24-hour monitoring of esophageal lumen)
Costochondritis or other musculoskeletal causes	Chest pain gradual or sudden; anterior chest; worse with deep breath, cough, sneeze, laughing or a single motion of the arm, neck or torso	Chest pain reproducible with point tenderness at the second and fourth intercostal space junctions; may have increased warmth, erythema, or edema at site	Chest x-ray: usually negative
Pneumonia	Pleuritic chest pain worse with cough or movement; recent URI; associated symptoms: fever, chills, dyspnea, tachypnea, and productive cough	Fever; increased dullness with percussion; late inspiratory crackles or coarse wheezes	Labs: WBC count elevated; may have hypoxia Chest x-ray: infiltrate
Pleurisy	Unilateral pain; sharp, knife-like, sudden onset; worse with deep breath, cough, laugh, sneeze Associated symptom: nonproductive cough	Low grade fever; pleuritic rub (disappears when holds breath)	Chest x-ray: may have pleural effusion
Anxiety	Usually tightness retrosternally for > 30 min Associated symptoms: fatigue, emotional strain, nausea, "lump" in throat, history of depression/anxiety	Hyperventilation	
Mitral valve prolapse	Usually asymptomatic Sudden onset of sharp stabbing pain that rarely radiates Associated symptoms: fatigue, palpitations, anxiety; lasting seconds to days	Usually positional; mid-to-late systolic click and late systolic murmur best heart at left MCL or left sternal edge.	Echocardiogram

(Table continued on next page.)

CAUSES OF CHEST PAIN	UNIQUE SYMPTOMS	UNIQUE SIGNS	DIAGNOSTIC TESTS FOR CONFIRMATION
Acute pericarditis	Onset: hours to days Pain: sharp, pleuritic, and positional; worsens with deep breaths, coughing, or reclining; improves with leaning forward	Pericardial rub (grating, scratchy noise when holding breath); distant heart sounds Associated symptoms: fever and tachycardia	EKG: ST-segment elevation in majority of leads; overall low QRS voltage Labs: WBC and ESR elevated
Acute aortic dissection	Sudden onset with maximal intensity immediately; tearing sensation radiating to back; little relieves pain Associated symptoms: nausea, vomiting, feeling of impending doom	Pain/decreased pulses in lower extremities; diaphoresis	Chest x-ray: widened mediastinum CT, MRI, TEE or angiography confirms diagnosis
Pulmonary embolism	Sudden onset of dyspnea with pleuritic chest pain Associated symptoms: syncope; history of DVT, tobacco use, OCP use, recent surgery	Tachycardia, tachypnea	V/Q scan, spiral CT, or pulmonary angiogram
Pneumothorax	Acute-onset dyspnea, moderate-to-severe unilateral sharp, stabbing chest pain	Absent or markedly diminished breath sounds on effected side	Chest x-ray

GERD = gastroesophageal reflux disease, CAD = coronary artery disease, GI = gastrointestinal, WBC = white blood cells, URI = upper respiratory infection, MCL = midclavicular line, DVT = deep vein thrombosis, OCP = oral contraceptive pill, CT = computed tomography, MRI = magnetic resonance imaging, TEE = transesophageal echocardiography, V/Q = ventilation-perfusion, ESR = erythrocyte sedimentation rate.

9. Is it necessary to obtain an EKG on every patient with chest pain? If not, when is it essential?

With the exception of obvious noncardiac chest pain (e.g., trauma), all adults presenting with chest pain should have a 12-lead EKG. If the patient has chest pain during the assessment, an EKG needs to be done within minutes of presentation. The EKG should not be postponed until after the history and physical exam are completed. The EKG, in combination with the history and physical exam, contributes greatly to the patient's risk stratification. In fact, the EKG is the most essential piece of objective data for assessing chest pain.

Abnormal EKGs are highly sensitive and specific for CAD. Previous EKGs for comparison or serial EKGs for patients who have continued chest pain increase the sensitivity of the test. However, a normal EKG does not rule out ischemic chest pain, although it does decrease the probability. In fact, 60% of patients with an acute MI have normal initial EKGs. Of patients with stable angina, ≤ 50% have normal EKGs.

10. What EKG findings help differentiate among ischemia, AMI, and noncardiac causes of chest pain?

Angina: EKG changes occur with pain, including ST-segment depression, T-wave inversion; EKG may be normal.

Unstable angina: ST-segment depression, transient ST-segment elevation, T-wave inversion; EKG may be normal.

AMI: ST-segment elevation, reciprocal ST-segment depression, significant Q waves, new-onset left bundle branch block (LBBB); EKG may be normal.

11. What pearls help in the interpretation of the 12-lead EKG?
- Acute ischemic changes cannot be determined for EKGs that show LBBB or 100% ventricular pacing.
- EKG monitoring via telemetry (or other cardiac monitors) does not accurately assess for ST-segment or T-wave changes indicative of ischemia; a 12-lead EKG is needed.
- The EKG must have at least two or more contiguous leads (next to each other) for ischemic "changes" to be significant.
- The aVR lead does not count on the 12-lead EKG to indicate ST-segment or T-wave changes.

12. Does the chest x-ray serve any purpose in the evaluation of chest pain?
Chest x-rays are usually unremarkable during acute ischemic episodes, with the exception of complications such as pulmonary edema. Abnormalities may take hours to days to become apparent. Chest x-rays are recommended for patients with signs/symptoms of the following:
- Congestive heart failure (to rule out infiltrates, acute pulmonary edema, or pleural effusions)
- Valvular heart disease (to assess for cardiomegaly)
- Pericardial disease (to assess for cardiomegaly)
- Acute aortic dissection or aneurysm (to assess for widened mediastinum)
- Pulmonary disease (to assess for infiltrates, pneumonia, or pleural effusions)
- Trauma (to rule out pneumothorax or fractures)

13. Under what situations should I request a stress test?
- Patients with "low probability" of coronary disease after risk stratification (see question 1)
- Stable patients with clearly noncardiac chest pain (see questions 5 and 7)
- Patients with stable predictable angina pattern (with no current or recently increase in symptoms)
- Intermediate- or high-probability patients who are stable and in whom AMI has been ruled out by cardiac enzymes and serial EKGs

14. Why would I order a stress test for a patient at low probability of CAD or clearly noncardiac chest pain?
Even when the probability that the patient is experiencing cardiac chest pain is low, you may consider ordering a stress test as the least invasive strategy to rule out CAD definitively. A negative stress test also may be invaluable for the patient who needs reassurance that chest pain is noncardiac in origin. In contrast, for patients experiencing chest pain who are at highest risk for CAD, are not stable, and/or are suspected to be experiencing an infarct, a stress test has great potential for injury by extending or inducing an infarction. Moreover, such patients are likely to require a more invasive diagnostic study to provide a definitive diagnosis, regardless of the results obtained through stress testing.

15. What is the role of laboratory testing in the office?
Routine ordering of lab tests (such as a complete blood count or chemistry panel) is unnecessary in otherwise healthy patients, adding little to the diagnostic process. However, lab tests may be helpful if the following are suspected: anemia, infectious processes (pneumonia), dysrhythmias, electrolyte imbalance, or AMI. Pulse oximetry, if available, may be useful in suspected hypoxia related to pulmonary or cardiac causes. Arterial blood gases (ABGs) and cardiac enzymes (total creatine kinase [CK], CK-MB, myoglobins, or troponin [I or t] are better suited for emergency department or inpatient settings. Patient transport to these facilities should *not* be delayed for the purposes of laboratory studies. In fact, most facilities require retesting upon arrival.

16. When I suspect or confirm that the chest pain is probably due to ischemia or sus-pected AMI, what are the most important actions to take?
- 12-lead EKG (within 5–10 minutes)
- Non–enteric-coated aspirin (clopidogrel in aspirin-allergic patients)
- Sublingual nitroglycerin or paste (in hemodynamically stable patients)
- Oxygen/cardiac monitor (if available)
- Call for urgent transportation to a local emergency department or hospital
- Intravenous access (if available and awaiting transport to the hospital)
- Serial EKGs if pain continues; compare with previous EKGs, if available

17. What is the appropriate treatment for various other causes of chest pain?

CAUSE OF CHEST PAIN	TREATMENT
GERD/esophageal reflux	Antacids or H_2 receptor antagonists If first-line treatment fails, try proton pump inhibitors (PPIs)
Musculoskeletal disorder	Local moist heat Nonsteroidal anti-inflammatory agents (NSAIDs)
Pneumonia	Antipyretics Antibiotics
Pneumothorax	Hospitalization Chest tube insertion
Pulmonary embolism	Hospitalization IV anticoagulation Long-term anticoagulation
Pericarditis	Aspirin or NSAIDs Corticosteroids and hospitalization if signs and symptoms of cardiac tamponade are present

GERD = gastroesophageal reflux disease.

18. When is it safe to evaluate/manage chest pain in an outpatient setting?
Patients who can be evaluated in an outpatient setting include those who, after risk strati-fication, have low probability for ischemic heart disease (patients with atypical symptoms, normal EKGs, and ≤ 1 risk factor).

19. Which patients should *not* be evaluated in an outpatient setting?
Patients who clearly should not be evaluated in an outpatient setting include patients at intermediate or high risk for CAD (see question 1) and patients with suspicious ischemic EKG changes not known to be longstanding, ongoing chest pain, or evidence of congestive heart failure.

20. Under what circumstance is it advisable to request a consultation or referral for chest pain?
The decision to refer depends on the care provider's expertise, available resources in the provider's setting, patient's clinical presentation, and status of the therapeutic relationship with covering physician. NPs must be proficient in understanding the clinical presentation and natural history of CAD, taking a focused history, performing a focused physical exam, and recognizing common ischemic changes of a 12-lead EKG for patients with chest pain.
Patients with stable angina, unchanged in pattern or frequency for several months, do not require referral or consultation. Cases that require referral or consultation with an internist or cardiologist include the following:
- Suspected ischemic chest pain
- Acute ischemia EKG changes, not known to be longstanding

• Hemodynamic instability
• Chest pain accompanied with syncope
• Suspected life-threatening conditions such as pulmonary embolism, aortic dissection, or pneumothorax

21. What controversies surround evaluation or treatment of chest pain? What are they and the pros and cons of each?

Controversy 1: aspirin dosing

• The American Heart Association/American College of Cardiologists recommend daily dosing of aspirin (81–325 mg).
• The most important concept is to administer some amount of aspirin.
• 162–325 mg of non–enteric-coated aspirin is the usual dose for patients with suspected MI in most large-scale, randomized, placebo-controlled trials.
• If the patient is unsure whether he or she has taken the aspirin, it is better to give it.
• For aspirin allergy another antiplatelet drug, such as clopidogrel, should be given.

Controversy 2: optimal cardiac enzyme markers to use for evaluation of suspected ischemic chest pain

ENZYME TEST	PROS	CONS

Creatine kinase-MB	May rise as early as 4 hours
	Currently in widespread use
	Values more readily interpreted
	  between agencies
		May be positive from other causes
		Not helpful in ischemia other than
		  AMI

Troponin (t and I)	More specific than CK-MB
	  for myocardial injury
	About the same amount of time
	  to rise
	Remains elevated for several
	  days so that events prior to
	  admission can be detected
	Available as a bedside assay
	More rapid turnaround than
	  CK-MB
	May become elevated in patients
	  with unstable angina at high
	  risk for complications
		Problem with hospital variations
		  (values cannot be compared for
		  hospital transfer patients)
		Serial testing not useful

BIBLIOGRAPHY

1. Beattie S: Management of chronic stable angina. Nurse Pract 24(5):44, 49, 53, 56, 59–61, 1999.
2. Desai B, Seaberg DC: The utility of routine electrolytes and blood cell counts in patients with chest pain. Am J Emerg Med 19(3):196–198, 2001.
3. Fallon EM, Roques J: Acute chest pain. AACN Clin Iss 8(3):383–397, 1997.
4. Gibbons RJ, Chatterjee K, Daley J, et al: ACC/AHA/ACP—ASIM Guidelines for the Management of Patients with Chronic Stable Angina: Executive Summary and Recommendations: A Report of the American College of Cardiology/American Heart Association Task Force on Practice Guidelines (Committee on Management of Patients with Chronic Stable Angina). Circulation 99:2829–2848, 1999.
5. Heatley R: The challenge of chest pain. Practitioner 243:249, 1999.
6. Hill B, Geraci S: A diagnostic approach to chest pain based on history and ancillary evaluation. Nurse Pract 23(4):20–47, 1998.
7. Lee TH, Goldman L: Evaluation of the patient with chest pain. N Engl J Med 342: 1187–1195, 2000.
8. Panju AA, Hemmelgarn BR, Guyatt GH, Simel DL: Is this patient having a myocardial infarction? JAMA 280:1256–1263, 1998.
9. Paraskos JA: Evaluation of the patient with nontraumatic chest pain. In Alpert JS (ed): Cardiology for the Primary Care Physician, 3rd edition. Philadelphia, Current Medicine, 2001, pp 37–46.

10. Ulstad VK: Cardiac testing. In Mladenovic J (ed): Primary Care Secrets, 2nd ed. Philadelphia, Hanley & Belfus, 1999, pp 115–120.
11. Uphold CR, Graham MV (eds): Clinical Guidelines in Adult Health, 2nd ed. Gainesville, FL, Barmarrae Books, 1999, pp 359–364.
12. Warner CD: Triaging and interpreting chest pain. J Cardiov Nurs 12:84–92, 1997.

18. CONGESTIVE HEART FAILURE

Leslie L. Davis, MSN, RN, CS, ANP

1. What are common precipitants of congestive heart failure (CHF)?
Common causes
- Coronary artery disease (CAD)—most common cause for Caucasians
- Hypertension—most common cause for African-Americans
- Idiopathic CHF
- Valvular dysfunction

Less common causes
- Endocrine (diabetes, thyroid dysfunction)
- Cardiotoxic substances (alcohol, cocaine, chemotherapy)
- Dysrhythmias (atrial fibrillation)
- Viral infections
- Restrictive cardiomyopathies (sarcoid, amyloid, hemochromatosis)
- Severe anemia
- Peripartum cardiomyopathy

2. What symptoms and signs should alert a provider to the likelihood of CHF?

Patients with suspected or known CHF may have some or all of the following signs and symptoms:

SYMPTOMS	SIGNS
Fatigue	Pallor
Decreased exercise tolerance	Unexplained weight gain
Anxiety	Jugular vein distention
Depression	Syncope
Dyspnea on exertion (DOE)	Orthostasis
Orthopnea	Rales or crackles that do not clear with cough
Paroxysmal nocturnal dyspnea (PND)	Tachypnea
Hemoptysis	Laterally displaced point of maximal intensity
Cough	Right ventricular heave
Palpitations	Extra heart sounds (S_3 or S_4)
Chest pain	Murmurs (mitral regurgitation and tricuspid
Nausea/vomiting	regurgitation most common)
Abdominal fullness or early satiety	Tachycardia
	Right upper quadrant tenderness
	Hepatomegaly or hepatojugular reflex
	Nocturia or oliguria
	Ascites
	Peripheral edema
	Decreased pulses

3. During the initial evaluation of a patient with CHF, what essential components should be included?
- Complete history and physical exam
- Initial testing to determine the cause of the CHF

• Measure left ventricular (LV) function (LV ejection fraction) to distinguish between systolic or diastolic dysfunction

4. What should be included in taking a history for a CHF patient?

The initial visit should include a complete history of the type, severity, and duration of symptoms. Typical symptoms at the patient's first presentation with CHF are dyspnea on exertion or fatigue at energy levels that normally are well tolerated. An assessment of how the symptoms impair activities of daily living (ADLs) is needed to determine the functional class, most commonly the New York Heart Association classification system (see question 5). Providers also should assess for chest pain, orthopnea, or paroxysmal nocturnal dyspnea (PND). In addition, other disorders that may possibly explain current symptoms (such as angina, pulmonary disease, musculoskeletal disorders, intermittent claudication, or endocrine disorders) should be excluded.

5. Describe the New York Heart Association (NYHA) classification system.

The NYHA classification system allows providers to grade the severity of symptoms on a subjective scale. It may be helpful in determining therapy options, evaluating patient response to treatment, or determining suitability for rehabilitation or employment.

NYHA CLASS	SYMPTOMS
Class I	No limitation; normal physical activity does not cause symptoms
Class II	Slight limitation of physical activity; comfortable at rest, but ordinary physical activity results in symptoms
Class III	Marked limitation of physical activity; comfortable at rest, but less than ordinary activity results in symptoms
Class IV	Inability to carry on any physical activity without discomfort; symptoms present at rest

6. How is NYHA classification best used?

• Although NYHA class predicts prognosis, it may not always correlate with severity of LV dysfunction.
• NYHA class may change at each visit; therefore, it should be assessed at each patient encounter.
• NYHA class may dramatically improve with initiation of correct medications at the correct dosages.
• Concurrent illnesses may worsen NYHA class, which improves when illnesses are treated or resolve.
• Patients with minimal symptoms (class I or II) also may have sudden death.

7. What diagnostic studies are helpful in narrowing down a differential diagnosis that includes CHF?

The single most useful diagnostic test for the evaluation of CHF is the two-dimensional echocardiogram. The following table reviews diagnostic studies that may help in determining the cause and type of CHF.

DIAGNOSTIC STUDY	PURPOSE
Two-dimensional echo-cardiogram with Doppler flow studies	Measure size of four heart chambers Measure function (LV ejection fraction) Assess valvular structures for stenosis or regurgitation Assess for ventricular thrombus Assess for presence of pericardial effusion

(Table continued on next page.)

DIAGNOSTIC STUDY	PURPOSE
Radionuclide ventriculography scan (RNV)	Measures myocardial viability Measure left and right ventricular function Measure size of chambers
Cardiac catheterization	Assess for ischemic cause of CHF LV angiogram measures LV ejection fraction Assess for mitral regurgitation or aortic regurgitation
Chest x-ray	Assess for cardiomegaly Assess for acute pulmonary edema Assess for pleural effusion or pneumonia
12-lead EKG	Assess baseline cardiac rhythm (rule out atrial fibrillation or LV conduction defects) Assess for left ventricular hypertrophy Assess for conduction defects (before starting medications) Assess for ischemia or old infarct (to determine cause of CHF)
Pulmonary function testing	To evaluate severity of pulmonary disease and to determine bronchodilator responsiveness
Laboratory testing	CBC to rule out anemia as a cause Thyroid function tests Potassium, blood urea nitrogen, creatinine to rule out renal insufficiency Liver function tests to rule out liver congestion or right sided heart failure.

8. In treating a patient who has previously been diagnosed with CHF, what are the most important facts to know about the specific patient's disease?
- Cause of CHF (ischemic vs. nonischemic)
- Most recent LV ejection fraction (LVEF)
- Whether the patient has systolic or diastolic dysfunction
- Current medications
- Current NYHA class

9. What is the difference between systolic and diastolic dysfunction?
Systolic dysfunction is the inability of the left ventricle to contract effectively (pump blood to the rest of the body). In systolic dysfunction, LVEF is below normal (< 50%). Diastolic dysfunction is the inability to fill and relax the left ventricle. Hypertension is the most common cause of diastolic dysfunction. In diastolic dysfunction, the LVEF is normal (≥ 50%).

10. Why is it important to determine whether a patient has systolic or diastolic dysfunction?
To determine the appropriate pharmacologic treatment and prognosis.

11. In treating a patient with CHF, what are the major goals of therapy?
- Identify and treat correctable etiologies.
- Control or reduce symptoms.
- Impede (or attenuate) the natural disease progression (even in asymptomatic patients).
- Improve survival.
- Reduce the need for rehospitalization.

12. What are the major pharmacologic treatments for CHF? What is the role of each?

MEDICATION CLASS	INDICATION FOR CHF	BENEFIT	CONTRAINDICATIONS
Ace inhibitors (If intolerant due to angioedema or intractable cough, try angiotensin II receptor blockers)	First line therapy for all NYHA Class patients with systolic dysfunction Possibly beneficial to patients with diastolic dysfunction	Prevents or delays disease progression Improved survival Reduction in hospitalization Symptoms relief	Renal failure with hyperkalemia (K+ > 5.5) Renal artery stenosis Pregnancy Angioedema Shock Moderate-to-severe aortic stenosis
Beta blockers	Systolic dysfunction, LVEF < 40%, stable class II–III	In combination with ACE inhibitor and diuretics: improved survival, reduction in hospitalization	Acute pulmonary edema Episodes of CHF decompensation or fluid overload Severe bradycardia or advanced heart block Reactive airway disease
Diuretics (Begin with thiazide diuretics; loop diuretics are first choice for patients with renal insufficiency; use lowest dose possible)	For symptoms of volume overload For those with systolic dysfunction, use in combination with ACE inhibitor; do *not* use as monotherapy!	Improvement of symptoms rapidly Spironolactone (Aldactone) for class III or IV patients adds mortality benefit	Caution with orthostatic hypotension Caution with worsening renal insufficiency
Digoxin (Lowest possible therapeutic range is best)	Systolic dysfunction that remains symptomatic after ACE inhibitor and diuretic Do *not* give to patients with diastolic dysfunction	No effect on mortality Improved symptoms and exercise tolerance Reduction in hospitalization	Worsening renal function increases toxicity risk Hypokalemia may induce toxicity
Angiotensin II receptor blockers	Patients with CHF intolerant to ACE inhibitors	Unknown clinical advantage over ACE inhibitors	Same as ACE inhibitors

ACE = angiotensin-converting enzyme.

13. What are the starting and target doses for each of the major classes of medications for CHF?

MEDICATION CLASS	EXAMPLES OF STARTING DOSE	TARGET DOSE OF EACH
ACE inhibitors	Captopril, 6.25 mg tid Enalapril, 2.5 mg bid Lisinopril, 5 mg qd Ramipril, 2.5 mg bid	Captopril, 50 mg tid Enalapril, 10 mg bid Lisinopril, 40 mg qd Ramipril, 5 mg bid
Beta blockers	Carvedilol, 3.125 mg bid Metoprolol XL, 12.5 mg qd	Carvedilol, 25–50 mg bid Metoprolol XL, 150 mg qd

(*Table continued on next page.*)

MEDICATION CLASS	EXAMPLES OF STARTING DOSE	TARGET DOSE OF EACH
Diuretics	Hydrochlorothiazide, 25 mg qd Furosemide, 20–40 mg qd Spironolactone, 12.5–25 mg qd	Lowest possible dose of furosemide is best, maximal dose = 120 mg bid Aldactone, 50 mg qd
Digoxin	Digoxin, 0.125 mg qd	Lowest possible therapeutic dose
Angiotensin II receptor blockers	Valsartan, 80 mg qd Candesartan, 16 mg qd Losartan, 25–50 mg qd	Unknown target; whatever is maximally tolerated

ACE = angiotensin-converting enzyme, qd = each day, bid = 2 times/daily, tid = 3 times/daily

14. How are ACE inhibitors used?

ACE inhibitors may be titrated to the target dose unless the patient has symptomatic hypotension (systolic < 90 mmHg) or renal status worsens markedly (potassium, blood urea nitrogen [BUN], creatinine levels). A potassium level < 3.5 or > 5.8 is a concern. An increased BUN level that is disproportionate to serum creatinine levels is usually corrected by reducing the diuretic dose and is not necessarily an indication to reduce or stop the ACE inhibitor.

Patients intolerant to ACE inhibition or angiotensin-II receptor blockers (ARBs) may be given a combination of hydralazine and isosorbide dinitrate. This substitution may have the same clinical benefit as ACE inhibitors or ARBs; however, the mortality benefit is not as great.

15. How are beta blockers used?

- With the target doses in mind, a general rule for upward titration of beta blockers (or ACE-inhibitors) is every 2–4 weeks.
- Initial doses of beta blockers should be given in a monitored setting, with assessment of orthostatic vitals within 1 hour after the first dose.
- Carvedilol must be given with food, with twice-daily doses at least 8–12 hours apart.
- Beta blockers doses may be doubled at each titration (for example, carvedilol, 3.125 mg twice daily, may be increased to 6.25 mg twice daily, then to 12.5 mg and so on).
- Do not titrate beta blockers upward if the following are present: systolic blood pressure < 90 mmHg, symptomatic orthostatic hypotension, heart rate < 50 beats/min, or evidence of marked fluid overload. If the patient experiences symptomatic hypotension, the doses of the beta blocker and ACE inhibitor should be separated by at least 1–2 hours.
- For patients in whom beta blockers are titrated upward, the diuretic dose may need to be increased for fluid overload at least a temporarily.
- The beneficial effects of beta blockade are often not evident for several months. CHF symptoms may even worsen temporarily. Symptoms usually are more pronounced in the first few titrations but improve as time goes on. Therefore, close follow-up is necessary during upward titrations. Upward titrations are not recommended via telephone follow-up.
- Beta blockers should not be stopped abruptly; taper downward over 1–2 weeks if possible.

16. How are diuretics used?

Diuretics should be prescribed at the lowest possible dosage and never be used as monotherapy for systolic dysfunction. Spironolactone is recommended for NYHA class III or IV patients with ejection fraction < 35%, creatinine < 2.5, and potassium < 5.0. It may be started at 12.5 mg daily with potassium levels checked every week for approximately 4–5 visits to ensure that the patient is not hyperkalemic.

17. How is digoxin used?

Digoxin should be started with the lowest possible therapeutic dose (0.125 mg/day). Digoxin levels of 0.8–1.1 are sufficient. There is no great therapeutic benefit with higher levels—only an increased chance of toxicity.

18. What are signs that the treatment needs to be adjusted?

CHANGE IN STATUS	TREATMENT ADJUSTMENT(S)
Significantly worsened renal function (potassium, blood urea nitrogen, creatinine levels)	If dehydrated, decrease (or stop) diuretic May need to decrease (or stop) ACE inhibitor Do not titrate beta blockers upward in this setting Watch for digoxin toxicity Instructions to avoid foods high in potassium
Hyperkalemia	Discontinue potassium supplementation Spironolactone: decrease (or stop if severe) Dietary instructions May induce digoxin toxicity ACE inhibitor: decrease dose
Hypokalemia	Add a potassium supplement Consider adding low-dose aldactone Consider adding low-dose magnesium oxide, especially if magnesium levels are low normal
Fluid overload	Increase diuretic(s) Do not titrate beta blocker upward in this setting Chest x-ray if acute pulmonary edema suspected
Symptomatic hypotension	Assess orthostatic vital signs Give fluids (oral or IV) May need to decrease (or stop) diuretics, beta blockers *or* ACE inhibitors
Marked bradycardia or advanced heart block	12-lead EKG to rule out arrhythmia Check digoxin level May need to decrease (or stop) beta blocker, digoxin, *or* ACE inhibitor

19. What causes an acute exacerbation of CHF?
- Overdiuresis
- Underdiuresis
- Uncontrolled hypertension
- Dysrhythmias
- Inadequate therapy
- Worsening CHF
- Dietary indiscretions, including excessive sodium or fluid intake
- Use of alcohol or cocaine
- Intentional or inadvertent changes in medications or dosages
- High doses of NSAIDs
- Noncardiovascular causes (severe respiratory infections, endocrine disorders, liver disease, renal disease)
- Financial problems
- Family or psychosocial issues

20. How does treatment differ for an acute exacerbation of CHF from chronic treatment?

During episodes of acute decompensation, the treatment goal is to identify and correct the precipitating event. Evidence of clinical deterioration may include increased body weight, increased jugular vein distention, increased liver size, rales, increased dyspnea, worsened NYHA classification, increased orthopnea, and pedal edema. The patient with CHF may need inpatient hospitalization for IV diuretics, vasodilators, and possibly IV inotropic agents. Beta blockers should *not* be titrated upward during this time. Referral to a cardiologist is needed (see question 20). The treatment goal for chronic CHF is to prevent the progression of disease and treat ongoing symptoms.

21. What are the nonpharmacologic treatments for CHF?
   • Low sodium diet (< 3 gm sodium; < 2 gm before giving large doses of diuretics)
   • Avoidance of excessive fluid intake
   • Avoidance of alcohol and other cardiotoxic substances
   • Tobacco cessation
   • Regular exercise (mild-to-moderate exercise, beginning at low levels)
   • Weight loss for obese patients

22. How often should follow-up visits occur for patients with CHF?
   For patients with NYHA class I or II, initial visits should be every 2–4 weeks until symptoms resolve or until the patient is on target doses of medications, if possible. Follow-up visits should occur every 3–6 months if the patient is stable. A careful evaluation for increased symptoms, increased dyspnea or tachypnea, increased weight, rales, or pulmonary effusions should be done at each visit. Lab values should be checked initially at 2- to 8-week intervals as medication adjustment occurs—otherwise, every 3–6 months if the patient is stable. An EKG should be done with a recent change in heart rhythm or for recent or prolonged episodes of angina. It is debatable how frequently echocardiography or chest x-rays should be done.
   For patients with NYHA class III or IV, follow-up visits may range from every 1–2 weeks up to every 1–3 months, depending on severity and stability of the patient. Every effort is made to prevent hospitalization. Home visits may be done in some settings. Most visits include laboratory assessment of potassium, blood urea nitrogen, and creatinine.

23. What information should the patient be taught about CHF?
   • General nature of the disease, prognosis, and compliance issues.
   • Self-monitoring of daily weights and checking for peripheral edema. Daily weights should be done at the same time every morning, with an empty bladder and on the same scales without clothing.
   • Signs and symptoms of worsening disease that patients should report to their provider (worsening dyspnea or exercise tolerance, orthopnea, weight gain > 3–5 pounds over baseline, or increased peripheral edema).
   • High sodium foods to avoid (canned or packaged foods; sports drinks are the worst).
   • Exercise beginning at low levels of speed and duration with gradual increase. Intense or isometric exercise (push-ups or weight lifting) is not recommended.
   • Importance of regular flu and pneumonia shots as indicated; avoidance of contact with other acutely ill people.
   • Avoid routine use or high doses of NSAIDs (affect diuretics and ACE-inhibitors and may cause fluid overload).

24. At what point should I consult a cardiologist or refer a patient with CHF?
   • When CHF has an unclear etiology
   • Possible underlying repairable heart disease (CAD or valvular problems)
   • Symptomatic dysrhythmias or conduction disturbances
   • NYHA class III or IV
   • Unstable course
   • Need for specialized cardiovascular testing

- Evaluation for heart transplantation (age < 65 yr for symptomatic CHF refractory to optimal therapy)
- Decompensation (especially if life-threatening or not responding to change in therapy in 1–3 days)
- Patients with hypertrophic cardiomyopathy who have symptomatic dysrhythmias or a family history of sudden death

25. How do I know when a patient with CHF needs to be admitted or sent to the emergency department for further evaluation and treatment?
- Patients experiencing moderate-to-severe heart failure for the first time
- Pulmonary edema
- Clinical or EKG evidence of myocardial ischemia or infarction
- Symptomatic hypotension
- Unexplained syncope, especially in patients with low LVEF
- New arrhythmia
- Hyperkalemia (potassium > 5.8)
- Fluid overload with any of the following that would prevent treatment as an outpatient: marked hypotension, worsened renal insufficiency, oliguria, mental status changes, or shock
- When chronic heart failure is refractory to outpatient therapy (e.g., large doses of diuretics no longer achieve adequate diuresis or the patient needs to be admitted for new medications or more aggressive IV medications [diuretics, vasodilators such as nipride or nitrates, or inotropes])
- Any other cause of acute decompensation (complicating medical illnesses such as pneumonia)

26. What factors affect the prognosis of a patient with CHF?
The most reliable physiologic measure of disease progression in CHF is the assessment of cardiac remodeling. Use of echocardiography or RNV to look at chamber size (degree of dilation) and to assess any change in EF. However, serial echocardiographies are not recommended. Otherwise poor prognostic indicators include the following:
- Advanced age
- Increased clinical severity of heart failure (decreased ejection fraction, increased chamber size, and/or worsened NYHA class)
- Ischemic cause of heart failure
- Tachycardia
- Hyponatremia
- Large palpable liver
- Poor or refractory response to optimal medical management
- Shorted intervals between hospitalization for IV inotrope therapy
- History of syncope or cardiac arrest

27. What controversies surround the treatment of CHF?

CLINICAL QUESTION	CURRENT ANSWER
Use of ACE inhibitors vs. angiotensin receptor blockers (ARBs)	ARBs should be used only for patients who are ACE inhibitor-intolerant (angioedema or cough). Ongoing studies are investigating this issue, but ARBs not yet FDA-indicated for CHF.
Pharmacologic treatment for diastolic dysfunction	Unclear which ACE inhibitor has clinical utility in patients with preserved LV function.

(Table continued on next page.)

CLINICAL QUESTION	CURRENT ANSWER
Therapeutic digoxin levels	Digoxin levels between 0.8–1.1 are adequate. Higher digoxin levels offer no more clinical benefit; in fact, they may be more likely to become digoxin toxic.
Routine use of chronic anticoagulation for low LVEF	Warfarin is no longer routinely indicated for low LVEF unless there is evidence of thrombus, a history of atrial fibrillation, or a known thromboembolic event.
Choice of antiarrhythmic agents	Before antiarrhythmic agents are started in patients with CHF, a cardiologist should be consulted. Asymptomatic arrhythmias should not be treated in patients with CHF. If an agent is required, amiodarone is preferred because of its less negative effect on contractility compared with other agents. However, routine use for all patients is not recommended because of the potential for increased serum digoxin levels and possible thyroid toxicity. Most regimens are started on an inpatient basis.

28. What other treatments on the horizon show promise for CHF?

Endolethin receptor antagonists (ERAs)

Phosphodiesterase inhibitors (PDEIs)

Recombinant human B-type natriuretic peptide (hBNP)

Vasopressin inhibitors

Tumor necrosis factor–alpha receptor blockers

There are ongoing studies to determine the optimal dosing and duration of therapy to maximize benefits. Another promising area of CHF therapy is the study of pharmacogenetics, which may provide insight into which therapies work best for which patients, based on identification of genetic basis of disease and treatment for the specific type of disease.

29. Discuss current and future surgical treatment options for CHF.

Coronary artery bypass grafting (CABG) remains the most common surgical therapy for patients with ischemic cardiomyopathy as the cause of the CHF. Biventricular pacing is a means of resynchronization therapy for patients with CHF and widened QRS intervals. Other surgical options include transmyocardial revascularization, left ventricular assist devices (as a bridge to cardiac transplantation), cardiac transplantation, cardiomyoplasty, transmyocardial laser revascularization, cellular transplantation, injection of growth factor (VEGF), and the total artificial heart. In addition, more noninvasive hemodynamic monitoring and extracounterpulsation therapies are currently being designed for patients with CHF.

BIBLIOGRAPHY

1. ACC/AHA Task Force on Practice Guidelines: Guidelines for the evaluation and management of heart failure. Circulation 104:2996–3009, 2001.
2. Beattie S: Heart failure with preserved LV function: Pathophysiology, clinical presentation, treatment and nursing implications. J Cardiovasc Nurs 14(4):24–37, 2000.
3. Branum K: Using beta-blockers in the treatment of heart failure. Nurse Pract 24(7):75-83, 1999.
4. Connolly K: New directions in heart failure management. Nurse Pract 25(7):23–41, 2000.
5. DeWald T, Gaulden L, Beyler M, et al: Current trends in management of heart failure. Nurs Clin North Am 35(4):855–875, 2000.
6. Fletcher L, Thomas D: Congestive heart failure: Understanding the pathophysiology and management. J Am Acad Nurse Pract 13(6):249–257, 2001.

7. Gheorghiade M, Cody R, Francis G, et al: Current medical therapy for advanced heart failure. Heart Lung 29(1):16–32, 2000.
8. Gomberg-Maitland M, Baran D, Fuster V: Treatment of congestive heart failure, guidelines for the primary care physician and the heart failure specialist. Arch Intern Med 161:342–352, 2001.
9. Leier CV: Evaluation of the patient with heart failure. In Alpert JS (ed): Cardiology for the Primary Care Physician, 3rd ed. Philadelphia, Current Medicine, 2001, pp 47–56.
10. McKelvie R: Community management of heart failure. Can Fam Physician 44:2689–2698, 1998.
11. Milfred-LaForest S: Pharmacology department: Pharmacotherapy of systolic heart failure: a review of the recent literature and practical applications. J Cardiovasc Nurs 14(4):57–75, 2000.
12. O'Connor C, Gattis W, Swedberg K: Current and novel pharmacologic approaches in advanced heart failure. Heart Lung 28(4):227–242, 1999.
13. Packer M, Cohn J: Consensus recommendations for the management of chronic heart failure. Am J Cardiol 83:1A–38A, 1999.
14. Richardson L: Women and heart failure. Heart Lung 30(2):87–97, 2001.
15. Uphold CR, Graham MV (eds): Clinical Guidelines in Adult Health, 2nd ed. Gainesville, FL, Barmarrae Books, 1999, pp 364–372.

19. ACUTE ABDOMINAL PAIN

Mary Jo Goolsby, EdD, MSN, APRN, ANP-C, and Laurie Grubbs, PhD, ARNP, ANP

1. What are the major classifications of abdominal pain?

When the immediate cause of abdominal pain is unknown, it can be classified by anatomic regions as well as type of pain. Abdominal pain is also often classified as acute or chronic.

2. How is the anatomic region helpful in classifying abdominal pain?

Nine anatomic regions are used to differentiate the locations of abdominal pain. Knowing which organs lie in each region can be helpful in considering the potential cause of pain that is limited to one region or another. The regions and the organs/structures included in each are identified below.

Right upper quadrant (RUQ): liver, gallbladder, tip of right kidney, diaphragm.

Epigastrium: stomach, pancreas.

Left upper quadrant (LUQ): spleen, pancreas, tip of left kidney.

Right flank: right kidney.

Midabdomen or periumbilical area: uterus, bowel, aorta.

Left flank: left kidney.

Right lower quadrant (RLQ): appendix, right ovary, bowel.

Hypogastrium or suprapubic area: bladder, uterus.

Left lower quadrant (LLQ): left ovary, bowel.

3. How is the type of pain helpful in classifying abdominal pain?

Three major categories are used to classify abdominal pain: visceral, somatoparietal, and referred. The patient's description of pain characteristics and associated symptoms, as well as physical signs, can help identify the type of pain, which, in turn, narrows the differential diagnosis.

Visceral pain typically is poorly localized, tends to be midline, and is rather vague. Patients appear restless and may writhe and shift positions in an attempt to achieve comfort. They often describe the pain as cramping or burning and may have other symptoms such as diaphoresis, pallor, or nausea. Visceral pain stems from inflammation or injury to the solid or hollow abdominal organs.

Somatoparietal (or peritoneal) pain is better localized and more intense. It is intensified by movement, including even deep respirations and/or cough. Patients remain quite still and guarded to minimize discomfort. Somatoparietal pain is experienced when the parietal peritoneum is inflamed.

Referred pain, as the name implies, is referred to the abdomen from an extraabdominal site.

The type and location of pain may change during the course of an illness, and such changes are important to note. For instance, the pain of appendicitis is usually visceral and located in the midline at onset. With progression and irritation of the parietal peritoneum, the pain shifts to the lower right abdomen and becomes intense and localized.

4. At what point is abdominal pain considered acute? When does it become chronic?

Acute abdominal pain generally refers to any pain of less than 24 hour's in duration. Chronic abdominal pain usually has persisted for a considerable time despite diagnostic studies and treatments. Glasgow and Mulvihill (1998) use the terms *chronic intractable abdominal pain* and *chronic undiagnosed abdominal pain* to refer to undiagnosed pain that has persisted for at least 6 months despite proper diagnostic studies.

5. Other than gastrointestinal or other intra-abdominal disorders, what are the other potential causes of abdominal pain?

Disorders of many systems can result in abdominal pain, including the neurologic, endocrine, cardiovascular, renal, musculoskeletal, hematologic, and respiratory systems.

Radiculitis stemming from spinal cord disorders may radiate to the abdomen. Pneumothorax or pneumonitis may cause abdominal pain. Abdominal pain can occur with myocarditis or myocardial infarction as well as hematologic disorders such as sickle cell anemia and hemolytic anemia. Adrenal disease, uremia, diabetes mellitus, and hyperparathyroidism may be accompanied by abdominal discomfort. This list of extra-abdominal causes is not exhaustive, and it is important to remember the broad potential causes of abdominal pain.

6. What is the best approach to the patient with abdominal pain?

The first step is to obtain a thorough history of the pain. The history should include all of the items normally considered as part of a symptoms analysis. You also should obtain a history of past health and current problems as well as a family history specific to the abdomen or other systems, depending on the potential causes as you develop the differential diagnosis. It is also important to ask key questions about the patient's habits, activities, and exposures.

7. What questions will help me to analyze fully the presenting symptom of abdominal pain?

The **PQRST** approach for symptom analysis helps to remember all of the dimensions that should be addressed:

P = palliative/provocative factors. What makes the pain worse? What makes it better? What have you tried to relieve the pain, and how did it respond?

Q = quality/quantity factors. Ask the patient to describe the pain in his or her own words. What does it feel like? Is it sharp, aching, crampy, dull, stabbing, or boring? On a scale of 1 to 10, how does the patient rate his or her pain?

R = region/radiation factors. Ask the patient to show you exactly where the pain is as well as other areas to which the pain seems to radiate or anywhere else the patient feels pain.

S = severity/associated symptoms. How does the patient describe the severity of the pain—mild, severe, excruciating, or agonizing? What, if any, other symptoms has the patient noticed? Ask about fever, nausea or vomiting, and shortness of breath. Ask female patients if they have had any vaginal discharge or other gynecologic symptoms. At this point you can start the review of the systems that you think may be involved.

T = timing, temporal sequence. When exactly did the pain start? Since it was first noticed, has it been constant or intermittent? What was the patient doing when he or she first developed the pain? Does the pain seem to occur in relation to particular activities, such as bending, eating meals, or taking deep breaths? Since the pain first occurred, has it become worse or better or stayed about the same? Has it changed in location since onset?

8. Of the symptoms that may accompany abdominal pain, are there any "red flags" indicating potential immediate threat?

- Pain of sudden, acute onset
- Pain that persists more than 6 hours and progresses in intensity and/or shifts location/distribution
- Pain that awakens the patient
- Pain that is associated with progressive intractable vomiting
- Pain associated with lightheadedness on standing or syncope
- Pain that radiates to the back or shoulder
- Pain associated with history of black, tarry stools
- Pain associated with decreased urine output

9. What information about past health is essential?

Ask about current conditions or diagnoses as well as any treatments. Ask about previous episodes of abdominal pain as well as specific illnesses commonly associated with abdominal pain, such as bowel obstruction, diverticulitis, pancreatitis, sickle cell anemia, kidney stones, and pelvic inflammatory disease. Ask about prior abdominal surgeries. It is important to learn which abdominal organs may have already been surgically removed (e.g., gallbladder or appendix) and to identify the potential for intra-abdominal adhesions. It is also helpful to ask the patient specifically about any abdominal diagnostic procedures.

10. What habits and sociocultural history should I include for patients with abdominal pain?

Ask about typical or recent diet and use of caffeine, tobacco, alcohol, or drugs. Ask about recent activities, exercise habits, occupation, and travel. Address sexual activity and practices. Ask whether the patient has been in contact with anyone else who is ill.

11. What components of the physical examination other than the abdominal exam, should I include?

The information learned from the history should help you to focus the examination. However, physical assessment should begin with a consideration of the general survey findings of the patient's appearance, posture, and demeanor as he or she gave the history of pain. Is the patient serious, guarded, and still (indicating possible peritoneal irritation) or more restless (indicating possible visceral irritation)?

Review the patient's vital signs, noting blood pressure, pulse, temperature, and respiratory rate. You should perform an examination of the heart and lungs and observe neurologic and musculoskeletal status. A rectal and vaginal examination should be performed with any complaint of acute abdominal pain. Determination of whether to perform a more detailed general assessment depends on the history and findings from the abdominal exam.

12. What are the five basic elements of the abdominal exam?

Auscultation, inspection, percussion, palpation, and special techniques.

13. How is auscultation performed?

The abdominal examination should begin with auscultation. Listen for bowel sounds in all quadrants and adventitious sounds such as bruits, venous hums, or hyperperistaltic bowel sounds (pops, tinkles, rushes, borborygmi). An abdominal bruit may indicate vascular narrowing, a venous hum over the liver may indicate hepatoma, and hyperperistaltic sounds may indicate obstruction or enteritis. When the peritoneum is inflamed, bowel sounds are often diminished.

14. What are the major elements of inspection?

As you auscultate, begin to inspect the abdomen. Observe the general contour and coloration of the abdomen, noting the condition of the overlying skin. Identify any scars, hyperperistalsis, or visible muscle rigidity. Hyperperistalsis may be visible with obstruction, whereas abdominal rigidity suggests peritoneal irritation with guarding. Bulges may be seen at the site of an abdominal hernia. Blue discoloration at the umbilicus is indicative of trauma, whereas blue discoloration of the flanks may occur with hemorrhage or pancreatitis.

15. Describe the approach to percussion.

Start percussion remote from the site of the pain to minimize discomfort. Note the general abdominal tones, considering the location of areas of dullness over organs and other areas. Later you will want to palpate carefully over any dull areas. Compare the areas of dullness overlying organs against the anticipated dimensions. Tympany may be noted over areas of abdominal gas. Ask whether percussion elicits discomfort, which is a sign of peritoneal irritation.

16. How is palpation performed?

Palpate the abdomen, beginning with light pressure applied generally over the abdomen remote from the site of pain. Notice any signs of discomfort; if the abdomen is tender and rigid, you may have limited success in palpating individual structures. If this step is tolerated, carefully palpate the abdominal organs and abdomen in general, using progressively deeper pressure and noting the characteristics of any palpable organs or masses.

17. What special techniques are used in the abdominal exam?

It is important to identify any signs of somatoparietal or peritoneal pain, which strongly suggest the need for urgent treatment. The most common of these techniques is the test for rebound tenderness. Rebound tenderness is tested by slowly pressing downward over the abdomen with your fingertips, holding the position until pain subsides or the patient adjusts to the discomfort, then quickly removing the pressure. Rebound pain, a sign of peritoneal inflammation, is present if the patient experiences a sharp discomfort over the inflamed site when pressure is released.

A simple test to elicit peritoneal pain involves asking the patient to take a deep breath and cough. This maneuver may trigger pain at the affected site in peritoneal irritation. Other techniques include heel strike, obturator, and psoas tests. During the pelvic or rectal examination, you should be able to palpate gently near the peritoneum and detect any localized pain. To assess for cholecystitis, check for Murphy's sign by palpating in the right upper quadrant as the patient takes a deep inspiration. Increased pain during this maneuver, although not highly sensitive, is indicative of gallbladder inflammation.

18. What physical findings should be considered "red flags" indicating the need for urgent diagnosis and treatment?

- Involuntary guarding
- Progressive abdominal distention
- Increased intensity of pain with movement, respirations, percussion, rebound
- Orthostatic hypotension
- Fever, leukocytosis, granulosytosis
- Decreased urine output
- Altered bowel sounds
- Pulsatile mass

19. When are laboratory studies indicated? Which should I include?

The answer, of course, depends to a great degree on the differential diagnosis based on earlier findings. However, acute abdominal pain should be assessed with a complete blood count (CBC) and differential as well as urinalysis. The CBC assesses the potential not only for infection or inflammation but also for anemia that may be associated with any GI bleeding. The urinalysis helps to establish hydration status as well as the potential for a genitourinary cause for the pain. You should consider the following studies, based on earlier findings: electrolytes, glucose, blood urea nitrogen and creatinine, liver functions, and amylase. You should perform a pregnancy test on *all* women who present with abdominal pain during childbearing years.

20. When are diagnostic images indicated? Which should I order?

Although the choice of whether to order diagnostic images depends on earlier findings, there are some recommendations about which studies are appropriate for complaints of acute abdominal pain.

Plain abdominal films. Abdominal films help to evaluate potential obstruction and to visualize renal calculi. They are also an inexpensive, useful study for general abdominal assessment. (See Chapter 4, Demystifying Radiology.)

Abdominal ultrasound. Ultrasounds are useful to assess or detect the possibility of gallstones, pelvic inflammatory disease, pancreatitis, and liver masses. The abdominal ultrasound is used to assess potential palpable abdominal masses as well as to assess potential appendicitis in children, pregnant women, and very thin patients.

Pelvic/transvaginal ultrasound. Pelvic ultrasound is useful in female patients if a problem with the uterus, ovaries, fallopian tubes, or bladder is suspected. It is more accurate than abdominal ultrasound for genitourinary lesions and may help to assess other lower abdominal lesions, including appendicitis and diverticulitis. In ordering an ultrasound, it is important to be specific about which type you want.

Computed tomography (CT). When an imaging study is required to assess further a complaint of lower right abdominal and possible appendicitis, CT is preferred over ultrasound for patients with rigid, noncompressible abdomens as well as obese patients. CT is more helpful than ultrasound in assessing potential abcesses associated with appendicitis and diverticulitis. CT is recommended when either mesenteric ischemia or a perforated ulcer is suspected.

21. What are the common intra-abdominal causes of acute abdominal pain?

Acute cholecystitis	Gastroenteritis
Small bowel obstruction	Acute pancreatitis
Acute mesenteric ischemia	Perforated ulcer
Hepatitis	Pelvic inflammatory disease
Acute appendicitis	Chronic problems (inflammatory bowel
Acute diverticulitis	disease, irritable bowel syndrome)
Abdominal aortic aneurysm	

The common findings for each of the listed disorders are discussed in the following questions. Remember that neither this list of abdominal pain disorders nor the list of findings is exhaustive.

22. What are the signs and symptoms of acute cholecystitis?

Onset of localized, persistent, constricting, or colicky RUQ pain is sudden and may follow a meal. Nausea, vomiting, and fever may be associated symptoms. The pain may radiate to the back, right shoulder, or right flank. Murphy's sign may be positive. White blood cell (WBC) count and total bilirubin may be elevated. RUQ ultrasound is highly sensitive in identifying stones in the gallbladder.

23. Describe the presentation of acute appendicitis.

Appendicitis usually evolves over a few hours; pain is initially poorly localized, midline, and vague. Associated symptoms include some degree of nausea and/or loss of appetite. In a matter of hours, the pain moves to the RLQ, becoming much more intense and well localized. At this point, temperature may be somewhat elevated. Percussion, palpation, and/or the various tests for peritoneal inflammation are positive. The WBC count is usually elevated. Although imaging is not necessary with classic findings, both ultrasound and CT are positive.

24. What findings suggest acute pancreatitis?

The classic symptom is sudden onset of intense pain in the epigastrium or LUQ, which may radiate to the back, flanks, or lower abdomen. Most patients have mild fever as well as loss of appetite, nausea, and vomiting and appear to be in much distress. Tachycardia and hypotension may be present. Rarely, discoloration may be seen around the umbilicus or flanks. The serum amylase level is usually elevated, as is the WBC count.

25. What symptoms and physical findings are typical of small bowel obstruction?

Most patients have sudden onset of sharp pain in the mid-abdomen, associated with nausea and vomiting. They may report that vomiting provides intermittent relief of pain. Patients are restless and appear distressed. Vital signs may include mild fever, tachycardia, and hypotension. The exam may identify sounds of hyperperistalsis and diffuse tenderness without peritoneal signs.

26. How does acute diverticulitis usually present?

Acute diverticulitis tends to evolve over time, like appendicitis. Patients often report an initial, vague discomfort in the mid-abdomen or suprapubic region that may be associated with loss of appetite, nausea, and/or vomiting. The pain later shifts to the LLQ, becomes much more intense, and is aggravated by movement. The patient may develop diarrhea and fever. Bowel sounds may be diminished, and peritoneal signs may be present. If imaging studies are performed, CT may identify not only the site of inflammation but also any related abcess. WBC count may be elevated.

27. Describe the signs and symptoms of a perforated duodenal ulcer.

The patient may describe an earlier history of duodenal ulcer symptoms. Perforation usually is associated with sudden onset of sharp, intense pain in the epigastrium, which soon extends to a large area of the abdomen and may radiate to the back. The patient has nausea and tends to be quite still, guarding a rigid abdomen. As chemical peritonitis develops, the pain may be greatest along the right side of the abdomen. Vital signs show fever, tachycardia, hypotension, and tachypnea. CT reveals the perforation.

28. Describe the typical history and presentation of acute mesentery ischemia.

The patient may describe a history of diarrhea and vomiting with associated weight loss. The patient's health history may include cardiovascular disease. The onset of the pain, described as intense cramping and located in the epigastrium and mid-abdomen, is usually sudden. As the ischemia and necrosis progress, peritonitis develops, the patient appears increasingly ill, the pain becomes excruciating, WBCs are elevated, and tachycardia and hypotension may be present. CT is recommended as the initial screening when mesenteric ischemia is suspected.

29. How does abdominal aortic aneuryms present?

There is usually sudden onset of a ripping, severe pain in the midabdomen or flank areas, which may radiate to the back. The patient feels faint and becomes diaphoretic and nauseated. Most patients present with a pulsatile mass and significant hypotension in addition to pain. The abdomen may be distended and the femoral pulses diminished.

30. What signs and symptoms are typical of pelvic inflammatory disease (PID)?

Most patients report a subacute onset of suprapubic, LLQ, and/or RLQ pain that is steady and moderate in severity and may radiate to the upper thigh. Loss of appetite, nausea, and/or vaginal discharge may be associated symptoms. The patient may be febrile. The abdominal and pelvic examination identifies tenderness over the lower abdomen and adnexa as well as cervical motion tenderness. Speculum examination may show an inflamed cervix and yellow or otherwise discolored discharge. Over time the patient may develop peritoneal signs.

31. What findings suggest the diagnosis of hepatitis?

The pain of acute viral hepatitis is usually limited to the RUQ and achy in nature. The patient may provide a history of preceding malaise, anorexia, and change in urine and stool. The examination identifies a tender and possibly enlarged liver as well as altered liver function tests. Similar findings, without the viral symptoms, often are present in hepatitis related to ischemia or drugs.

32. Describe the typical presentation of gastroenteritis.

The pain associated with gastroenteritis may be acute in onset and usually is diffuse and crampy. Associated symptoms include anorexia, nausea, vomiting, and/or diarrhea. Exaggerated bowel sounds (borborygmi) may be auscultated. The abdomen may be distended and guarded. Patients may have symptoms of an infection, including fever and malaise. Depending on the amount of diarrhea or vomiting, the patient may develop signs of dehydration.

33. What symptoms and historical findings may suggest inflammatory bowel disorders (IBD)?

IBD includes both Crohn's disease and colitis. The pain associated with IBD can be unrelenting or intermittent and is a chronic problem. It ranges from mild to severe and from vague to colicky. Associated symptoms such as diarrhea are often present. However, because the associated abdominal pain may be recurrent and the patient may develop associated peritonitis, IBD is one consideration in patients with acute abdominal pain. The history of recurrent intestinal symptoms is helpful in identifying the cause as chronic in nature. For complaints of acute changes in pain or other symptoms, the assessment should include efforts to identify related peritoneal inflammation.

34. When should you suspect irritable bowel syndrome (IBS)?

IBS is another problem characterized by either persistent or recurrent bouts of abdominal pain and typically is accompanied by diarrhea and/or constipation. The pain or discomfort is often relieved with defecation. The pain of IBS is typically vague, and patients may complain of flatulence, bloating, and/or "gurgling." Associated pain may be severe, especially with the onset of an acute bout. For this reason, IBS should be considered in assessing acute abdominal pain. It is thought to be related to abnormalities in motility, mediated by the central nervous system. Although IBS is not identifiable by structural or biochemical abnormalities, mucosal or motility changes may be seen with flexible sigmoidoscopy.

35. What should I do if I have examined the patient and the cause of the pain is not evident?

The answer depends on the patient's condition. If the patient has signs of severe illness (e.g., significant fever, tachycardia, pallor, diaphoresis, severe localized pain) and you do not identify a problem that you can treat, refer the patient to a surgeon for further evaluation. If, however, the patient appears stable and findings are vague, you may consider performing frequent, serial examinations and/or diagnostic studies. In this case, you may ask the patient to return later in the day for a repeat examination. An old adage says, "Real diseases declare themselves"; with time the symptoms and/or physical findings should point to a diagnosis. However, up to 50% of patients with abdominal pain are diagnosed as "nonspecific"; it is not unusual to have a patient with some degree of abdominal discomfort but no identified cause. Nonspecific pain is a diagnosis of exclusion. Make sure that the disease is not trying to declare itself at a time when you are not understanding the declaration! When deciding whether to proceed with serial assessments or referral, you should weigh carefully the risks and benefits of both approaches, erring on the side of safety. When in doubt, do *not* use a shotgun diagnostic approach. Consider requesting a telephone consultation with a surgeon or other specialist to help determine what further route to take.

36. When should a patient be referred for acute abdominal pain?

A patient should be referred if surgical intervention is necessary; most of these patients need urgent or same-day referrals. Examples include appendicitis, cholecystitis, bowel obstruction, perforated ulcer, acute mesenteric ischemia, and abdominal aortic aneurysm. Immediate transport to the hospital is indicated for all patients in whom pain is believed to indicate an abdominal aortic aneurysm, and all patients whose condition is unstable.

Conditions that can be managed medically and, therefore, are not urgent include gastroenteritis, inflammatory bowel disease, diverticulitis (unless perforated), hepatitis, pancreatitis, and PID. However, if intractable pain, nausea, vomiting, or diarrhea is present, the patient may need hospitalization for pain management or hydration.

Patients in whom abdominal pain and/or other associated symptoms fail to respond to early, appropriate treatment also should be referred, including those with IBD, diverticulitis, and PID. For management of hepatitis B and C, chronic pancreatitis, or IBD, referral to a gastroenterologist or infectious disease specialist is usually warranted. The treatment for these diseases is complex, and the patient will benefit from the specialist's care.

BIBLIOGRAPHY

1. Adelman A: Abdominal pain. In Mengel MB, Schwiebert LP (eds): Ambulatory Medicine: The Primary Care of Families. Stamford, CT, Appleton & Lange, 1996.

2. Dains JE, Baumann LC, Scheibel DB: Advanced Health Assessment and Clinical Diagnosis in Primary Care. St Louis, Mosby, 1998.
3. Glasgow RE, Multihill SJ: Abdominal pain, including the acute abdomen. In Felman M, Sleisinger MH, Scharschmidt BF (eds): Sleisinger and Fordtran's Gastrointestinal and Liver Disease: Pathophysiology/Diagnosis/Management, 6th ed. Philadelphia, W.B. Saunders, 1998.
4. Hurst JW (ed): Medicine for the Practicing Physician. Stamford, CT, Appleton & Lange, 1996.

20. ERECTILE DYSFUNCTION

Susanne A. Quallich, APRN, BC, NP-C, CUNP

1. What is erectile dysfunction?

Erectile dysfunction (ED) is defined as the inability to achieve and maintain an erection sufficient to permit satisfactory sexual activity.

2. What is the estimated prevalence of ED in the United States?

Some estimates indicate that ED affects as many as 10–20 million men in the U.S. This number increases to up to 30 million if men with moderate-to-complete erectile dysfunction are included. ED increases in prevalence with age.

3. What is the physiology of a normal erection?

A normal erection requires the coordination of both neural and vascular events that control arterial flow to and venous return from the penis. Sympathetic innervation originates within the T11–L2 spinal tracts, whereas parasympathetic and sensory innervation arise from S2–S4. As arousal begins, the smooth muscles in arterioles that supply the paired corpora cavernosa and the corpora spongiosium relax and allow increased flow of blood into the penis. The trabecular smooth muscle in the cavernous spaces also relaxes to allow filling of the sinusoids and expansion of the penis. The combination of these two processes traps the blood within the penis by compressing the subtunical venous plexus against the tunica albuginea, which prevents venous outflow and results in a rigid erection. During intercourse, inflow and outflow of blood slow down because of the contraction of the muscles surrounding the base of the penis. After ejaculation or removal of erotic stimuli, sympathetic nervous system control again becomes dominant, the trabecular smooth muscles relax, and the trapped blood is able to flow out of the penis, which becomes flaccid.

4. Is there more than one type of erectile dysfunction?

Yes. ED can be organized into several categories, based on the suspected cause.

CATEGORY	CAUSES	PROPOSED PHYSIOLOGIC MECHANISM
Psychological	Performance anxiety, depression, psychological stress, relationship issues, psychotic disorders, misinformation or ignorance of normal anatomy/function	Possible increased sympathetic outflow or elevated catecholamine levels Possible direct inhibition of spinal erection center by CNS
Neurologic	CVA, SCI, radical pelvic surgery, pelvic irradiation, diabetes, Alzheimer's disease, pelvic trauma, CNS tumors, diabetes mellitus, alcohol abuse, vitamin deficiency, Parkinson's disease, spina bifida, multiple sclerosis	Direct damage to the areas of CNS that control erections Prevention of initiation of erection Damage to pelvic or sacral nerves that control erection Diabetic polyneuropathy
Endocrinologic	Hypogonadism, hyperprolactinemia, hyperthyroidism, hypothyroidism, diabetes mellitus, orchiectomy	Decreased nocturnal erections Decreased libido Decreased circulating testosterone

(Table continued on next page.)

CATEGORY	CAUSES	PROPOSED PHYSIOLOGIC MECHANISM
Arteriogenic	Atherosclerosis, hypertension, hyperlipidemia, smoking, pelvic trauma, diabetes mellitus	Penile artery insufficiency Damage to or stenosis of common penile or cavernous artery due to trauma
Cavernosal (venogenic)	Age, Peyronie's disease, diabetes mellitus, insufficient trabecular smooth muscle contraction	Failure of venous occlusion Venous leakage Decreased compliance of penile sinusoids
Medication-induced	Antihypertensives, antidepressants, antipsychotics, alcohol abuse, smoking, antiandrogens, alpha-adrenergic blockers, beta blockers, tranquilizers, thiazide diuretics, centrally acting sympatholytics, cimetidine, estrogens, polypharmacy, marijuana	Blockage of central neurotransmitter pathways Chronic alcohol abuse: hypogonadism, polyneuropathy Vasoconstriction (smoking, illicit drugs) Depression of testosterone levels (marijuana) Polypharmacy
Systemic disease-induced	CRF, coronary heart disease, COPD (fear of inducing exacerbation), CHF, hepatic failure, scleroderma, recent myocardial infarction, chemotherapy, cirrhosis	Increased refractory period Decreased force of ejaculation Less turgid erections Increased length of time from stimulation to erection CRF: decreased testosterone, autonomic neuropathies, vascular disease

CVA = cerebrovascular accident, SCI = spinal cord injury, CRF = chronic renal failure, COPD = chronic obstructive pulmonary disease, CHF = congestive heart failure.

5. What are the pertinent aspects of the history in evaluating a patient for ED?
- Patient's age
- Onset and duration of ED
- Psychosocial factors, including the nature of current relationship(s), details of current techniques, and patient's knowledge of anatomy and physiology of sexual response
- Patient's current medications
- Comorbidities, including psychiatric issues or depression
- History of back, retroperitoneal, or pelvic surgery
- Changes in penile sensation
- Nature of dysfunction (i.e., whether the problem is attaining or sustaining an erection, insufficient rigidity, penetration, or ejaculation)
- Presence or absence of nocturnal erections and their quality
- Remedies that the patient has tried
- Previous exposure to chemotherapy or radiation
- Previous traumatic sexual experiences
- Patient's social history, including smoking, alcohol, and recreational drug use
- Degree to which ED has affected the patient's quality of life, as assessed by the Sexual Health Inventory for Men (SHIM), a short questionnaire that has been validated for assessment of ED

6. What other considerations are important when a patient presents with the complaint of ED?

ED typically exists with comorbidities and can be an indicator of more serious diseases. If a patient presents with ED in the absence of conditions such as diabetes mellitus, hypertension, or neurologic disorders, the history and work-up must be targeted to evaluate the risk factors and manifestations of conditions that can contribute to ED. If the patient has newly diagnosed medical conditions, they should be managed before initiating therapy for ED. Successful management of other conditions may change the nature of the patient's complaints and possibly reverse ED.

7. What is the focus of the physical examination in evaluating a patient with ED?
- Blood pressure
- Evaluation of secondary male sex characteristics and testicular size
- Evaluation of lower extremity and femoral pulses
- Neurologic examination that focuses on perineal and penile sensation as well as anal sphincter tone
- Digital rectal exam in men older than 50 years
- Examination of the penis to evaluate for structural abnormalities, such as Peyronie's disease

8. What lab work is indicated for the work-up of ED?
Initial lab work includes urinalysis and total testosterone level. If the patient complains of low libido or if findings include decreased testes size, a free testosterone level should be included. If a low testosterone level has been documented, a serum prolactin level should be drawn to evaluate for a prolactinoma. Other tests may include complete blood count (CBC), blood urea nitrogen (BUN), or creatinine, but selection should be based on clinical findings and history. In the context of suspected diabetes, a serum glucose or glycosylated hemoglobin level may be indicated. A lipid profile also may be included. Thyroid-stimulating hormone (TSH) or thyroid profile may help if the patient has symptoms of hyper- or hypothyroidism.

9. What is the value of serum testosterone level in the initial work-up for ED?
There is some controversy over the value of a testosterone level. Most experts agree that a total serum testosterone is indicated. However, because up to 97% of serum testosterone is bound to protein, total and free (bioavailable) testosterone levels are necessary. Testosterone should be measured before 10:00 AM, because it is secreted according to a diurnal rhythm. A low afternoon testosterone must be redrawn, because it does not conclusively indicate the true level. Testosterone levels typically begin to decline in the seventh decade but rarely to the point of causing ED.

10. If the testosterone level is low, are other tests indicated?
When the morning total testosterone level is low, the test should be repeated, along with measurement of free testosterone, leutinizing horomone (LH), and follice-stimulating hormone (FSH) levels. Low total and free testosterone levels and a high LH level suggest testicular failure. If hypogonadism is the suspected cause of ED, prolactin and LH levels should be drawn. A pituitary adenoma should be suspected if the bioavailable testosterone level is < 20 ng/dl, the LH level is low or normal, and prolactin is elevated; the patient should be screened for with a magnetic resonance imaging scan.

11. What diagnostic studies are available? What do they evaluate?

TEST	DESCRIPTION
Nocturnal penile tumescence and rigidity (NPTR)	Screens for neurologic integrity by measuring changes in the circumference of the penis for 3 consecutive nights in a sleep lab
Penile duplex ultrasound	Evaluates penile arteries and hemodynamics
Penile brachial pressure index	Screens for penile arterial disease

(Table continued on next page.)

TEST	DESCRIPTION
Penile arteriography	Evaluates penile arteries in the setting of trauma
Cavernosometry/ cavernosography	Evaluates cavernosal artery pressure and integrity of the veno-occlusive mechanism
Intercavernosal pharmacologic testing	Screens for possible causes of ED based on the time it takes for a patient to attain an erection and how long it is maintained

Routine use of these tests is controversial; usually they are ordered at the discretion of a urologist.

12. What other considerations affect the treatment plan for patients with ED?

It is important to determine the patient's expectations for the outcome of the treatment as well as his preferences for the type of treatment. In appropriate situations, the patient's partner also should be considered in determining the treatment plan, because his or her expectations also affect success of treatment. It is important to emphasize to the patient and his partner that the goals of ED treatment are to provide an erection that is sufficient for penetration and thus allow the patient to perform without anxiety during sexual activity. No treatment for ED affects the patient's libido, with the possible exception of men treated for hypogonadism.

13. How is psychogenic ED distinguished from organic ED?

PSYCHOGENIC ED	ORGANIC ED
Sudden onset	Gradual and insidious onset
Selective ED	Persistent ED
Normal erections during masturbation	Absent nocturnal and morning erections
Normal pattern of nocturnal and morning erections	Inability to achieve satisfactory erection under any circumstances
Associated with emotional stress, fear, guilt, anxiety, religious inhibition, parental inhibition, traumatic past experience	

14. When should a patient with ED be referred to a specialist?

Patients with a history of pelvic or perineal trauma or curvature of the erect penis (Peyronie's disease) are appropriate referrals to a urologist. Patients suffering from endocrinopathies can be referred either to a urologist (hypogonadism, testicular failure) or endocrinologist. Patients with psychiatric disorders, psychosexual disorders, or premature ejaculation should be referred to a sex therapist, counselor, or psychiatrist. Patients suffering from lumbar disc disease or lumbar stenosis can be referred to a neurosurgeon or orthopedist, and patients with suspected vascular disease may be a candidate for vascular surgery referral.

15. What is the initial pharmacologic treatment for ED?

Once potentially reversible conditions have been appropriately treated, the initial pharmacologic treatment for ED is sildenafil (Viagra). Several studies have shown that sildenafil improves the quality of erections and increases satisfaction with intercourse, but its success requires that the penile nervous system is at least partially intact. For sildenafil to be effective, the patient also must be sexually stimulated. Sildenafil has been shown to be effective in patients with a variety of systemic conditions, including diabetes, coronary artery disease, hypertension, pulmonary vascular obstructive disease, depression, and spinal cord injury as well as in patients who have undergone nerve-sparing radical prostatectomy or transurethral resection of the prostate. Sildenafil also has proved effective in patients taking other medications that typically contribute to ED.

In administering any pharmacologic treatment for ED, however, it is important to remind the patient that the treatment may not work with the initial dose (because of anxiety). Only a single sildenafil dose daily is recommended, regardless of the dose that is effective for a particular patient. Sildenafil is approximately 69% effective overall.

16. What are the contraindications to sildenafil?

Patients using any form of nitrates, including sublingual, transdermal, transnasal, or oral formulations as well as recreational "poppers" (amyl nitrate), are not candidates for sildenafil. Relative contraindications to the use of sildenafil include myocardial infarct or stroke in the past 6 months, serious arrhythmia, history of heart failure, coronary artery disease, or poorly controlled hypertension.

17. Are there second-line pharmacological therapies for the treatment of ED?

Yes, but because they involve injecting medication into the corpora of the penis, they are significantly more invasive. Either alprostadil or papaverine can be used alone, but they typically are used together and sometimes in combination with phentolamine. Alprostadil is available in a prefilled injectible form called Caverject or Edex. Only three intercavernosal injections per week are recommended, and the injections must be at least 24 hours apart, regardless of the formulation. Instruction in the proper technique for injection is vital. Success rates range from 60% to 100%. Alpostadil also can be prescribed as an interuretheral suppository (MUSE) that is administered via a plunger-like device, but this method has less consistent results than injections. It does, however, provide an option for anticoagulated patients.

Both yohimbine and trazodone have been reported to improve ED, but little research has been done to support these claims or to establish safety and dosing regimens.

18. What are the contraindications to second-line therapies?

Any patient who is anticoagulated is not a candidate for vacuum erection devices (VEDs) or injection therapies. Injection therapy also is contraindicated for patients with poor vision or poor manual dexterity as well as patients at risk for priapism, such as those with sickle cell or those taking monoamine oxidase inhbitors. Gross obesity also may make it difficult for the patient to visualize the correct place to inject.

19. What nonpharmacologic treatment options are available?

Other alternatives are available to patients not interested in pharmacologic management. VEDs work by generating negative pressure on the penis and thus drawing blood into the penis. Once the penis is erect, a thick elastic band is slipped from the base of the device onto the base of the penis to prevent outflow of blood. This band should be left in place for no more than 30 minutes. An additional option is psychosexual therapy, which may involve the patient alone or the patient and his partner.

20. Define priapism. What are its causes?

Priapism is a persistent erection, lasting more than 1 hour, that is not necessarily the result of sexual activity and does not subside after orgasm. It occurs idopathically as well in patients diagnosed with sickle-cell disease or neoplasm; it is also a risk of penile injection therapy. Any patient complaining of an erection lasting more than 2 hours should be directed to the nearest emergency department, because priapism is a urologic emergency and can result in fibrosis of the corpora and impotence if not treated in a timely fashion.

21. Discuss the role of testosterone replacement in the treatment of ED.

Testosterone replacement is appropriate in only a small number of men: those with hypogonadism documented by a low testetrone level. Exogenous testosterone therapy, however, creates the risk of aggravating lower urinary tract symptoms by contributing to benign prostatic hyperplasia or accelerating the progression of occult prostate cancer. The response rate to testosterone therapy is low, and patients must be monitored with prostate specific antigen

(PSA), liver function tests, complete blood count, and rectal examinations every 6 months for 2 years after the initiation of therapy and yearly thereafter.

22. What are the treatment options for patients who fail first- and second-line treatments for ED?

Penile prostheses remain the primary surgical option for patients who have failed pharmacologic treatment. Single-piece malleable prostheses and two- or three-piece inflatable prostheses are available.

It is also possible to treat ED with penile artery revascularization surgery, although this option usually is available only for younger patients (age < 50 years) with arteriogenic ED due to pelvic or perineal trauma.

23. What risks are associated with penile prosthesis surgery?
- Infection
- Risk of erosion of a cylinder of the prosthesis into the urethra or through the corpora
- Risk and highly invasive nature of the surgery itself
- Possibility of prolonged postoperative pain
- Potential need for reoperation if the device fails
- Problems related to a poorly sized prosthesis
- Risk of needing to remove the device, which alters the natural function of the corpora and diminishes the likelihood of successful drug-assisted erections after the device is removed.

24. What are the advantages of penile prostheses?

Prostheses allow spontaneity and the highest documented degree of patient and partner satisfaction of all treatment modalites for ED. They do not affect libido, orgasm, penile sensation, ejaculation, or urination. A three-piece inflatable prosthesis is the preferred treatment for patients with ED due to Peyronie's disease.

25. Describe the follow-up after initiation of treatment for ED.

It is important to evaluate a patient within 6 months after beginning treatment to determine (1) the success of and patient satisfaction with the chosen treatment modality, (2) the presence of possible side effects, and (3) the nature of continued ED (if other medical conditions exist, their continued management can effect both ED and the success of its treatment). The successful treatment of ED may uncover other sexual dysfunctions, such as premature ejaculation, that also respond to evaluation and management. Regular follow-up visits can be scheduled every 6–12 months.

26. What are the possible side effects of the pharmacologic treatments for ED?

MEDICATION	SIDE EFFECTS
Sildenafil (Viagra)	Headaches, nausea, flushing, dyspepsia, nasal congestion, abnormal vision, dizziness
Vacuum erection devices	Penile irritation, pain, numbness, and brusing; retarded antegrade ejaculation; penile distention and edema
Alprostadil injection	Priapism, scar tissue formation with chronic use, painful erection, infection at injection site, hypotension, seizures, bradycardia, tachycardia
Papaverine injection	Headache, nausea, diaphoresis, flushing, infection at injection site
Combination alprostadil, papaverine, phentolamine injection	Penile bruising, transient dizziness, fibrosis at injection site, painful erection, priapism, infection at injection site, flushing, nasal congestion
Interuretheral alprostadil	Penile pain, prolonged erection, urethral pain/burning, hypotension, dizziness, low response rate

BIBLIOGRAPHY

1. American Urological Association Erectile Dysfunction Clinical Guidelines Panel: Report on the Treatment of Organic Erectile Dysfunction. Baltimore, American Urological Association, 1996.
2. Korenman SG: New insights into erectile dysfunction: A practical approach. Am J Med 105(2):135–144, 1998.
3. Laumann EO, Paik A, Rosen RC: Sexual dysfunction in the United States. JAMA 281:537–544, 1999.
4. Lewis JH: The role of the NP in the diagnosis and management of erectile dysfunction. Nurs Pract 25(Suppl):14–18, 2000.
5. Lewis R: Surgery for erectile dysfunction. In Walsh PC, Retik AB, Stamey TA, Vaughn ED (eds): Campbell's Urology. Philadelphia, W.B. Saunders,1998, pp 1215–1236.
6. Lue TF: Male sexual dysfunction. In Tanagho EA, McAnincho JW (eds): Smith's General Urology. New York, Lange Medical Books, 2000, pp 788–810.
7. Mobley DF, Baum N: A proactive approach to the contemporary ED environment. Cont Urol 12 (12):12–19, 2000.
8. Montague DK, Lakin MM: Erectile dysfunction. In Kursh ED, Ulchaker JC (eds): Office Urology: The Clinician's Guide. Totowa, NJ, Humana, 2001, pp 343–351.
9. Moskowitz MA: The challenges of diagnosing erectile dysfunction in the primary care setting. Nurs Pract 25(Suppl):1–3, 2000.
10. National Institutes of Health Consensus Development Panel on Impotence: Impotence: NIH consensus conference. JAMA 270:83–90, 1993.
11. Stanley GE, Bivalacqua TJ, Hellstrom JG: Penile prosthetic trends in the era of effective oral erectogenic agents. South Med J 93:1153–2000, 2000.
12. Wilson SK, Delk JR: Inflatable penile implant: Predisposing factors and treatment suggestions. J Urol 153:659–661, 1995.

21. HEMATURIA

Susanne A. Quallich, APRN, BC, NP-C, CUNP

1. Define hematuria.
   Microscopic hematuria denotes the presence of more than three red blood cells (RBCs or erythrocytes) per high power field (HPF) in two of three properly collected urine specimens. **Gross hematuria** results when the number of erythrocytes is significant enough for the patient or clinician to perceive a color change in the urine.

2. How common is hematuria?
   Microscopic hematuria is quite common and should prompt referral to a urologist for further evaluation of the urinary tract. It may be present in 9–18% of otherwise normal people and can result from both urologic and nonurologic conditions. Gross hematuria also should prompt a urologic evaluation. Malignancy is found in up to 40% of patients with gross hematuria, and hematuria is often the only sign of the malignancy. Because hematuria can be intermittent, serial urine collections may be indicated to establish the diagnosis. When in doubt, the clinician should not hesitate to refer for a full urologic evaluation.

3. What are the risk factors for developing hematuria?
   Recent trauma, urologic surgery or instrumentation, family history of renal disease or renal calculi, history of pelvic radiation, or recent febrile illness can cause hematuria. Vigorous exercise, such as marathon running, can lead to transient hematuria. Risk factors for the development of urologic malignancies—such as smoking; employment in chemical, petroleum, or printing industries and age > 40 years; or a history of a urologic disorder or disease—are also considered risk factors for hematuria.

4. What are the keys to preliminary urinalysis interpretation?
   In evaluating hematuria, it is mandatory to include both urine dipstick and microscopic evaluation. Urine dipstick is 90% sensitive for hematuria and is a quick, inexpensive screening tool, although its specificity is somewhat lower than its sensitivity and false positives are possible. Microscopic evaluation confirms the presence of RBCs and details their morphology.

URINALYSIS COMPONENT	INTERPRETATION
Color	Bright red in patients with urologic or anatomic cause
	Tea-colored or brown urine may be due to old clots, glomerulonephritis
Specific gravity	May see low specific gravity with hydronephrosis, intrinsic renal disease
Protein	3–4+ may indicate glomerulonephritis
Leukocyte esterase	Positive test suggests infection within urinary tract
Erythrocyte casts	Indicates glomerular source for hematuria
Crystalluria	May indicate stone disease
Nitrite	Positive test suggests infection within urinary tract

5. What other laboratory tests are helpful for evaluating hematuria?
   Serum creatinine and blood urea nitrogen (BUN) provide information about kidney function. They are useful in patients with suspected stone disease and possible obstruction due to benign prostatic hyperplasia (BPH), kidney stones, or ureteral stones.

Hemoglobin and hematocrit are not routinely indicated, because microhematuria rarely causes enough blood loss via the urinary system to alter values. Both are indicated in the evaluation of severe gross hematuria or suspected hemorrhagic cystitis.

Urine cultures are indicated in patients with suspected urinary tract infection (UTI). Urine dipstick shows positive leukocyte esterase and > 3–5 white blood cells per HPF.

Urine cytology is part of a routine hematuria work-up, and positive cytology may indicate bladder, ureteral, or renal pelvic malignancy. This test sent should be sent from a first-voided morning urine on 3 separate days.

6. What can cause a false-positive test for blood?

A false-positive test can result from hemoglobin (due to intravascular hemolysis) or myoglobin (due to massive muscle breakdown) in the urine. The sample lacks RBCs on microscopic examination. Oxidizing agents such as povidone or contamination of the collecting container with bleach also can cause a falsepositive test. Some vegetables (e.g., beets, rhubarb, blackberries) can also discolor urine. Highly concentrated or very dilute urine also distorts the concentration of RBCs as a result of RBC osmotic lysis. Medications, such as pyridium, can discolor urine. Menstrual bleeding, in the context of poor urine collection, also can create a false-positive sample; in this context, bladder catheterization helps to obtain a clean specimen.

7. What drugs can cause hematuria?

Antibiotics (reported but unusual): penicillins, cephalosporins, sulfa drugs, rifampin, polymycin.

Analgesics: nonsteroidal anti-inflammatory drugs, aspirin, aminosalicylic acid.

Diuretics (reported but unusual): furosemide, thiazides, ethacrynic acid.

Anticoagulants: warfarin, heparin, enoxaparin, clopidogrel, ticlopidine.

Others: antineoplastics (e.g., cyclophosphamide)

8. What information should be included in the history when a patient presents with hematuria?

- Patient's age and sex
- Current medications
- Past episodes of hematuria
- Timing of the hematuria as well as its onset, duration, and color of urine (bright red, pinkish, tea-colored, transparent, opaque)
- History of recent trauma to abdomen or pelvis
- Description of any pain associated with urination and its location
- Presence of irritable bladder symptoms (urgency, frequency, dysuria)
- History of tobacco use
- Complete urinary history, including recent urinary tract surgery, instrumentation, catheterization, sexual history, and history of sexually transmitted diseases
- Presence of renal disease
- Recent prostate-specific antigen (PSA) or history of prostate disease in men
- Family history of urologic malignancy
- Current regimen of intermittent self-catherization, if appropriate

9. On what does the physical examination focus?

The physical exam should focus on areas of the urinary tract that are the suspected source of the blood. The examination may include the abdomen, pelvic region, and external genitalia. A rectal examination in men is also appropriate, as is a pelvic examination in women.

10. Does the timing of the hematuria during urination have clinical significance?

Yes. The point in the urine stream when the hematuria is most noticible can help establish possible sources for the blood in the urine.

DESCRIPTION OF HEMATURIA	POSSIBLE SITE	POSSIBLE CAUSE
Microscopic hematuria	Any site within upper or lower urinary tract	Urinary tract infection; prostatitis; urethritis; medical renal disease; bladder, ureteral, or renal malignancy; stone disease
Initial gross hematuria	Anterior urethra	Stricture, meatal stenosis, urethritis, urethral cancer
Total gross hematuria	Source above bladder neck: bladder, kidney, ureter	Renal, ureteral, or bladder stone; renal, ureteral, or bladder tumor; trauma; vigorous exercise; renal tuberculosis; hemorrhagic cystitis; interstitial cystitis; sickle cell disease; nephritis; autosomal dominant polycystic kidney disease; poststreptococcal glomerulonephritis
Terminal gross hematuria	Bladder neck, prostate, posterior urethra	Benign prostatic hypertrophy (BPH), regrowth BPH after transurethral resection of the prostate, bladder neck polyps, posterior urethritis, tuberculosis

11. How does one begin to differentiate among the potential causes of hematuria?

If the patient has microscopic hematuria in the context of a suspected or confirmed UTI, treating the UTI should cause the hematuria to resolve. Other benign causes of microscopic hematuria should be excluded, such as menstruation, sexual activity, or recent instrumentation of the urinary tract. If a benign cause is suspected, a repeat urinalysis can be performed 48 hours after cessation of the activity; if it is negative, no further evaluation is required.

Hematuria also can be temporary and has been reported in athletes, especially long-distance runners. It is thought to be caused, in part, by repetitive trauma to the dome of the bladder. Hematuria in this context usually resolves spontaneously in 24–48 hours, and no further evaluation is warranted.

Gross hematuria or persistent microscopic hematuria can be a sign of prostate, bladder, kidney, or ureteral malignancy. Obtain an intervenous pyelogram (IVP) to evaluate upper tracts, and refer to a urologist for cystoscopy and/or ureteroscopy, which visually evaluates for bladder or upper tract lesions.

A patient with persistent microscopic hematuria or a patient with gross hematuria should be referred for a IVP to evaluate for filling defects in the collecting system and ureters. A referral for a urologic evaluation is required.

The initial evaluation for an episode of gross hematuria should occur in a more urgent manner, because it is more often associated with malignancy. Referral for an IVP and consultation with a urologist should be initiated.

12. Describe the difference between urologic hematuria and medical renal hematuria.

Urologic hematuria results from nonglomerular bleeding and leads to circular RBCs, a lack of erythrocyte casts, and little proteinuria. Medical renal hematuria results from glomerular bleeding due to various causes and is suggested by dysmorphic RBCs, erythrocyte casts, and significant proteinuria (> 300 mg/dl) and should prompt a complete evaluation or referral to a nephrologist.

Possible Causes of Urologic and Medical or Renal Hematuria

UROLOGIC HEMATURIA	MEDICAL RENAL HEMATURIA
Stone disease (renal, ureteral, bladder)	History of analgesic abuse
Prostate cancer	Bleeding disorder
Bladder tumor	Bleeding dyscrasias/sickle cell disease
Ureteral tumor	Human immunodeficiency virus
Renal tumor	Diabetes mellitus
Ureteropelvic junction obstruction	Atrioventricular fistula
Phimosis	Infections such as hepatitis
Vesicoureteric reflux	Exercise (marathon running)
Bladder diverticula	Berger's disease (IgA nephropathy)
Renal cysts	Benign familial hematuria
Benign prostatic hypertrophy	Sytemic lupus erythematosus
Urethral stricture disease	Drug-induced interstitial disease
False urethral passage in a patient	Postinfectious glomerulonephritis
who is self-catheterizing	Familial glomerulonephritis
Genitourinary or gynecologic surgery	Mesangioproliferative glomerulo-
and procedures	nephritis
Family history of renovascular, stone,	Vascular disease (e.g., renal artery
renal cystic disease	embolism)

13. What tests should be completed before referral to a urologist?

The patient should be evaluated with urinalysis (to rule out benign causes of microscopic hematuria), urine cytology, and the appropriate imaging study.

14. What is the role of plain abdominal films in the hematuria work-up?

Kidney, ureters, and bladder (KUB) study is the simplest uroradiologic work-up. It can be helpful as a screening or preliminary test, especially if clinical suspicion points to possible renal or ureteral lithiasis. KUB often shows calcified abnormalities, both within the urinary tract and skeletal system, and also may demostrate large soft tissue masses.

15. Which radiologic test is most helpful as an initial study in patients with hematuria?

IVP, also known as intravenous urogram (IVU) or excretory urography, remains the initial and preferred study for evaluation of the pelvis and ureter, in part because of its moderate cost and ease of administration. This test demonstrates a wide variety of upper tract lesions and is well tolerated by most patients, although it is recommended that the patient have a serum creatinine level ≤ 1.6. Most commonly used to screen for filling defects, IVP may miss small filling defects because of the bolus of dye. Because plain abdominal films are taken after the dye injection, they require bowel preparation to help ensure the quality of images. The number of films, volume of dye injection, and speed of the injection depend on the institution as well as on the patient's age, comorbidities, and physical condition. IVP also provides a crude estimation of renal function. Its use is complicated by possible allergy to the dye (which can be treated with preprocedure steroids), modest soft-tissue contrast resolution, possible contrast-induced renal toxicity, and potential cardiovascular issues related to the osmotic load. No special training is required for its administration; thus, IVP is widely available. Its utility, however, is coming into question with the advent of computed tomography (CT) and ultrasound.

16. Does abdominal ultrasound have a role in the evaluation of the hematuria patient?

Ultrasound is a noninvasive, relatively inexpensive, and widely available procedure that avoids radiation exposure and the risk of intravenous contrast. Ultrasound is superior to IVP for the evaluation of small lesions and is more sensitive in the evaluation of renal masses than IVP. It has limited utility for upper tract filling defects but can be useful for differentiating between medical and urologic renal disease. Ultrasound is also limited by the patient's body habitus and the skill of the operator.

17. What is the role of CT scanning in the evaluation of hematuria?

CT also can demonstrate filling defects, but it is not cost-effective as a screening tool or as an initial step in the evaluation of microscopic hematuria, unless stone disease is highly suspected. Its main role in the evaluation of the urinary tract is in staging malignancies. CT scan is a superior imaging method for evaluating of renal and retroperitoneal pathology and is indicated when bladder or renal malignancy is suspected and when the IVP or ultrasound indicates a mass. Unenhanced helical CT scan is also superior for the evaluation of suspected or actual stone disease because thin 3-mm slices are used.

18. What is the relationship of hematuria to trauma?

Microscopic or gross hematuria after trauma indicates damage to the urinary tract, usually as the result of rapid deceleration injury or penetrating trauma. Imaging studies are sometimes indicated for persistent hematuria. Hematuria due to trauma should be managed by a urologist because emergent surgery to repair intra-abdominal structures may be indicated.

19. Does anticoagulation contribute to the incidence of hematuria?

Therapeutic anticoagulation should not lead to hematuria. Anticoagulation does not necessarily predispose to hematuria, unless the patient becomes excessively anticoagulated. It is important to remember, however, that patients who are anticoagulated may have coexisting urologic malignancies, and an episode of hematuria in anticoagulated patients warrants an evaluation.

20. What sort of follow-up is appropriate for patients with hematuria?

A great deal of controversy surounds this subject. Many patients are likely to continue to exhibit hematuria after a complete work-up, especially in the context of preexisting medical renal disease. Some studies cite the incidence of genitourinary tumors manifesting within the 2–5 years after a negative workup at 0–3%. Many authorities recommend yearly monitoring of urinalysis until the hematuria is absent or for 2–3 years. Patients who are a greater risk for urologic malignancies (such as smokers) should be followed more closely; some authorities recommending repeat urinalysis, urine cytology, and blood pressure at 6, 12, 24, and 36 months. A significant increase in the degree of hematuria, a new episode of gross hematuria, abnormal urine cytology, or new irritative voiding symptoms (in the absence of UTI) demands reevaluation.

BIBLIOGRAPHY

1. Grossfeld GD, Wolf JS, Litwin MS, et al: Asymptomatic microscopic hematuria in adults: Summary of the AUA best practice policy recommendations. Am Fam Physician 63:1145–1154, 2001.
2. Kreder KJ, Williams RD: Urologic laboratory examination. In Tanagho EA, McAnincho JW (eds): Smith's General Urology. New York, Lange Medical Books, 2000, pp 50–64.
3. Licht MR: Urologic history, physical examination, and urinalysis. In Kursh ED, Ulchaker JC (eds): Office Urology: The Clinician's Guide. Totowa, Humana, 2001, pp 77–87.
4. Mariani AJ: The evaluation of adult hematuria: A clinical update. AUA Update Series 27:186–191, 1998.
5. Williamson MR, Smith AY: Fundamentals of Uroradiology. Philadelphia, W.B. Saunders, 2000.

22. JOINT PAIN

Paula J. Watt, PhD, FNP

1. People of all ages present with the chief complaint of joint pain. Do the causes differ among the various age groups?

In any age group the initial assessment should focus on the common reasons for the complaint with careful attention to history to identify any unusual circumstances or potentially offending factors. The age group should remind you of typical behavior and a potential differential diagnosis based on common complaints. With any group be sure to inquire about environmental, traumatic, viral, and insect exposures, genetic history, and school or work problems.

2. What are the most common causes of joint pain and aches in children?

Children present with a multitude of varied complaints related to joint pain. They have a tendency toward falls, outdoor exposures, traumatic injury, and viral insults due to frequent exposure and growth and development issues. Because children are generally poor historians, a careful history and physical examination are crucial to establishing a clear differential diagnosis. In children, separations of the growth plate and fractures are more common than ligament injuries. The most common and misused diagnosis, according to Paget et al., is "growing pains." True growing pains peak at 4–5 years of age and occur only at night; They are benign and self-limiting. Rheumatic diseases are varied; pathogenesis is unclear but probably associated with a combination of genetics, autoimmunity, and environmental factors. Formally called juvenile rheumatoid arthritis, idiopathic childhood arthritis is now the umbrella term for at least eight subtypes of noninfectious or traumatic rheumatic diseases in children. In addition, growth issues lead to common avascular necrotic issues such as Legg-Calve-Perthes disease (capital femoral) and Osgood-Schlatter disease (tibial tubercle).

3. What causes of joint pain should be considered in adolescents?

Adolescents frequently present with sports-related arthropathies because they, too, are active and tend to be accident-prone. Adolescents are risk takers and tend to engage in self-destructive behaviors as well as multiple sports that contribute to pain. The sports physical exam is an opportune time to observe adolescents for any potential problems. Marfan's syndrome has received much attention because of sudden death associated with the risk of dissecting aortic aneurysms. Physical characteristics include ligamentous laxity, hypermobile joints, arm span greater that height, and leg length greater than trunk.

4. Summarize the common causes of joint pain in adults.

Adults may have work- or exercise-related overuse syndromes and injuries as well as the beginning of various genetic rheumatic diseases. Three of the most common rheumatic conditions are rheumatoid arthritis, systemic lupus erythematosus, and fibromyalgia.

5. How does advanced age affect the differential diagnosis?

Seniors are susceptible to all of the previous disorders, which may be complicated by osteoporosis. All seniors with joint pain should be evaluated for signs and symptoms of osteoporotic changes. Falls and spontaneous fractures are also common and can cause multiple fractures of the spine, extremities, and hips.

6. What true emergencies may be associated with joint pain?

In addition to the obvious need for referral of patients with traumatic malalignment fractures and dislocations, several situations require immediate referral for evaluation and management because of the potential complications:

1. **Osteomyelitis** or infections of the bones and joints can result from penetrating wounds, open fractures, and hematogenous spread of infection from other sites. Early diagnosis and prompt treatment reduce the likelihood of complications, but any delay can cause permanent bone loss and possible growth abnormality.

2. **Pyogenic arthritis** can result from adjacent osteomylelitis or underlying systemic infection. Antibiotics, aspiration, and surgical drainage may be indicated.

3. **Avascular necrosis** is interruption of the vascular supply of bone due to rapid growth, trauma, or infection. Although complete recovery is often possible, complications such as compromised function and permanent deformity necessitate referral for careful management and follow-up.

Various **malignant diseases** may present with rheumatologic syndromes. Any persistent musculoskeletal pain, pain that is unusually intense for the amount of objective findings, atypical pain or symptoms, and sudden onset of musculoskeletal deviations should be evaluated carefully.

7. What are the most important questions to ask a patient with joint pain?

The single most important part of the assessment for musculoskeletal disorders is the history. Questions should include the following:

1. **Reason for consultation and duration of complaints**: chronologic review of present illness with emphasis on locomotor system, relationship of time and disease, present functional assessment, and symptom analysis (how the pain started, inciting events, pattern and progression).

2. **Present medical care**: any current medical treatment, other therapies, alternative treatment.

3. **Past medical, surgical, and trauma history**: any history that may affect or has an association with musculoskeletal disorders; skin disorders, chronic diseases, medications; pertinent work history of overuse or exposures; sexual history and exposure to sexually transmitted diseases; recent trips or exposure to animals; emotional and physical stress.

4. **Family history**: anyone in the family with musculoskeletal disorders, recent illness.

5. **Review of systems**: general health, eyes, skin, gastrointestinal and genitourinary systems.

8. What parts of the physical exam are essential for patients with joint pain?

The careful musculoskeletal exam should begin with observation and proceed methodically and gently:

- Observe for appropriate height and weight distribution related to the condition.
- Observe attitude, comfort, apparent state of nutrition, ease of undressing, method of rising and sitting.
- Examine patient in standing, sitting, and supine positions, relying mainly on inspection.
- When palpitation and manipulation are used, be gentle and forewarn of potentially painful maneuvers.

Five aspects of the physical examination should be emphasized in patients with rheumatic disease:

1. **Gait**: identify assistance appliances; notice any favoring of one side or lurch.

2. **Spine**: observe posture, pelvis, alignment, and flexion and extension capabilities and limitations.

3. **Muscles**: assess grip, shoulder movement, leg movement, sitting, squatting, toe-walking, tone, symmetry, and tender points in muscle belly and insertion points.

4. **Upper extremities**: observe movement, strength, symmetry, structure, and tissue changes. For differentiation, pay particular attention to the joints in the hand (distal interphalangeal, proximal interphalangeal, thumb interphalangeal, and metacarpophalangeal)

5. **Lower extremities**: observe movement, strength, symmetry, structure, and tissue changes.

9. How can I differentiate between the major common causes of joint pain?

Two key components are important to guide the evaluation and development of the differential diagnosis: whether symptoms are acute or chronic and the pattern of joint involvement. Age also can be an indicator, especially in illness typical of childhood.

10. What causes of joint pain are associated with acute and chronic episodes?

Acute episodes: infection, crystal-induced spondyloarthropathies, trauma, acute manifestations of connective tissue disorders.

Chronic episodes: rheumatoid arthritis, seronegative spondyloarthropathies, osteoarthritis, chronic sequelae of trauma and degenerative disorders.

11. What joint involvement patterns are typical of specific diseases?
- Symmetric: rheumatoid arthritis.
- Asymmetric: spondyloarthropathies, injury, overuse, plant thorn.
- Migratory: rheumatic fever, infectious processes.
- Polyarticular: rheumatic disease.
- Monoarticular: osteoarthritis, infectious disease, crystal-induced synovitis.
- Intermittent: infectious disease, Tick-borne disease.
- Location: overuse syndromes, injury, sciatica.

12. What causes of joint pain are most common at specific ages during childhood?

Osteochondrosis syndromes often affect specific sites at certain ages:

Age (yr)	Ossification
3–5	Capital femoral
6	Tarsal navicular
8–9	Calcaneus
9–11	Capitellum
11–13	Tibial tubercle
12–14	Second metatarsal head
13–16	Vertebral ring

13. Is it necessary to do an x-ray for every complaint of joint pain?

X-rays may not be necessary or appropriate for every complaint of joint pain. According to Paget et al., the use and sequence of imaging techniques depend on their sensitivity and specificity for the particular problem. Consider the potential sensitivity and specificity of all imaging techniques, along with their availability, cost, and associated risks. Select the imaging study with the potential to contribute to a confident diagnosis in the shortest amount of time at the least cost and risk to the client—but only if the results will affect the course of action. Initial joint pain may be managed with rest, ice, and nonsteroidal anti-inflammatory drugs; if it does not resolve, further evaluation with imaging is indicated.

14. What diagnostic studies are most helpful in differentiating among common causes of joint pain? When is each appropriate?

IMAGING TECHNIQUE	APPROPRIATE FOR
Plain roentgenography	Bone and joint
Fluoroscopy	Surgery, invasive procedures
Tomography	Subtle fracture, spinal fusions
Radionuclide scanning	Metastatic disease
Computed tomography	Soft tissue, pelvis, spine
Magnetic resonance imaging	Soft tissue
Ultrasonography	Differentiation of masses

15. Describe the typical features and initial treatment for each major cause of joint pain.

DISEASE	FACTORS	TREATMENT	PRECAUTIONS
Back pain (generalized or localized back pain due to multiple potential factors, such as vertebral body process, intervertebral disk, joints, ligaments, nerve roots, paraspinous musculature, referred pain from adjacent structures, malignancy, disease [sickle cell])	Associated symptoms and patterns of pain are key to the diagnosis. Fever raises suspicion of infectious process. Weight loss, chronic cough, and bowel changes suggest malignancy. Similar pain elsewhere may suggest more general rheumatologic or endocrine condition. Fatigue or sleep disturbance suggests fibromyalgia. Morning stiffness or improvement with exercise suggest seronegative spondyloarthropathy.	Based on etiology; commonly includes rest, ice, NSAIDs, muscle relaxants, physical therapy or disease modification.	
Fractures (spontaneous or traumatic disorders which may be frank, microfiber, or stress fracture)	Often cannot be detected through physical examination; suspect when excessive swelling and bruising are present.	Based on alignment/ stabilization; initial pain control, immobilization, initial reduction in swelling, physical therapy after healing has occurred.	Growth-plate separation fractures in children can lead to premature closure of plate with resultant deformity.
Sprains (injury to ligamentous structures as a result of sudden or prolonged stress to supporting structures)	Classified by degree of injury: Grade I: minimal tear, joint stable Grade II: severe tear, joint stable Grade III: complete tear, unstable joint	Based on initial stabilization, anti-inflammatory/pain control, rapid rehabilitation.	Recovery time of 2 weeks to 6 months, depending on severity. 10–40% of patients experience chronic sprains.
Strains (injury involves overstretching or tears of muscles or tendons)	Classified by degree of injury: Grade I: no significant structural damage Grade II: partial disruption of fibers and increased laxity Grade III: complete tear, unstable joint	Same as for sprains.	

(Table continued on next page.)

DISEASE	FACTORS	TREATMENT	PRECAUTIONS
Degenerative joint disease (degenerative disorder with deterioration of articular cartilage and formation of new excessive bone at joint surfaces)	Distinguished by morning stiffness of < 1 hour duration, limitation of movement, bony overgrowth. Most commonly affects weight-bearing joints such as knee and hip, DIP, PIP, MTP.	Focuses on preserving function and decreasing pain, weight control, exercise; aspirin and NSAIDs, cartilage repair.	Surgical replacement may be necessary when activity is severely limited or pain is uncontrolled.
Fibromyalgia (widespread pain and diffuse tenderness without inflammation)	May be separate entity or found in association with other rheumatologic conditions. Distinguished by presence of tender points in 11 of 18 specifically identified sites.	Based on presence of sleep cycle alteration (sleep agents, low-dose antidepressants), improvement of exercise tolerance and physical conditioning, pain relief of occasionally troublesome tender points.	
Rheumatoid arthritis (systemic disease of symmetric inflammatory polyarthropathy involving primarily small joints of hands and feet)	Distinguished by morning stiffness of > 1 hour duration Systemic features such as fatigue and weight loss, and rheumatoid nodules. PIP, MCP most commonly affected.	Consists of education, disease modification, maintaining joint function, prevention of deformities; NSAIDs, DMARDs.	Joint repair or replacement may be necessary.
Bursitis/tendinitis, overuse syndromes (inflammation of synovial membrane lining in any of 160 bursal sacs or tendon or tenosynovial sheath)	Result of trauma, overuse, systemic disorders, or sepsis. Distinguished by localized pain elicited by movement of specific motor units.	Rest, ice, NSAIDs, steroid injection, and antibiotics if sepsis is determined to be present.	

NSAIDs = nonsteroidal anti-inflammatory drugs, DIP = distal phalangeal, PIP = proximal interphalangeal, MTP = metatarsophalangeal, MCP = metacarpophalangeal, DMARDs = disease-modifying antirheumatic drugs.

16. What are the major pharmacologic and natural botanical treatments of joint pain and their considerations?

See table on page 148 and 149.

17. What sources may provide NPs with updated knowledge about musculoskeletal issues?

The *Manual of Rheumatology and Outpatient Orthopedic Disorders* is quite valuable (see bibliography). The *Journal of Musculoskeletal Medicine*, provides an excellent way to keep up with current issues and to review common disorders.

Pharmaceutical Treatment of Joint Pain

DRUG	USE	PRECAUTIONS
NSAIDs	Most common initial treatment for mild-to-moderate pain. Antipyretic, anti-inflammatory, and analgesic. Selection is based on clinical experience, patient convenience, side effects, and cost with great variability in individual response; tendency for certain drugs to work well for one complaint and not another. After failure of adequate trial with one drug switch to a different class.	Recommendations are against combinations of drugs because of the possibility of counter or side effects. Not uncommon for rheumatologists to combine drugs or exceed usual recommended doses at specialist level Consult rheumatologist about combinations of rheumatic drugs.
Intra-articular injection	To deliver corticosteroids to inflamed joints, bursae, or tendons. Injections should be limited to: Large joints, 3–4 times/year/10 times cumulatively Small joints, 2–3 times/year/4 times cumulatively	Must not be used until infection has been ruled out. Repeated injections into small joints of the hand may lead to deformity; injections into tendon sheaths may result in rupture.
Sleep disorder/ stage 4	Rheumatic complaints may begin with or include sleep cycle alterations. May include either tricyclic antidepressants at subtherapeutic doses or sleep agents.	Watch for potential habituation of drugs such as zolpidem (Ambien).
DMARDs	Alter disease effects, primarily in rheumatoid arthritis or destructive inflammatory arthritides.	Serious potential side effects. Monitor CBC; differential; platelets; CXR; hepatic, renal, and pulmonary function. Rheumatology referral.
Antimalarials	Used primarily in rheumatoid arthritis, systemic lupus erythematosus, skin and joint disease.	Deposition of pigment in the macula usually associated with prolonged use.
Corticosteroids	Potent anti-inflammatory agents that suppress many disease manifestations. When indicated, use at the lowest dose controlling symptoms.	Controversial ability to alter significantly disease process. Undisputed severe side effects when used long term or at high doses
Cytotoxic agents	Reserved for severe inflammatory arthritis unresponsive to other therapies and as last-line treatment, preferably in elderly.	Prescribed only in consultation/referral with rheumatologist.

(Table continued on next page.)

Pharmaceutical Treatment of Joint Pain (cont.)

DRUG	USE	PRECAUTIONS
Hypouricemic agents	Lowers serum uric acid by decreasing production (allopurinol) or increasing excretion (probenecid) as prevention of gouty conditions	Should not be prescribed until acute attack has subsided because they have no effect in acute process.
Vasoactive agents	Management of systemic and pulmonary hypertension, Raynaud's, and congestive heart failure associated with rheumatic conditions.	
Tumor necrosis factor receptor blocker	Reduction in structural damage. Used as adjunct to DMARD or alone to reduce signs and symptoms	May increase susceptibility to infection; supervise first dose, and monitor infections carefully. Rheumatologist referral.
Glucosamine	Constituent of cartilage and synovial fluid with a variety of not yet fully understood pharmacologic actions. Findings of reduced joint space narrowing, potential cartilage reformation, and reduced pain.	Limited scientific data.

NSAIDs = nonsteroidal anti-inflammatory drugs, DMARDs = disease-modifying antirheumatic drugs, CBC = complete blood count, CXR = chest x-ray.

BIBLIOGRAPHY

1. Hay W, Groothuis J, Hayward A, Levin ML (eds): Current Pediatric Diagnosis & Treatment, 13th ed. Stamford, CT, Appleton & Lange, 1997.
2. Light L: Glucosamine sulfate for osteoarthritis. Integr Med Consult 3:4, 25, 29, 2001.
3. Murphy J (ed): Nurse Practitioners' Prescribing Reference. New York, Prescribing Reference, Inc., 2001.
4. Paget S, Gibofsky A, Beary J (eds): Manual of Rheumatology and Outpatient Orthopedic Disorders, 4th ed. Philadelphia, Lippincott Williams & Wilkins, 2000.
5. Ruddy S, Harris E, Sledge C, et al (eds): Kelley's Textbook of Rheumatology, 6th ed. Philadelphia, W.B. Saunders, 2001.
6. Tierney L, McPhee S, Papadakis M (eds): Current Medical Diagnosis and Treatment, 38th ed. Stamford, CT, Appleton & Lange, 1999.

23. ACUTE WOUND MANAGEMENT

Karen Koozer Olson, PhD, FNP-CS, and
Louise A. Autio, PhD, FNP, BC, RN

1. What are the most common causes of lacerations and acute wounds?

Each year more than 12 million patients in the U.S. sustain traumatic lacerations necessitating repair. Wounds and traumatic injuries account for about 25% of all emergency department visits. Wounds due to blunt trauma are most common; non-glass shearing injuries are the second most common. Bite injuries, most frequently from dogs, account for about 6% of all traumatic wounds. Patients are treated in a variety of clinics for lacerations and wounds on a daily basis, most without complications or significant implications for the patient. However, treatment and care of wounds and lacerations involve complex clinical decision, such as wound assessment and cleaning, closure and dressing selection, and antibiotic and immunization considerations.

2. What are the goals of acute wound management?

- Maintain homeostasis by minimizing bleeding and preventing infection
- Preserve the function of the wounded area
- Maintain the appearance of the wound area and minimize scarring

3. What portions of the history are essential when a patient presents with an acute wound or laceration?

The essential history for wound management includes the age of the wound and details about how the injury occurred. Problematic wound mechanisms include animal or human bites, punctures, decubitus ulcers and crush injuries with burst lacerations. You should determine whether the wound contains foreign bodies and whether the wound was cleaned at the injury site. Obtain a history of allergies and tetanus immunization. Determine whether any risk factors for poor or delayed wound healing are present, such as multiple trauma, peripheral vascular disease, insulin-dependent diabetes, or history of keloid formation or scar hypertrophy. A history of radiation to the wound site may complicate healing time. Immunodeficient patients and patients taking steroids also may experience delayed healing.

4. How do I perform a thorough wound assessment?

The basics of posttraumatic assessment include evaluation of airways, breathing, and circulation as well as any evidence of disability from the injury. Once these parameters are assessed the practitioner's attention should focus on the wound. In many cases, wound assessment may be done without the use of anesthesia. Good lighting, however, is essential. The wound needs to be assessed for nerve, tendon and vascular integrity, and imaging may be necessary to determine whether any foreign bodies are present in the wound. Anesthesia may still be needed to ensure adequate wound cleansing and for the patient to tolerate the overall assessment procedure. If it is necessary to apply anesthesia for cleansing, be sure to assess motor and sensory function before the anesthesia is applied.

Wounds at increased risk for poor cosmetic results are located in the vermilion border of the lip, the mucosa, or natural hair. Wounds in the palm of the hand are also at high risk for neurologic involvement.

5. What are the guides for selecting and using anesthetics?

Anesthetic selection should consider the location, size, and extent of the wound. Three major categories of anesthesia are commonly used:

1. Topical gels containing mixtures of lidocaine or cocaine, epinephrine, and tetracaine. Topical gels require about 20 minutes of contact to obtain effective patient comfort and have a duration of about 30 minutes.

2. Wound infiltration and field blocks are accomplished by direct injection of anesthetic into either the tissue directly surrounding the wound or the nerve in the area. Wound infiltrations work well in wounds that are small and relatively clean.

3. Nerve blocks are suggested in grossly contaminated and more extensive wounds.

6. What is the role of epinephrine in managing an acute wound?

Epinephrine is a powerful vasoconstrictor that decreases bleeding in the wound; because of this same characteristic, however, it is contraindicated in wounds in areas of end artery flow (fingers, toes, tips of the nose, pinna of the ear, and penis). Because it can cause palpitation and tremors, it is relatively contraindicated in patients with coronary artery dsease.

7. When should diagnostic studies be considered in response to an acute wound?

Diagnostic studies are indicated in wounds associated with dysfunction distal to the injury and when a foreign body or underlying trauma to the bone, blood supply or nervous system is suspected. Radiographs should be ordered for crushing wounds or deep penetration wounds and also may be used to locate foreign bodies or debris. Cultures are not normally done unless healing is delayed.

8. After the assessment, what should be the first step in care of the wound?

Complete and thorough cleansing and debridement of the wound are the most important first steps. Cleaning and debridement are accomplished through both mechanical (copious irrigation or washing with normal saline) and chemical means (e.g., antimicrobial washes). A water pick with low power can be used to clean wounds.

9. For which wounds is open management recommended?
- Superficial wounds
- Abrasions and wounds that involve a large loss of superficial skin
- Wounds with a great deal of tissue damage
- Wounds grossly contaminated with feces, human or animal saliva, or soil and dirt
- Puncture wounds
- Large, nonapproximated flap wounds, which can be stabilized with Steri-Strips but should not be closed with sutures
- Wounds with low infection risk that are 12–24 hours old
- Wounds with high infection risk that are older than 6 hours

10. How do I differentiate between wounds with a low risk of infection and wounds with a high risk of infection?

The risk for infection at a wound site depends on several variables, including the patient's overall health, comorbidities, and other current treatments. For situations in which the risk of infection is higher, see question 26.

11. Describe the approach to open wound management.

Open wound management must start with wound hygiene. Wounds should be completely irrigated, and all debris should be removed. Wound dressings serve two major functions. The first is to protect the wound from further insult and to keep it clean; the second is provide a moist environment that promotes healing. Commercial products that serve this function include the hydrocolloid gel and foam. Nonadhesive occlusive dressings also can be used; examples include Telfa, Duo Derm, and Opsite. Bulky dressings or splints may be used to immobilize wounds over joints. Wounds should be kept clean and dry for the first 48 hours.

12. If it is determined that closure is appropriate, what are the available options?

Four closure options are currently used: staples, sutures, Steri-Strips, and surgical glue; sutures and Steri-Strips are the most common. Steri-Strips is the brand name of an adhesive tape. The two types of sutures are absorbable and nonabsorbable (e.g., nylon, prolene). Staples are metal clips, most commonly used in surgical closings. Dermabond, a relatively new surgical glue approved by the Food and Drug Administration (FDA) for laceration closure, is gaining in popularity; its strength is comparable to that of a 5-0 suture.

13. What are the advantages Steri-Strips?

Steri-tape works best in superficial, straight, low-tension wounds; flap wounds; and lacerations; they also can be used in patients who have a high potential for infection, patients who are currently steroid dependent, and elderly patients with frail skin. Advantages include low cost, ease of application, relatively pain-free application, and application by a variety of health care providers. Steri-Strips can be used to provide support to wounds after sutures are removed, to distribute tension across the wound, to eliminate closure technique scarring, to minimize follow-up visits, to secure flap lacerations better than sutures, and to provide greater resistance to infection than sutures.

14. What are the disadvantages of Steri-Strips?
- They do not adhere well to oily or hairy skin.
- They do not support lacerations well in lax skin.
- They do not provide adequate support for large wounds and wounds under significant tension.
- Confused patients, young children, and uncooperative patients may remove the Steri-Strips.
- They do not adhere well in wounds that have significant drainage.
- They should be used with caution around a digit because they may cause constriction and loss of circulation to the distal portion of the digit.

15. How should Steri-Strips be applied?

Wounds that are 4–5 cm in length can be taped with $\frac{1}{4}$-inch tape; wounds > 5 cm are most likely to need $\frac{1}{2}$-inch tape. Benzoin may be applied to the area to increase adhesion. The strips should overlap the wound about 2–3 cm on each side. Start at the midpoint of the wound, approximate the sides, and then work outward to the edges of the wound. Wound tape should be placed about 2–3 cm apart. Additional wound tape can be placed over the cross-tapes to prevent loosening of the ends. Wounds heal at the same rate, regardless of the type of closure method; therefore, the tape remains in place for the same amount of time as sutures in similar situations.

16. What are the advantages and disadvantages of using sutures?
Disadvantages
- Expensive to use
- Require the use of local anesthesia
- Must be done by a skilled clinician
- Require the patient to return for follow-up removal
- Placement takes longer than Steri-Strips or surgical glue
Advantages
- Areas of high tension
- Large or very long wounds
- Areas of oily or hairy skin
- Areas exposed to twisting, turning, or frequent washing

17. How do you determine the type of suture to use?

Suture selection is a complex clinical decision. Sutures are available in various sizes and materials as well as in absorbable and nonabsorbable forms. The nonabsorbable suture retains strength, whereas the absorbable suture loses strength as it remains in place. The natural absorbable suture loses tensile strength more quickly than the synthetic absorbable suture. Nonabsorbable suture is normally used for skin repairs. Colored sutures can be used for lacerations in the hair for easier identification and removal.

The size of the suture depends on various factors, including whether the suture material is natural or synthetic, how the suture will be tied or placed, the site of the wound, and the tensile strength needed to keep the wound closed. The thinner the suture, the more zeros (e.g., 4-0 is smaller than 3-0). The larger suture materials have greater strength but also create larger entry and exit wounds. The clinician must consider all of these factors in selecting suture materials.

18. How long should sutures remain in place?

Wounds heal most quickly in areas of dense vascularization such as the face. In the extremities wound healing takes longer. Sutures that are removed before 7 days do not normally retain scars, whereas sutures left in place longer than 14 days almost always leave scars. Scar formation tends to be greater in oily, pigmented skin than in dry pale skin. Movement around joints also increases the time necessary for healing. Generally sutures may be removed from the face in 3–5 days, from the scalp and extremities in 7–8 days, and from mobile joints, chest, palms of the hands, and feet in 10–14 days.

19. What can be done to minimize the scarring effect of sutures?

Suture placement causes small puncture wounds that develop small plugs of keratinized epithelium. The appearance of these small plugs is called railroad tracking. This appearance can be minimized if the sutures are removeed in less than 7 days. Wound tape can be used to support the wound.

20. Although staples are used primarily to close surgical wounds, what should a practitioner in ambulatory care know about following a patient who has been discharged with staples?

Staple manufacturers make implements that facilate staple removal. They resemble a cross between a pair of pliers and common paper-staple removers. Staples are removed in the same time frame as sutures and with sterile technique, using the manufacturer's removal equipment.

21. Do surgical glue and over-the-counter glues serve the same purpose?

Currently, Dermabond is the only FDA-approved surgical adhesive. Dermabond is available in pharmacies and through medical suppliers. Super Glue and Krazy Glue, which have been used for quick, inexpensive relief from paper cuts, are considerably cheaper than the FDA-approved glue and readily available in local drug and grocery stores. When patients use these products at home, they run the risk of allergic reactions to the glue, poor cosmetic appearance from poorly approximated edges, infections from improper cleansing and retained debris, and lack of proper tetanus coverage. Home treatment may delay practitioner assessment and consequently may result in higher treatment cost and poorer outcomes. There is also the risk that patients may inadvertently glue their fingers together. If this happens, the manufacturer of Krazy Glue recommends that the patient roll the fingers back and forth to loosen the bonds, soak the fingers in warm water, or apply acetone (found in fingernail polish remover). Acetone is an effective solvent but may cause pain in an open wound as well as skin irritation.

22. What are the advantages of using surgical glue to close a wound?

- Inexpensive cost
- Ease of application
- Minimal clinician learning time for application

- Shortening of wound closure time by 20–50% compared with sutures
- No need for anesthesia
- No need for follow-up or removal visits
- No risk of needlestick injury
- Shelf life in solution as long as 2 years
- Functional tensile strength comparable to that of 5-0 sutures

Because the first-day strength of Dermabond is much less than sutures, however, application is limited to wounds on the face, extremities (but not over joints), and selected areas over the torso.

23. What are the disadvantages of surgical glue?

- It is brittle and subject to fracture when used on long lacerations or over skin creases.
- Adhesive washes off in few days if exposed to repetitive washings before healing has occurred.
- Movement weakens the bond.
- For the above reasons Dermabond should not be used on hands, joints, or other areas that requiring frequent washing.
- Small children may pick it off prematurely.

24. What should the practitioner know about the application of surgical glue?

Dermabond is painted over opposed edges for the entire length of the wound. Allow time to dry between applications. A minimum of three applications is recommended. Dermabond polymerizes on contact with moisture on the skin surface and forms a strong, flexible bond to the uppermost layer of skin in approximately 45 seconds. This bond holds the wound edges together. Heat is released during the exothermic reaction and may cause a slight burning sensation for some patients. The adhesive acts as a protective dressing against moisture and infection. Dermabond can be used on any size of length laceration with intact epidermis, but subcutaneous sutures are strongly recommended in extremity lacerations, and good wound cleansing is needed. Tissue adhesive has been effectively used on scalp lacerations.

On day 1 the breaking strength in tissue adhesive is only about 10–15% that of a wound closed with 5-0 monofilament sutures. But wound breaking strength at 5–7 days equals that of suture-repaired wounds. The use of adhesive is restricted to low-tension areas. Wound adhesive can be used on all facial lacerations and selected torso and extremity lacerations. On the face and areas of less movement, the adhesive stays in place for 7–14 days and sloughs off with the epidermis.

25. What about tetanus status should the clinician consider?

About 35% of all tetanus develops from what initially appears to be a trivial injury. Puncture wounds of the foot are at highest risk for developing tetanus. Children and young adults are most likely to have tetanus immunity, whereas elderly patients are the least likely. Generally recognized recommendations include immunizations for clean minor wounds if the last tetanus shot was longer than 10 years; for all other wounds, immunization is recommended if the last known tetanus shot was longer than 5 years.

26. In what circumstances is prophylactic antibiotic therapy warranted?

Only 5–10% of all patients with an uncomplicated laceration develop an infection, and antimicrobials are often overused. Small, uncomplicated, non-bite wounds do not require systemic antimicrobial therapy. Topical antibiotics can be used on open or sutured wounds. The following wounds should be assessed for systemic antimicrobial treatment:

- Wounds in the hands and feet and wounds older than 6–8 hours
- Facial and other wounds older than 24 hours
- Puncture or crushing wounds for which extensive debridement is indicated
- Wounds contaminated with soil or vegetable matter

- Wounds that result from bites
- Wounds in tendon, cartilage, bones, or joints
- Wounds in immunocompromised patients
- Wounds in areas of impaired circulation or patients with cardiovascular disease

27. How is antibiotic selection determined?

Antibiotic selection should be based on suspected microorganism. Over 90% of wound infections result from *Staphylococcus aureus* or streptococcal bacteria. Antimicrobials effective for these organisms include first-generation cephalosporins (Keflex) and Augmentin. Erythromycin may be given to patients with penicillin allergies. Antibiotics for wound prophylaxis should be initiated as soon as possible. Many clinicians prefer to use intramuscular administration in the clinic to ensure timely treatment. If oral antibiotics are used, the prescription should be filled and taken at the earliest possible time.

Other Common Wound Contaminants

CONTAMINATION VEHICLE	LIKELY MICROORGANISM	ANTIMICROBIAL
Soil	Clostridium sp. and gram-negative organisms	Augmentin, doxycycline
Fresh water	*Aeromonas hydrophilia*	Ciprofloxacin, Bactrim, or Septra
Salt water	*Vibrio vulnificus*	Doxycycline

28. What patient education is necessary for each type of closure?

Patient education should include the need to assess and report any signs or symptoms of infection, such as increased redness, heat, streaking, increase in drainage or pain, or odor. Patients with sutures or staples need to be aware of the timeline for removal. All patients require information about the care specific to the type of closure. Patients with wounds that have a potential for scar formation should be cautioned to minimize exposure to the sun, which may increase the risk of scarring. Patients should be told to return if the wound reopens.

29. What follow-up is required for each closure type?

Follow-up care is related to the extent of the wound, wound location, and type of closure. Aftercare includes wound maintenance, removal of closure staples and sutures, and patient education about the continuing process of wound healing. Education should include a discussion of the return of normal tensile strength vs. visual healing of the area. In areas of cosmetic concern, when sutures are removed as soon as possible to prevent railroad track scarring, Steri-Strips or glue may be applied during the aftercare visit to support wounds for an additional time.

The wound-healing process occurs over a period of months. The period between 7 and 10 days is most vulnerable to unwanted opening. The wound has only about 5% of normal tensile strength after 2 weeks. At 2 months the wound has retained about 35% of normal tensile strength.

30. How does age affect caring for wounds and lacerations?

Lacerations in children are always problematic. It is difficult to clean and debride the wound, and sutures are frightening for a child. When necessary, consider using absorbable sutures so that the child does not have to return for suture removal. Skin tapes and surgical glue are effective with children because application is painless and follow-up care may be optional. However, children may pick at the tape and remove it. Elderly frail skin also presents a challenge for the clinician because it is difficult to close. Such wounds should not be closed under a lot of tension. Steri-Strips are often effective.

31. What are the commonly applicable CPT and billing codes?

CPT and billing codes for wound care are extensive and depend on the location of the wound and the extent of closure methods. Codes 12001–12021 are used for simple laceration repair; codes 12031–12057 for moderate lacerations; and codes 13100–13300, for lacerations requiring extensive repair. About 300 codes describe laceration repair.

BIBLIOGRAPHY

1. Bruns TB, Robinson BS, Smith RJ, et al: A new tissue adhesive for laceration repair in children. J Pediatr 132:1067–1070, 1998.
2. Hollander JE, Singer AJ, for the Stony Brook Octylcyanoacrylate Study Group: Application of tissue adhesives: Rapid attainment of proficiency. Acad Emerg Med 5:1012–1017, 1998.
3. Knight J: Proper use of skin adhesives for wound repair. J Am Acad Nurse Pract 13(1):13–14, 2001.
4. Maw JL, Quinn JV, Wells GA, et al: A prospective comparison of octylcyanoacrylate tissue adhesive and suture for the closure of head and neck incisions. J Otolaryngol 26:26–30, 1997.
5. Penoff J: Skin closures using cyanoacrylate tissue adhesives. Plast ReconstrSurg 103:730–731, 1999.
6. Pfenninger J, Grant F: Procedures for Primary Care Physicians. St Louis, Mosby, 1994.
7. Quinn J, Maw J, Ramotar K, et al: Octylcyanoacrylate tissue adhesive versus suture wound repair in a contaminated wound model. Surgery 122:69–72, 1997.
8. Trott A: Wounds and Lacerations: Emergency Care and Closure, 2nd ed. St. Louis, Mosby, 1997.
9. Uphold C, Graham M: Clinical Guidelines in Family Practice, 3rd ed. Gainesville, FL, Barmarrae Books, 1998.

24. CHRONIC WOUND MANAGEMENT

Anna S. Beeber, MSN, RN, CRNP, and Sarah H. Kagan, PhD, RN, CS, AOCN

1. How are chronic wounds classified?

Wounds are generally classified by cause (venous, arterial, or pressure ulcers) and level of tissue involvement (partial or full thickness).

2. How do you differentiate among the classifications?

Chronic wounds are classified by etiology. Assessment of the patient and the wound determines how a wound is classified. The cause of a wound may be an underlying disease, as in diabetic foot ulcers or peripheral vascular ulcers. Wound etiology also may be the mechanism of injury, as in a pressure ulcer or skin tear.

Wounds also may be classified by level of tissue involvement. Partial-thickness wounds involve epidermal and possible dermal injury. The epidermal loss appears as a wound without depth that has a red or pink base. Such wounds are sharply painful. Full-thickness wounds involve the epidermis, dermis, subcutaneous tissues, and, possibly, fascia, muscle or bone. Full-thickness wounds also may involve damage to nerve and vascular structures, which alters sensation.

3. What are the differences between arterial and venous wounds?

	ARTERIAL WOUNDS	VENOUS WOUNDS
Source	Ischemia	Venous insufficiency
Assessment	Cool extremities Pallor with elevation Decreased or absent pulses	Warm extremities (if no underlying arterial disease) Palpable pedal pulse Edema
Location	Distal lower extremities, including toes, ball of foot Pretibial skin	Gaiter area (the area of soft tissue from just above the malleoli to just below the popliteal, circumferentially) Medial or lateral malleoli
Skin appearance	Atrophic skin Loss of hair Thickened nails Dependent rubor/elevational pallor	Stasis dermatitis (xerosis, scaling, pruritus) Brawny edema (pigment changes with brown or red color) Lymphedema Lipodermatosclerosis
Wound appearance	Ulcers with "punched-out" margins Pale wound bed Nonhealing edges	Irregular margin Beefy red wound base Exudative wound
Pain	Pain, often severe and unrelieved, secondary to ischemic pattern	Pruritus and possible burning or "itching" pain

4. What diagnostic studies are important for arterial and vascular wounds?

Diagnostic studies aid in determining the extent of disease and in ruling out acute processes (e.g., deep vein thrombosis). The vascular study most used for arterial ulcers is pulse volume recordings. This noninvasive measurement of segmental blood pressure determines the ankle-brachial index (ABI). The ABI is computed by dividing the systolic blood pressure in the ankle (posterior tibialis) by that in the arm (brachialis). A reading of 0.7 or less indicates arterial disease. The patient should be referred to a vascular surgeon for consultation. Several studies are of use in venous disease. Doppler studies rule out acute deep vein thrombosis, whereas photoplethysmography and air plethysmography are used to determine peripheral vascular resistance in venous disease. Photoplethysmography uses infrared light to determine venous filling time. Air plethysmography determines venous volume, reflux, and refill by placing an air-filled cuff around the calf.

5. How does the treatment of arterial and venous wounds differ?

	ARTERIAL WOUNDS	VENOUS WOUNDS
Nonsurgical treatments	Avoid constricting garments Diet and lifestyle management Smoking cessation Supervised exercise (develops collateral circulation)	Edema management (lower extremity elevation, diuretics as indicated) Compression therapy (Unna's boots, elastic compression stockings) Exudate management (absorptive dressings) Debridement as indicated
Surgical treatments	Restore perfusion (angioplasty or arterial bypass grafts as indicated) Split-thickness skin grafts	Split-thickness skin grafts

6. What is a pressure ulcer?
    A pressure ulcer is a wound caused by pressure-related tissue ischemia. Pressure ulcers most often occur over bony prominences (e.g., occiput, scapulae, sacrum, ischial tuberosities, calcaneus). Pressure ulceration occurs when increased tissue pressure closes capillaries, causing a decrease in blood flow. The amount and duration of pressure and the ability of the tissue to tolerate injury vary on an individual basis. Mobility, nutritional status, age, and comorbid conditions are individual factors that may place a patient at higher risk for developing pressure ulcers.

7. What specific factors predispose to development of a pressure ulcer at one site instead of another?
    For the bed-bound patient lying supine, pressure ulcers most often occur on the occiput, scapula, elbow, sacrum, and calcanei. For the patient lying prone (i.e., the surgical patient on the operating table), the areas most likely to incur pressure ulceration are the submentum, breasts, iliac crest, patellae, and dorsum of the feet. The seated patient may develop pressure ulcers at the ischial tuberosities, popliteal fossae, and possibly the elbows.

8. How do you stage a pressure ulcer?
    Pressure ulcers have been categorized by the National Pressure Ulcer Advisory Panel according to the level of tissue involvement. Stage I pressure ulcers are defined as nonblanchable erythema of intact skin. They appear as a red area over a bony prominence that does not blanch when palpated. Stage II pressure ulcers are classified as partial-thickness tissue loss. Stage III is full-thickness tissue loss that extends to the fascia. Stage IV pressure ulcer is a full-thickness injury extending to the muscle and bone and sometimes causes tissue necrosis. A nonstageable pressure ulcer has eschar formation so that the extent of the injury cannot be determined.

9. What are the keys to pressure ulcer management?
    The first priority is to remove the source of pressure. This strategy depends on the mobility of the patient. Moving the patient off the affected area decreases tissue pressure.

Recommended positioning routines depend on each patient's tissue pressure threshold; however, a change in position should occur at least every 2 hours for bed-bound patients. Patients with lower thresholds for pressure, may need repositioning more often. The use of pillows and other positioning devices is helpful. Consultation with physical and occupational therapy may help to identify positions and schedules for turning and seating that optimize the patient's abilities while providing functional exercise. Avoid "positioning" aids, such as "donut cushions" that serve as tourniquets, creating venous congestion and limiting perfusion.

10. What are the keys to successful wound management?
Wound management involves minimizing any underlying cause and providing systemic and/or local treatment, as indicated:

Removal of causative factors in wound management is essential to prevent further injury. For example, pressure must be relieved in a pressure ulcer to achieve healing. Similarly, tissue perfusion must be optimized through strategies that restore arterial circulation (e.g., angioplasty) to heal an arterial ulcer.

Systemic control of underlying or potential conditions that can affect wound healing is mandatory. For instance, glycemic control must be achieved in diabetic patients for healing to occur. Nutritional deficits must be corrected in malnourished patients for the phases of wound healing to progress normally.

Local care of a wound should be guided by assessment. The goal of local therapy is to maintain a clean, moist, protected wound. For example, if the wound has exudate and drainage, use of absorptive dressings is appropriate. If the wound is covered by eschar, debridement is usually necessary.

11. Do different types of wounds heal differently?
Wound healing is characterized by primary, secondary, and tertiary intent.

Primary intent is seen after a surgical or traumatic wound that receives prompt closure.

Secondary intent occurs when a wound is left open and allowed to heal without closure. The body corrects the tissue deficit, developing granulation tissue, and closes the skin through re-epithelialization. Healing time depends on the extent of the tissue defect. The wound that heals through secondary intent is considered to be colonized by normal skin flora. Chronic wounds of long standing, in patients who live in institutions or are hospitalized frequently, may be secondarily colonized with pathogens common to institutions (e.g., methicillin-resistant *Staphylococcus aureus*).

Tertiary intent occurs when a wound is initially left open to heal through secondary intent for a certain period and then is closed surgically. Such wounds may produce less scaring than a secondary wound because of the primary closure.

12. What physiologic stages occur through the three phases of wound healing?

PHASE OF HEALING	GOAL	ACTION	INDICATOR/ ASSESSMENT
Inflammatory phase	Contain the injury Control blood loss Initiate immune response Remove or neutralize debris	Neutrophils and macrophages remove cellular debris Immune cascase Begin fibroblast migration	Serous exudate Local inflammation May see proteinaceous slough
Proliferative phase	Restore tissue defect Re-epithelialization	Development of collagen-capillary matrix Fibroblast migration Epidermal cell migration	Granulation tissue Wound contraction

(*Table continued on next page.*)

PHASE OF HEALING	GOAL	ACTION	INDICATOR/ ASSESSMENT
Remodeling phase	Scar formation	Alignment of collagen fibers along lines of tension Collagen cross-linking Capillary bed remodeling	Scar tissue

13. How does nutrition affect wound healing?

Specific macro- and micronutrients are essential for wound healing. Replacing absent nutritional stores or supplementing deficiencies is necessary for optimal wound healing. Patients with chronic wounds are at high risk for protein malnutrition because of the increased metabolic state needed to regenerate tissue. They are also often at risk for protein malnutrition from poor intake and comorbid conditions. Low protein stores impair inflammatory function, tissue regeneration, and infection fighting. The serum albumin measurement indicates the long-standing protein status (up to 3 weeks), whereas the prealbumin level measures protein stores within the past 14 days.

Fluid status is also important in patients with chronic wounds. Patients with large fluid loss through exudate can become dehydrated. In addition, fluid intake is imperative to wound healing. Fluid intake should be monitored but not avoided in patients with pulmonary or cardiac problems. Often when a wound has large exudative loss, the need for oral fluids increases. Fluid status can be monitored through serum sodium level and blood urea nitrogen-to-creatinine ratio.

Micronutrients such as vitamin A and zinc assist with the synthesis of albumin, whereas vitamin C and copper are linked with collagen production. Vitamin E may suppress the inflammatory phase of healing and should be taken into account for patients with chronic wounds.

14. What supplementation is appropriate for patients with a chronic wound?

Zinc sulfate (220 mg/day with 10–15 mg of elemental zinc) has been linked to protein synthesis and production of collagen. It is often depleted in patients with weight loss.

Vitamin C supplementation is associated with improved collagen production and can be safely prescribed for patients who do not have nephrolethiasis or renal failure. The dosage for vitamin C supplementation is 500–1000 mg/day. Steroids often decrease the production of collagen.

Vitamin A supplementation (25,000 IU orally or 10,000 IU intravenously) for 10 days has been found to increase wound healing. Vitamin A can be toxic if given for longer than 10 days or at a higher dose than indicated.

15. What are the key components of wound assessment?

To determine the etiology of a chronic wound, examination and assessment cannot be underestimated. When examining the wound and periwound area, note the size and location of the wound along with the color of the wound bed. As mentioned before, location of a wound often offers clues to the cause of the wound itself (e.g., pressure ulceration on the sacrum or a gaiter area venous stasis ulcer).

Periwound tissue should undergo the same careful examination as the wound itself. Of particular interest is erythema of the periwound tissue. Erythema can be characterized in people with white skin as a pink or red color to the tissue surrounding a wound. Erythema in people of color may look purple or brown.

The **color of the wound bed** may indicate the perfusion status of the involved tissue. A red or pink wound bed indicates perfused tissues, whereas pale or dusky coloring idicates tissue hypoxia. For further assessment of the wound and periwound tissue, use palpation and percussion for ballottement. Note induration, fluctuance, masses, exudate consistency, and pain upon palpation.

Exudate consistency reveals information about phase of wound healing as well as microbial overgrowth and infection. Note the characteristics of any exudate, including amount, odor, color, and consistency. Most importantly, odors may be indicative of bacterial overgrowth or frank infection. Anaerobic overcolonization smells strongly putrid, whereas fungal overgrowth smells like bad yeast bread. Necrotic tissue may have a pronounced odor as it liquefies.

Assessment of the **wound edges** is important to determine the existence of healing. A wound with pink pearly edges is healthy and ready to begin re-epithelialization, whereas dusky or pale edges may indicate an hypoxic wound bed. Black or dark edges generally indicate advancing tissue necrosis.

16. When should patients with wounds be referred? To whom?

The types of wounds for which you most often refer a patient or request a consultation include wounds of vascular origin, significant pressure ulcers, or wounds with necrotic tissue or infectious overgrowth. A registered nurse (RN) wound care specialist is a great resource for dealing with chronic wounds. The wound care specialist can recommend an appropriate plan of care, assuming the care of the wound, or suggesting the appropriate referral. Examples of the types of wounds for which you commonly consult another provider are described in the table below, along with the appropriate action, including the discipline to which the patient may be referred.

PHYSICAL EXAM FINDING	DIAGNOSTIC EXAM	ETIOLOGY	REFERRAL OR ACTION
Pale lower extremity ulcer	Peripheral volume recorder (PVR)	Arterial vs. venous ulcer	Vascular surgery
Bright blanchable erythema with satellite lesions in skin folds	Potassium hydroxide (KOH) preparation test	Fungal overgrowth	Dermatology
Nonblanchable erythema located over bony prominence		Pressure ulcer	Plastic surgery Physical therapy Occupational therapy
"Beefy-looking" red wound bed without edema		Healthy granulation tissue	Maintain clean, moist environment
Black, yellow, or gray tissue in wound		Tissue necrosis	Plastic surgery
Maceration		Pooling of fluid on skin surface, usually from exudate or fluid source (i.e., urine in incontinent patient)	Manage fluid source or use absorptive dressing
Dermal–epidermal separation	None	Friction injury of blister/bullae rupture	Replace epidermis as possible; create clean, moist protected environment

17. How do you determine the size of a wound?

Determine the size of the wound through routine measurement. The mode of measurement should be consistent across assessments. Modes of wound measurement include using a ruler, tracing the external borders of a wound with tracing paper, and photography at a measured distance from the wound bed. For wounds with irregular borders, tracing and photography are often the best modes of measurement.

18. How do you assess wound healing?

Healing is best determined by repeated assessments and measurements of the wound. The frequency of assessments depends on the individual situation. An acutely infected dehiscent surgical wound may be assessed several times per day (in an acute care setting), whereas a more stable, healing pressure ulcer may be assessed weekly. Wound healing should be assessed at least once each week, preferably by the same clinician(s), and as needed for any significant change in the patient's status or perception of wound symptoms (e.g., pain, edema, exudate). Wounds healing by secondary intent should exhibit granulation, contraction, and then re-epithelialization that is easily visualized.

19. How do you know when a wound is infected?

Wound infections can be characterized as either localized or systemic, including bacteremia and risk of sepsis. Cardinal signs of local infection must be assessed. The presence of localized edema or a "boggy" sensation on palpation, erythema, warmth, purulence, and acute pain greater than baseline are characteristic of an infected wound. The threat of systemic infection mandates examination of the patient's overall status, including comorbid conditions and nutritional status. Laboratory values, including a complete blood count with differential and electrolyte assays, are essential. Swab cultures of a chronic wound are not a sensitive diagnostic test for the presence of infection, because wound flora may cause false-positive results. Surgical biopsy or aseptic aspirations of a fluid collection are definitive, quantitative procedures that may be used to determine infection. However, culture is often unnecessary if systemic and local assessments are correctly interpreted and empirical or data-based interventions are initiated. Rapid referral to clinicians in infectious disease or other appropriate disciplines is essential if a patient does not respond to empiric therapy.

20. Why is moisture important to wound healing?

Moisture is important in wound healing because fibroblasts cannot migrate and may die if dessicated. Wound bed hydration also facilitates endogenous enzyme release so that dead cells can be removed. In contrast, excessive moisture inhibits healing.

21. Define eschar and slough.

Eschar is devitalized, necrotic tissue. **Slough** is proteinaceous exudate at the base of a wound. The wound bed obscured by eschar or slough cannot be fully assessed. For wound assessment and healing to occur, eschar usually should be debrided. However, intact, dry eschar overlying the calcaneus may be maintained and used as a "biologic dressing," under which the wound granulates and re-epithelializes. Eschar that overlies and protects critical structures (e.g., carotid artery) should not be removed without specialty surgical consultation.

22. Why is debridement important to wound management?

Debridement removes necrotic tissue and allows granulation to occur. When eschar forms, the inflammatory cells (neutrophils and macrophages) are unable to keep up with the cellular debris. The wound bed becomes filled with devitalized tissue. When the devitalized tissue is removed, the wound bed undergoes a renewed immune response for healing. Wound debridement is mandatory in infection because immediate removal of purulent material and microbial colonies is essential to successful treatment. Surgical incision and drainage of an infected wound also relieves pain by reducing pressure on surrounding structures.

23. What nonsurgical debridement techniques can be used?

Mechanical and chemical means may be used for nonsurgical wound debridement. Use of cytotoxic agents and hypertonic solutions are often used but should be avoided because of the potential for tissue injury. Agents that rely on enzyme or chemicals are both effective and atraumatic.

METHOD	ACTIVE INGREDIENT	MECHANISM OF ACTION	INDICATION	CONTRAINDICATION	APPLICATION	SPECIAL CONCERNS
Accuzyme	Enzymatic debridement with papainurea	Proteolysis	Debridement of eschar or slough, desire to avoid sharp debridement	Papaya allergy, clinical wound infection	Ointment applied once each day after cleansing with NSS	Contact dermatitis of periwound tissue is common; protect with moisture barrier (e.g., zinc oxide paste, petrolatum)
Panafil	Enzymatic debridement with papainurea/chlorophyllin–copper	Mild proteolysis with possible promotion of fibroblast migration	Debridement of slough, inability to use sharp debridement, promotion of granulation	Papaya allergy, clinical wound infection	Ointment applied once each day after cleansing with NSS	Contact dermatitis of periwound tissue is common; protect with moisture barrier (e.g., zinc oxide paste, petrolatum)
Autolytic debridement	Endogenous proteolytic, fibrinolytic, and collagenolytic enzymes	Produced by the body during inflammatory phase of healing	Naturally occuring process		Maintain wound moisture; patient should have adequate leukocyte and neutrophil counts	Requires use of adhesive moisture barrier, such as hydrocolloid or semipermeable film dressings
Wet-to-damp dressing	Coarse mesh gauze with saline solution	Mechanical removal of necrotic tissue	Removes necrotic tissue and absorbs exudate	Wounds with large amount of exudate	Saline moist gauze is packed in wound and changed 3 times daily	Wet-to-dry dressings not indicated; this method is nonselective and causes tissue desiccation and trauma
Calcium alginate	Seaweed-based product; exchanges calcium and sodium ions	Debrides fibrinous exudate, absorbs liquid exudate, maintains wound moisture	Wounds with large amounts of exudate	Nonexudative wounds	Product loosely packed in wound and covered with a dry dressing; change 2 times/day	May decrease odor

NSS = normal saline solution.

24. How do you choose the correct dressing for a particular chronic wound?

Dressing choice should be guided by four principles.

1. Wound moisture must be maintained.
2. The wound must be cleansed of gross and microscopic debris and kept clean.
3. The site must be protected from further injury.
4. The plan of care should promote optimal patient comfort.

A fifth principle involves considering the ease of application by care providers. The advanced practice nurse should investigate what dressings are appropriate. For example, some brands of hydrocolloid are easy to use, promote autolysis, and maintain a clean wound. However, clinical utility may vary from brand to brand and should be investigated on an individual basis. Transparent film dressings (e.g., Tegaderm) are semipermeable waterproof dressing useful for superficial wounds with no exudate. Wet-to-damp dressing are an effective means of maintaining wound moisture, but they must be changed frequently (3 times/day or more), and care must be taken to avoid trauma from tape or other adhesives.

BIBLIOGRAPHY

1. Agency for Health Care Policy and Research, Public Health Service, U.S. Department of Health and Human Services: Pressure Ulcers in Adults: Prediction and Prevention. Clinical Practice Guideline. Washington, DC, Agency for Health Care Policy and Research, Public Health Service, U. S. Department of Health and Human Services, 1992.
2. Agency for Health Care Policy and Research, Public Health Service, U.S. Department of Health and Human Services: Treatment of Pressure Ulcers. Clinical Practice Guideline. Washington, DC, Agency for Health Care Policy and Research, Public Health Service, U. S. Department of Health and Human Services, 1994.
3. Chang H, Wind S, Kerstein M: Moist wound healing. Dermatol Nurs 8(3):174–176, 204, 1996.
4. Compher C, Kim JN, Bader JG: Nutritional requirements of an aging population with emphasis on subacute care units. AACN Clin Issues 9:441–450, 1998.
5. Cooper DM: Assessment, measurement, and evaluation: Their pivotal roles in wound healing. In Bryant RA (ed): Acute and Chronic Wounds: Nursing Management. St. Louis, Mosby, 2000, pp 51–83.
6. Doughty D, Waldrop J, Ramundo J: Lower-extremity ulcers of vascular etiology. In Bryant RA (ed): Acute and Chronic Wounds: Nursing Management. St. Louis, Mosby, 2000, pp 265–300.
7. Hampton S: Wound assessment. Profess Nurse 12(12 Suppl):S5–S7, S12, S17, 1997.
8. Kosiak M: Etiology and pathology of ischemic ulcers. Arch Phys Med Rehabil 40:62–69, 1959..
9. Rolstad BS, Ovington LG, Harris A: Principles of wounds management. In Bryant RA (ed): Acute and Chronic Wounds: Nursing Management. St. Louis, Mosby, 2000, pp 85–112.
10. Singhal A, Reis ED, Kerstein MD: Options for nonsurgical debridement of necrotic wound. Adv Skin Wound Care 14(2):96–103, 2001.
11. Waldrop J, Doughty D: Wound-healing physiology. In Bryant RA (ed): Acute and Chronic Wounds: Nursing Management. St. Louis, Mosby, 2000, pp 17–40.

25. MENOPAUSE

Arlene Pericak, FNP, MS

1. Define menopause.

Menopause is the cessation of menstrual periods, which generally signals an end to fertility. Although menopause occurs with the last menstrual period, it is diagnosed when menses have ceased for 12 consecutive months.

2. Define perimenopause.

Most women begin perimenopause around age 47 years. Perimenopause is the period before menopause when hormonal levels decrease and/or fluctuate; it usually occurs 3–5 years before menopause. During this period many symptoms develop, including hot flashes, insomnia, fatigue, headache, irritability, depression, inability to concentrate, and premenstrual symptoms. Menstrual flow changes in amount and duration. The menstrual cycle changes in length, and some cycles are skipped. Patients need to be educated that they are still ovulating; therefore, conception is possible.

3. At what age does menopause begin?

Menopause usually occurs around 51 or 52 years of age, and most women reach menopause by age 55.

4. Can you identify the onset of menopause when a woman has had a hysterectomy?

If the ovaries are removed during surgery, the woman immediately enters surgical menopause. However, if at least one ovary is left, the woman needs to be questioned about signs and symptoms of menopause. In many cases, she may have symptoms that indicate the onset of perimenopause. After hysterectomy, it is necessary to obtain follicle-stimulating hormone (FSH) levels to determine actual hormonal status. FSH should be measured annually beginning with the onset of any symptoms of hormonal fluctuations or at the age at which menopause would be expected and continued until menopause is established.

5. How should menopause be viewed?

Nurse practitioners should view menopause as a natural passage of life. Because of advanced medical and nursing knowledge, women are living longer. Twenty-five years or more are spent in a postmenopausal state.

6. What nonpharmacologic measures or behaviors are helpful during menopause?

Women experiencing menopause need to take time to care for themselves. At menopause, the risk of several health problems increases, including osteoporosis and heart disease. Menopause is a good time for women to reconsider their lifestyle and initiate positive healthful behaviors. Such behaviors include exercise, diet, relaxation, and tobacco cessation.

Exercise is important in minimizing cardiovascular and osteoporosis risk and increasing the sense of well-being. Ideally, women should take 20–30 minutes every day to exercise and include both weight-bearing and low-impact aerobic exercise. They should be encouraged to select a combination of enjoyable activities, which may range from out-of-doors walking to work-outs following a home video. Routine exercise works best, and women should choose a time of day that is convenient so that a routine can be established.

Diet contributes to weight management, cardiovascular risk reduction, and even calcium maintenance. Weight management contributes to a sense of well-being and positive body image/self-concept. A diet high in protein and low in sugars and carbohydrates increases energy. Fat should be limited to 30% or less of total caloric intake. Eight glasses of water per day are helpful to combat bloating and maintain skin integrity. A multivitamin supplement is important, along with 1500 mg of calcium.

Relaxation may take the form of meditation, yoga, or simply reading a book. Menopause is a good time for women to learn to pamper or reward themselves, and often they can do so at low cost. Inexpensive facials and manicures can be obtained from training schools.

Substance use. Tobacco should be eliminated or at least minimized. Alcohol and caffeine should be used sparingly.

7. Discuss the role of spirituality.

Spiritual practices may help to alleviate anxiety and depression. Spirituality includes organized religion, meditation, or beliefs in a higher power. Spiritual practices are not only relaxing but also give a sense of hope and strength. Menopause may be a time of great turmoil, with responsibilities to adolescents and/or older parents. Religious or spiritual beliefs can strengthen the soul to help cope with uncooperative adolescents or ill parents.

8. What is the role of hormonal replacement therapy?

Hormonal replacement therapy (HRT) includes estrogens, progestogens, and sometimes androgens. Progestogens are prescribed only to women with an intact uterus; they prevent estrogen-induced endometrial cancer.

9. When should you prescribe HRT? How long should you keep the patient on HRT?

In general, it is best to start HRT in the first 1–2 years after menopause to optimize protection from bone loss and heart disease. The benefits of HRT end with its discontinuation; therefore, it is best to stay on HRT indefinitely. It is important to know the patient's history and prescribe the length of time accordingly. Benefits of taking HRT should always outweigh risks.

10. What benefits are commonly associated with estrogen replacement?

Estrogen replacement therapy (ERT) can relieve atrophy of the urogential area, maintain bone density, and reduce hot flashes. Estrogen may reduce the risk of Alzheimer's disease. Estrogen-takers are less likely to get colon cancer. The cardiovascular benefits of estrogen are currently being debated (see question 20).

11. What are the available forms of estrogen?

The table below lists the most common forms of estrogen. Other medications include intranasal and injectable forms. It is best to start at the lowest possible effective dose; individual risks and characteristics should be used to determine the appropriate route and dose.

Estrogen Replacement Therapy

ESTROGEN	BRANDS	RECOMMENDED DOSAGES
Conjugated estrogen	Premarin	VM = 0.625–1.25 qd, cyclic OP = 0.625 qd, cyclic UG = 0.3–1.25 mg qd
Estradiol, transdermal	Climara, Estraderm, Vivelle, Alora, FemPatch	VM = 0.025–0.05 mg applied twice/wk, weekly, cyclic OP = 0.05 mg, applied twice/wk, weekly, cyclic
Estradiol, oral	Estrace	VM = 1–2 mg/day OP = 0.5 mg/day, cyclic UG = 1–2 mg/day, cyclic
Esterified estrogens	Estratab, Menest	VM = 0.3–1.25 mg qd OP = 0.3–12.5 mg qd UG = 0.3–1.25 mg qd

(Table continued on next page.)

Estrogen Replacement Therapy (cont.)

ESTROGEN	BRANDS	RECOMMENDED DOSAGES
Estropipate	Ogen, Ortho-Est	VM = 0.625–5 mg qd, cyclic
		OP = 0.625 mg qd, cyclic
		UG = 0.625–5 mg qd, cyclic
Ethinyl estradiol	Estinyl	VM = 0.05 mg qd, cyclic*
Synthetic conjugated estrogens	Cenestin	VM = 0.625–1.25 mg qd*
Vaginal applications*		
Estradiol	Estring	UG = 2 mg, inserted every 90 days
Conjugated estrogen	Premarin	UG = 0.5–2 g qd, cyclic
Estradiol hemihydrate	Vagifem	UG = 1 tablet qd × 2 wk, then 2 ×/wk

qd = each day.
VM = use for moderate-to-severe vasomotor symptoms; attempt to taper and/or discontinue dosage after 3–6 months of therapy.
OP = use for osteoporosis prevention; continued therapy is recommended, because rate of bone loss increases without therapy.
UG = use for urogenital symptoms; attempt to taper and/or discontinue when possible.
* Not indicated for prevention of osteoporosis.
Source: Drugfacts A-Z: Estrogens. Retrieved June 10, 2001: http://www.drugfacts.com/DrugFacts/home/home.jhtml.

12. What characteristics are considered to determine the route of administration?

For patients at risk for cholelithiasis or with hypertriglyceridemia or hypertension, prescribe transdermal estrogen. Oral estrogen doses pass through the liver and increase the synthesis of triglycerides, globulins, and angiotensinogens, which may lead to cholelithisasis, hypertriglyceridemia, and hypertension. Many different types of patches are available. Some contain only estrogen, whereas others contain estrogen and progestin. Some are applied twice weekly, others once weekly. Most patches are indicated to prevent moderate-to-severe symptoms of menopause.

If the patient experiences primarily urogenital symptoms, select vaginal creams, rings, or inserts, which are approved by the Food and Drug Administration for atrophic vaginitis.

13. What is the most commonly prescribed HRT regimen for women with an intact uterus? Why?

The most commonly prescribed HRT is 0.625 mg of estrogen and 2.5 mg of medroxyprogesterone acetate daily. The most popular prescribed regimen is the continuous regimen because patients report little or no bleeding. Alternatively, a cyclic dose of 5–10 mg of medroxyprogesterone may be prescribed for 10–14 days/month (usually the last part of the month), along with a continuous dose of estrogen. Premphase is a packaged, cyclic product containing 14 conjugated estrogens tablets (0.635 mg) and 14 tablets combining conjugated estrogen (0.625 mg) and medroxyprogesterone acetate (5.0 mg). The tablets are taken once daily in the directed sequence. Prempro provides combined, continuous doses of estrogen (0.625 mg) and progesterone (2.5 or 5.0 mg).

14. Does continuous hormonal therapy prevent interval bleeding?

No. Although patients who want to avoid bleeding should receive continuous therapy, they should be told that spotting may occur. Abnormal pathology must be ruled out by obtaining an endometrial biopsy if bleeding persists with either continuous or intermittent therapy.

15. What kind of exam and diagnostic tests should be completed before prescribing HRT?

A nurse practitioner needs to take the time for a thorough history and physical exam. Appropriate diagnostic studies should be obtained. Most importantly, the patient needs to be given the facts about HRT. Together you and the patient can decide what the best treatment plan will be. Time spent initially helps to prevent later problems.

16. What history is necessary?
- Past and present history of chronic diseases, including personal history of heart disease, breast and endometrial cancer, and diabetes. Careful attention should be paid to the most commonly accepted contraindications for ERT, which include a history of thrombophlebitis related to estrogen and embolism, unexplained abnormal vaginal bleeding, and active estrogen-dependent cancer or active liver disease.
- Prior hormonal therapy and response/tolerance
- Family history of heart disease and breast cancer
- Current medications
- Current habits, including use of tobacco, alcohol, caffeine, and other substances as well as physical activity

17. What physical exam should be obtained?
- Thyroid: Determine size, symmetry, and texture.
- Breasts: Assess for lumps, discharge, skin changes, and nodes.
- Lungs: Assess for rales or other adventitious sounds.
- Heart: Assess size and murmurs, clicks, or abnormal heart sounds.
- Abdomen: Ensure that the abdomen is soft and that no organomegaly is present.
- Pelvic: Rule out atrophic vaginitis, prolapses, urethra caruncle, uterine fibroids, and enlarged adnexas. In postmenopausal women you should not be able to feel the ovaries or uterus. Atrophy of the ovaries and uterus begins in perimenopausal patients. If enlargement of the ovaries or uterus is present, order a pelvic ultrasound and refer the patient to a specialist.
- Extremities: Rule out edema.
- Musculoskeletal system: Observe posture, with special attention to the spine.

18. What, if any, diagnostic studies are warranted?
When you are unsure of menopausal status, assessment of FSH is the most helpful study; FSH is usually > 40 mIU/ml in menopause. As ovulation declines and hormonal levels drop, FSH levels rise. Other helpful diagnostic studies should be considered before initiating hormonal therapy include pap smear, mammogram, and bone density. The usefulness of estrogen, progesterone, androgens, thyrotropins, or other diagnostic studies varies and should be considered on an individual basis:
- Estradial hormones fluctuate during perimenopause and are usually of little help in the diagnosis of menopause.
- Pap smear rules out cervical cancer.
- Mammogram helps to rule out breast cancer.
- Bone density measurement should be ordered for women with known risk factors for osteoporosis and older women.
- Progesterone level, although not usually obtained, can identify signs of ovulation.
- Androgen tests (testosterone, free testosterone, and dehydoepiandrosterone sulfate [DHEAS]) should be obtained for signs of hyperandrogenism.
- Serum thyroid-stimulating hormone (TSH) test, as indicated, to rule out hypothyroidism, which may be confused with menopause.
- Baseline chemistry may be ordered to rule out any underlying disease, including liver disease or electrolyte disturbance.
- A lipid profile is important to determine risk for cardiac disease.
- Endometrial biopsy is performed to evaluate abnormal bleeding, with possible referral to a specialist.
- Pelvic ultrasound to evaluate any pelvic mass, with possible referral to a specialist.

• Human chorionic gonadotropin (urine or serum) is important to rule out pregnancy as the cause of amenorrhea.

19. What patient education is important during the initial visit?

Patients should take time to review ERT/HRT literature and possibly view a video about the treatment regimens for menopause. A second appointment may be necessary after the patient has taken some time to understand the benefits and risks of HRT. Major areas of education include the following:

1. The facts about the ongoing controversies regarding breast cancer and established heart disease. It is important to include the patient in a discussion so that an informed decision can be made, with the determination that the benefits of taking hormones outweigh the risks. Women worry about the links between hormone use and heart, breast, and gallbladder disease. Individualize any discussions to patients' personal and family history of diseases or associated risks so that they can make decisions with adequate, relevant information.

2. Patients need to be educated about the side effects of HRT/ERT and the importance of reporting side effects instead of simply discontinuing therapy. Women who elect to try HRT need to know that side effects can be managed. The most common reasons that women discontinue HRT include breast tenderness, bloating, headaches, and unwanted bleeding.

20. What is the relationship between heart disease and ERT?

The most significant findings relate to women with known heart disease: a mildly increased incidence in heart attacks and stroke was found during the first 1–2 years of therapy, followed, perhaps, by a lessening of risk with continued therapy. One possible reason for these findings may be increased development of thrombi. According to the HERS trial, women who have established heart disease or are at high risk for cardiovascular disease (e.g., women with diabetes) should not be prescribed HRT.

Older observational studies not specifically involving women with known heart disease supported the belief that ERT is protective, because ERT users were less likely to die of heart disease than women who did not take ERT. ERT may reduce heart disease development by decreasing low-density lipoprotein and increasing high-density lipoprotein. Although progesterone alters this affect, combined HRT still has an overall favorable outcome on lipid levels. This favorable outcome persists despite a potential increase in triglyceride levels

Currently, there is much debate about how to interpret the results of these many studies. Clearly more randomized, ongoing trials are needed to study the role of ERT in cardiovascular disease. Trials are under way to provide data about HRT/ERT therapeutic interventions. At this point, it is recommended that ERT not be initiated when the intent is specifically to prevent cardiovascular disease.

21. What are the facts about breast cancer and ERT/HRT?

Clearly the association between breast cancer and ERT/HRT remains a hot topic. Some studies have shown a small increased relative risk of breast cancers among ERT users, and it is not unlikely that breast tumors grow at a faster rate with hormone induction. However, HRT users also have been determined to have a decreased breast cancer mortality rate with early diagnosis of breast tumors. Meta-analyses of earlier observational studies give little support to the belief that short-term ERT is associated with increased risk of breast cancer. A randomized study is needed to help explain the controversy surrounding hormones and breast cancer. Observational data are not as reliable as data from randomized studies.

22. What are hot flashes?

Women describe hot flashes in many different ways. The characteristics and severity of hot flashes vary from woman to woman. They are often described as a feeling of warmth in the face, neck, and chest, during which the woman may look flushed and perspire. The intensity and duration of the warmth vary, as does the resultant degree of disruption of daily activities and sleep. Some patients also report palpitations and anxiety. Hot flashes are triggered by caffeine, alcohol, nicotine, stress, anxiety, certain spicy foods, and a warm environment (heat outside or inside).

23. How can hot flashes be avoided or treated nonpharmacologically?

Encourage the patient to stop smoking and to engage in daily exercise and some form of relaxation. Dietary measures may help to prevent hot flashes, such as avoidance of hot spicy food, hot liquids, caffeine, and alcohol.

24. When patients taking estrogen complain of continued hot flashes, what other measures can be added?

Patients taking Premarin (0.625 mg) who complain of hot flashes should be questioned carefully. If the hot flashes affect sleep and/or activities of daily living, encourage the measures listed above. If this plan is not successful, increase the estrogen dose. However, you should later attempt to decrease the dose, when possible. Vitamin E, 400–800 IU/day, may be helpful.

25. What nonhormonal pharmacologic therapy is available for hot flashes?

Clonidine, an adrenergic receptor agonist, may reduce the frequency of hot flashes. Doses range between 0.05 and 0.4 mg/day. Patients need to be educated about the frequent side effects, which include dry mouth, palpitations, drowsiness, dizziness, and hypotension.

Bellergal, which is a combination of phenobarbital, belladonna alkaloids, and ergotamine tartrate, also is used to reduce hot flashes. Bellergal has significant side effects, including sedation. The phenobarbital in Bellergal can be addicting. With this in mind, Bellergal is prescribed for a short time only.

26. What herbal remedies are commonly used for menopausal symptoms?

For women experiencing emotional disturbances, vaginal dryness, or hot flashes attributed to menopause, the following herbs may be considered:

- Black cohosh (*Cimicifuga racemosa*) is believed to alleviate the symptoms of hot flashes, vaginal dryness, and depression. No long-term studies of its use are available.
- Kava-kava (*Piper methysticum*) has been used for anxiety and insomnia. Studies have shown improvement on the Depression Status Inventory Scale (DSI).
- St. John's wort is taken to decrease depression. It is a popular herb in Germany with studies to support its use.
- Soy/phytoestrogens are compounds with a structure similar to that of estradiol found in the body. Some evidence suggests that soy may help to decrease hot flashes and vaginal dryness. Soy products range from soy protein drinks to soy hot dogs. Studies of soy/phyoestogens are small and limited. Additional research is needed.

27. If the patient complains of sexual dysfunction, dyspareunia, or decreased libido, does HRT help?

It may. ERT relieves vaginal dryness. HRT/ERT also can help with mood, which indirectly increases libido.

28. Is testosterone useful in HRT?

Testosterone can restore libido, increasing the patient's sense of well-being. The addition of androgen therapy (testosterone) to HRT/ERT has gained much attention for postmenopausal women. Testosterone is produced in the ovaries and adrenal glands. During menopause, women lose testosterone as well as estrogen. Androgen may be added to estrogen therapy in many different forms. It can be prescribed in oral, topical, genital or nongenital, and sublingual forms; as subcutaneous pellets; and as combined estrogen-androgen pills. The most beneficial starting oral dose is 0.50 mg of methytestosterone. Side effects include facial hair, acne, lowered voice, muscle aches, irritability, weight gain, and clitoral enlargement.

These side effects can be eliminated if the oral dose is kept between 0.25 mg and 0.8 mg of methytestosterone per day. Blood levels of methytesterone should be checked when the patient is taking oral therapy. A large, long-term study of women taking testosterone therapy clearly is needed. If the testosterone is not successful, it should be discontinued.

29. What if a patient has risk factors for osteoporosis or contraindications to HRT or does not desire to take it?

There are other options to prevent osteoporosis in patients who cannot or do not want to take HRT. The need for calcium to affect bone density is well documented from randomized, controlled clinical trials. The following options may be considered:

1. Dietary supplements of 1500 mg of calcium are needed in the postmenopausal state to prevent osteoporosis. Patients should be encouraged to take calcium supplements long before menopause. Patients also should take a vitamin D supplement.

2. Calcitonin-salmon is a nasal spray for postmenopausal women. It is recommended for women who are more than 5 years postmenopausal with low bone mass compared with healthy premenopausal woman. More efficacy data are needed.

3. Evista (raloxifene HCl) is a selective estrogen receptor medication (SERM) that prevents and treats osteoporosis in postmenopausal women. The dose is 60 mg once daily. Evista is a good choice for patients who have a negative history for active or past venous thromboembolic events. Evista is given to women who no longer have vasomotor symptoms, are at risk for osteoporosis, and are not taking HRT. Side effects include hot flashes, leg cramps, and thrombophlebitis (rare). Evista is less effective for the treatment and prevention of osteoporosis than ERT/HRT and Fosamax.

4. Fosamax (bisphosphonate, alendronate) is indicated for bone disorders and the prevention and treatment of osteoporosis in postmenopausal women. The Fosamax tablet must be swallowed whole and taken in the morning with a full glass of water. A woman cannot take food before taking Fosamax and should not lie down, eat, or take any other medications within 30 minutes after taking it. Adverse reactions to Fosamax include acid regurgitation, esophagitis, esophageal ulcer, stricture, and erosions. Fosamax should not be prescribed for women with esophageal abnormalities or disease. The dose to treat osteoporosis is 10 mg/day or 70 mg/week; the dose to prevent osteoporosis is 5 mg/day or 35 mg/week.

BIBLIOGRAPHY

1. Andrews WC, Weisman C, et al: Guidelines for Counseling Women on the Management of Menopause. Washington, DC, Jacobs Institute of Women's Health, 2000, pp 14, 19, 22, 24, 26, 27, (http://www.jiwh.org)
2. Archer D, Boggs P, et al: Menopause Core Curriculum Study Guide, United States. Cleveland, OH, North American Menopause Society (NAMS), 2000, pp 174, 180, 208, 212, 214.
3. Archer D, Wulf H: Decisions in prescribing HRT. Patient Care Nurse Pract 4(5):56, 2001
4. Benson MD: Gynecologic Pearls. Philadelphia, F.A. Davis, 2000.
5. Carlson E, Li S: Androgen therapy for menopausal women. Clin Excell Nurse Pract 2(6):324–327, 1998.
6. DRUGFACTS A-Z: Estrogens. Retrieved June 10, 2001 at http:// www.drugfacts.com/DrugFacts/home/home.jhtml.
7. Murphy J, Burke J, et al: Nurse Practitioners Prescribing Reference. New York, 2001, pp 197, 223, 255.
8. Rakel R, Bope E: Conn's Current Therapy. Philadelphia, W.B. Saunders, 2001, p 1105.
9. Shoupe D: Practical strategies for treating hot flashes. Womens Health Prim Care 4(2):170–172, 2001.
10. Speroff L: A clinician's perspective on the research data. Womens Health Prim Care 2:(5):15–18, 1999.
11. Speroff L: Myths and misperceptions: Breast cancer and HRT. Womens Health Prim Care (2 Suppl):6, 1999.
12. Villablanca A: HRT and cardiovascular risk in women: Where do we stand? Womens Health Prim Care 4(2):122, 2001.
13. What's New in Endocrinology: Managing menopause: New practice guidelines. Womens Health Prim Care 3(8):547–548, 551, 2000.
14. Wysocki S, Speroff L, et al: Hormone replacement therapy and breast cancer. Am J Nurse Pract 4(10):51, 2000.

26. MANAGING NONOBSTETRIC HEALTH PROBLEMS IN PREGNANT PATIENTS

Jill C. Cash, MSN, APRN, BC

1. Various health problems may occur during pregnancy. Should the pregnant patient be treated by her primary care provider or her obstetrician for acute/chronic conditions?

The patient should be treated holistically, and all providers should be aware of all treatment regimens. Primary care providers and obstetricians may provide prenatal care for the low-risk client. Common acute problems such as upper respiratory infections and gastroenteritis can easily be treated by the obstetrician and/or primary care provider. An obstetrician should care for high-risk patients with chronic conditions such as hypertension and heart disease.

For some health problems during pregnancy, the primary care provider and/or specialist should be consulted for treatment. For example, a pregnant patient who has been diagnosed with a skin disorder but does not respond to therapy should be referred to the dermatologist for evaluation and treatment.

2. What types of acute health problems are commonly seen in primary care settings in pregnant patients?

Acute health problems commonly seen during pregnancy include upper respiratory infections, vaginitis, gastroesophageal reflux disease, urinary tract infections, and anemia.

3. How should pregnancy be ruled out before treatment of nonobstetric problems in women of child-bearing age?

All women of child-bearing age should be considered pregnant until proved otherwise. The patient's verbal history of her last menstrual period, proper use of contraception (e.g., oral contraceptive pills, condoms, foam) or sexual inactivity are methods to rule out pregnancy as long as the patient is reliable. Other methods of ruling out pregnancy include a urine or serum human chorionic gonadotropin pregnancy test in the office. It is imperative to know that the patient is not pregnant before prescribing teratogenic agents.

4. How can I tell if a medication is safe to use during pregnancy?

The *Physicians' Desk Reference* (PDR) lists all medications along with the classification of the drug for use during pregnancy and lactation. Medications are classified as follows:

Category A: Well-controlled studies in human subjects indicate no known fetal risks.

Category B: Studies performed in animals have disclosed no fetal risks, but adequate studies have not been performed in women.

Category C: Animal studies reveal adverse fetal effects; no adequate studies have been performed in women.

Category D: Fetal risk is documented. Use is recommended only if the benefits of the medication outweigh the risk (life-threatening events).

Category X: Fetal abnormalities have been documented in animal and human studies. Such drugs are contraindicated in pregnancy.

5. How should Pap smear results be handled during pregnancy?

Pap smears should be performed at the initial prenatal physical examination if the last Pap smear was performed 1 year ago or longer. Abnormal results (atypical cells of undetermined significance) should be treated appropriately (e.g., infections), and the Pap smear should be repeated in 4 months. Dysplastic or repeated abnormal results should be further evaluated with colposcopy and biopsy, as indicated. The only difference for evaluation of cervical cells during pregnancy is avoidance of endocervical curettage.

6. Should women be encouraged to exercise during pregnancy?

Yes. Women should be encouraged to exercise 3–4 times per week, performing weight-bearing activities (walking, step aerobics, treadmill activity) for approximately 20–30 minutes. Studies have shown that weight-bearing activities are associated with an increase in fetal and placental growth in normal pregnancies. Regular exercise during pregnancy also increases stamina during labor activity.

7. What is a safe maximum heart rate for pregnant patients during exercise?

The target heart rate should not exceed 120 beats per minute.

8. Should a patient with chronic hypertension continue the same antihypertensive medications during pregnancy?

Patients with chronic hypertension should be followed by an obstetrician or perinatologist during pregnancy. Early prenatal care should be established to monitor blood pressure values and to change medications and dosages as appropriate. The patient may continue the same antihypertensive medication as long as it has no known teratogenic effects. If the current medication is teratogenic, it should be discontinued and a substitute medication should be started.

9. Does chronic hypertension pose a risk to the mother or fetus during pregnancy?

Yes. Women with chronic hypertension are at greater risk for complications during pregnancy. Pregnancy-induced hypertension and abruptio placentae are two examples. The fetus is at great risk for intrauterine growth retardation due to the poor vascular supply and perfusion to the placenta and fetus.

10. What is the effect of thyroid disease on pregnancy?

Patients with thyroid disease that is adequately treated before and during pregnancy usually do well. Patients diagnosed with hyperthyroidism with inadequate treatment have a higher incidence of fetal and neonatal mortality and low birth weight. Uncontrolled thyroid disease also can predispose the patient to other endocrine disorders such as diabetes. Women with hypothyroidism are commonly infertile because of anovulation. Pregnant women with untreated hypothyroidism are at risk for anemia, pregnancy-induced hypertension, placental abruption, stillbirth and postpartum hemorrhage. Risks of undertreatment for the fetus include a higher spontaneous abortion rate (2 times the normal rate), low birthweight, and hyperthyroidism.

11. What is the effect of pregnancy on thyroid disease?

Hyperthyroidism may be exacerbated in the early stages of pregnancy but usually improves as the pregnancy progresses. One symptom of hyperthyroidism is severe hyperemesis. Undiagnosed women with severe hyperemesis gravidarum should be evaluated for hyperthyroidism.

12. How do serum thyroid studies change during pregnancy?

During pregnancy levels of thyroid-stimulating hormone (TSH) and free thyroxine (T_4) remain the same. Increases in total T_4 and Triiodothyronine (T_3) result primarily from the influence of estrogen on thyroid-binding globulin.

13. What medication is safe to treat thyroid disease during pregnancy?

Propylthiouracil (PTU) is the drug of choice to treat hyperthyroidism during pregnancy and lactation. If iodide or methimazole treatment is needed after pregnancy, breast-feeding is not recommended. Thyroxine replacement (Synthroid) is used to treat hypothyroidism during pregnancy. Thyroid levels (TSH and free thyroxine) should be monitored periodically because levels may change during pregnancy.

14. Which medications alter the serum TSH level?

All medications should be reviewed with the patient. Common medications that may alter serum thyroid levels are listed below.

THYROID HORMONE	MEDICATION	CHANGE
T_4	Iodine	Increased or decreased
TSH	Phenytoin	Decreased T_4
	Phenobarbital	Decreased T_4
	Ferrous sulfate	Decreased T_4 or increased TSH
	Prenatal vitamins	Decreased T_4 or increased TSH
	Aluminum hydroxide	Decreased T_4 or increased TSH
	Androgens	Decreased TBG
	Estrogens	Increased TBG
	Corticosteroids	Decreased TBG, decreased TSH, blocks conversion of T_4 to T_3
TBG	Salicylates	Decreased TBG

T_3 = triiodothyronine, T_4 = thyroxine, TSH = thyroid-stimulating hormone, TBG = thyroxine-binding globulin.

15. How does pregnancy affect a patient with asthma?

It is difficult to predict how pregnancy will alter the course of asthma. One-third of patients improve, one-third worsen, and one-third have no change during pregnancy. However, most bronchiole changes are similar in subsequent pregnancies.

16. What medications can be used safely to care for patients with asthma?

Oral and inhaled bronchodilator medications may be used prophylactically during pregnancy. Treatment of acute asthmatic episodes may include inhaled beta-adrenergic agents and steroids.

17. How much alcohol is considered safe during pregnancy?

There is no known safe level of alcohol consumption for the mother during pregnancy; therefore, abstinence is recommended.

18. What harmful fetal effects result from alcohol consumption during pregnancy?

Small amounts of alcohol may cause intrauterine growth retardation and developmental delay. Excessive and frequent exposure to alcohol causes fetal alcohol syndrome. Symptoms include central nervous system abnormalities, mental retardation, developmental delay, facial abnormalities, and congenital anomalies of the heart, skeleton, and urogenital system.

19. Is it necessary to screen all patients for urinary tract infections during pregnancy?

Yes. Approximately 7–10% of pregnant women have asymptomatic bacteriuria during pregnancy. Approximately 20–30% of untreated women have pyelonephritis by the third trimester. Therefore, routine prenatal urine cultures and sensitivities should be performed in all pregnant women at the initial prenatal visit.

20. Should car seat belts be worn by pregnant patients?

Yes. Seat belts should be worn at all times while the woman is in a moving vehicle to reduce the possibility of ejection from the vehicle if an accident occurs. The patient should be instructed in proper placement of the lap belt below the abdomen, along with the use of the three-point shoulder harness for proper restraint.

21. What conditions should be considered when the pregnant patient presents with complaints of abdominal pain?

Round ligament pain, ectopic pregnancy, appendicitis, cholecystitis, hernia, trauma, domestic violence, urinary tract infection, pyelonephritis, kidney stones, abruptio placentae, and premature labor.

22. Is a heart murmur normal in pregnant patients who had no cardiac abnormalities or murmurs before pregnancy?

Yes. The increase in total blood volume during pregnancy commonly results in a systolic murmur. Innocent systolic murmurs along the left sternal border should be no louder than grade III–IV.

23. Does pregnancy complicate sickle cell disease?

Yes. Sickle cell disease is commonly aggravated by the increased metabolic demands of pregnancy. The patient's hematologist should be involved in her care during the pregnancy. Blood work should be closely monitored every 2 weeks to detect severe anemia. Transfusion may be needed for severe anemia. The mother is at risk for sickle cell crisis and its sequelae, anemia, infection, and pregnancy-induced hypertension.

24. Which antibiotics are safe and commonly used for bacterial infections during pregnancy?

Penicillin, cephalosporins (Keflex, Ceclor), erythromycin, nitrofurantoin (Macrodantin, Macrobid), and clindamycin.

25. Should common vaginal infections, such as bacterial vaginosis and candidal infection, be treated during pregnancy?

Yes. Bacterial vaginosis can be treated safely with clindamycin throughout pregnancy and with metronidazole after the end of the first trimester. Candidal infection can be treated safely with Monistat or Terazol during pregnancy.

BIBLIOGRAPHY

1. Cash JC, Glass CA: Family Practice Guidelines. Philadelphia, Lippincott Williams & Wilkins, 2000.
2. Clapp JF, Kim H, Burciu B, Lopez B: Beginning regular exercise in early pregnancy: Effect on feto-placental growth. Am J Obstet Gynecol 183(6):1484–1488, 2000.
3. Mooney C, James D, Kessenich C: Diagnosis and management of hypothyroidism in pregnancy. JOGNN 27:374–382, 1998.
4. Scoggin J, Morgan G: Practice Guidelines for Obstetrics and Gynecology. Philadelphia, Lippincott-Raven, 1997.
5. Seltzer V, Pearse W: Women's Primary Health Care: Office Practice and Procedures, 2nd ed. New York, McGraw-Hill, 2000.

27. LESBIAN HEALTH CARE

Betsy Shank Pless, PhD, FNP

1. Why is it important for practitioners to be knowledgeable about lesbian health?

Lesbians have continued to receive relatively little attention despite the growing attention to women's health. The Institute of Medicine (IOM) Committee on Lesbian Health Research Priorities identified three broad reasons for studying lesbian health:

1. To gain knowledge and improve the health status and health care of lesbians
2. To confirm beliefs and to counter misconceptions about the health risks of lesbians
3. To identify health conditions for which lesbians are at risk or tend to be at greater risk than heterosexual women or women in general.

2. How is the term *lesbian* defined?

There is no standard definition. Usually, sexual orientation includes the dimensions of behavior (sexual activity with with other women), affect (desire and/or attraction to other women), and cognition or identity (self-identification as lesbian). Women exhibit different degrees of each dimension. In a national sample, more than 90% of women who are self-identified as lesbian also reported both same-sex behavior and desire for other women. However, many women who reported desire for other women or same-sex behavior did not identify as lesbians. Lesbians do not constitute a homogeneous group and vary in many dimensions, including race, ethnicity, socioeconomic status, and age.

3. What aspects of the health care system may reduce lesbians' access to services?

Substantial numbers of lesbians have described hostile, intimidating, and humiliating experiences with health care providers. In 1973 the American Psychiatric Association removed homosexuality as an illness or pathologic condition. However, research still suggests that lesbians avoid seeking health care because of negative attitudes from providers, particularly in the specialties of obstetrics/gynecology, family practice, and surgery. The routine presumption of heterosexuality has been identified as the most common manifestation of bias among health professionals and the biggest barrier to obtaining quality health care. Among 110 gynecologists surveyed in 1976, one-half said that they had never treated a woman whom they knew or thought to be a lesbian.

4. What other major barriers to care are faced by lesbians?

1. **Structural barriers** include availability of services and access to services. Lesbian relationships usually are not afforded the same legal status as heterosexual marriages. The general lack of availability of family health insurance coverage for lesbians makes it especially difficult for all family members to see the same providers and to enjoy the multiple benefits that they can provide. In addition, in some cases there is a legal refusal to honor the lesbian partner of a patient as her health care proxy, to allow them to stay with their partner during treatment, or to include them in discussion about their partner's treatment.

2. **Financial barriers** include lack of insurance coverage, although domestic partner benefits are increasingly available through some employers. According to the National Lesbian Health Care Study, 16% of lesbian respondents stated that they did not receive health care because it was unaffordable, and 27% reported that they lacked health insurance.

3. **Personal and cultural barriers** relate primarily to disclosure to health care providers and their cultural competency. Several studies have found that lesbian patients are reluctant to disclose their sexuality to providers because of fear of inadequate care or embarrassment. In most studies, lesbians say they would not disclose their sexual orientation to any health care

provider. Reported responses of health care providers and health care students to learning that the patient is lesbian include voyeuristic curiosity, shock, withdrawal, physical roughness, insults, and breaches of confidentiality.

5. What are the specific risks and protective factors of lesbians for various health problems?

Specific health risks for lesbians include a lower rate of screening for cervical cancer and inadequate knowledge of the risks of sexually transmitted diseases caused by vaginal secretions or objects used during sexual activity. On the other hand, cervical cancer is less common among lesbians, especially lifetime lesbians, given the primary risk factors of early age of first heterosexual coitus and heterosexually transmitted diseases such as human papilloma virus (HPV). The transmission of HPV to a female sexual partner must be considered, and the female partner should be evaluated and treated as indicated. Several studies have revealed frequent cases of vaginitis in lesbians, some of which can be transmitted through hand-genital contact. There is no notable risk for transmission of AIDS specifically as a result of sexual activity with other women. Guidelines for safe sex for lesbians are lacking.

Nulliparity, increased prevalence of smoking, and lower use of oral contraceptives are reported to put lesbians at higher risk for breast and endometrial cancer. However, no epidemiologic studies support the conclusion that lesbians are at increased risk for breast or other cancers. More lifetime lesbians than heterosexual women have a body mass index > 27, indicating obesity. However, evidence also indicates that lesbians are less likely than heterosexual women to be overly concerned about their weight. Although smoking and higher BMI are two risk factors for cardiovascular disease, there are no population-based data about cardiovascular disease among lesbian women.

Factors that are suggested as protective of lesbian health include involvement in the lesbian community, strong family ties, and the support and socialization of lesbian friends.

6. Are lesbians at a higher risk for specific mental health disorders?

Although risk factors specifically related to mental health of lesbians are largely unexplored, stress has been hypothesized to exert an influence. This hypothesis is based on information about the stress effects of discrimination in other groups. Common manifestations of the increased stress felt by lesbians include serious depression, alcohol abuse, and suicidal ideation. It is suggested that alcohol problems and suicide among lesbians are overestimated because of the disproportionate sampling from gay bars. In addition, mid-life lesbians report not only high levels of stress but also overall satisfaction with their lives. No evidence indicates that lesbians as a whole have a greater tendency toward mental health problems such as depression, anxiety, psychotic disorders, dissociative disorders, and personality disorders than heterosexual women.

7. How can the practice environment be welcoming and respectful of women of all sexual orientations?

A number of professional associations have developed statements about the care of people of all sexual orientations. The Healthy People 2010 Companion Document for Lesbian, Gay, Bisexual, and Transgender Health is designed to make the information from Healthy People 2010 more pertinent to targeted populations. Clinic-specific factors also can offer an environment of acceptance. The waiting room of any practice can easily convey an open, nonjudgmental atmosphere by the presence of educational materials specifically related to sexual orientation. The following suggestions have been offered in the literature:

1. Increased knowledge base of health practitioners with respect to lesbian health care, including training and programs for all staff on diversity, antidiscrimination, and basic gay, lesbian, bisexual, and transgender issues. There also should be provision of training for direct care staff on how, when, and where to make appropriate referrals for lesbian clients and their families. The development of relationships with agencies and providers with expertise in lesbian health issues is important.

2. Review of routine office forms for heterosexual assumptions, particularly related to marital status and birth control. Inclusion of phrases, such as "living with a spouse/sexual partner" instead of simply "married," signals openness on the part of the practitioner to sexual orientation and ensures that the needs of lesbian clients and their families are met. On the health history form, inclusion of neutrally worded questions about sexual activity and past heterosexual activity of patients indicating current relationships only with women are also important.

3. Written sign-off policies that are posted in the agency and communicate an inclusive, nondiscriminatory work place environment. These policies should be reviewed annually and discussed with job applicants during the interview process. It is also important to include all policies in orientation materials.

4. Assurance of confidentiality of client data, including information about sexual orientation. All clients should be informed about data collection that includes references to sexual orientation and/or gender identity and in what circumstances such data may be disclosed. The intake form also should note that answering questions about sexual orientation and gender identity is the client's option. Procedures should be developed and implemented for intake, assessment, and treatment of minors that is sensitive to sexual orientation.

8. What are the current thoughts and practices about assisted reproduction for lesbians?

Recent studies indicate that slightly less than one-third of lesbians surveyed have borne children, most commonly through previous heterosexual marriage. Evidence indicates that approximately 30% of lesbians who do not currently have children but desire them have attempted artificial insemination. Some lesbians have reported opposition on the part of physicians to their attempts to conceive through artificial insemination. It is speculated that this lack of medical support contributes to the low success rate reported by lesbians who have attempted the procedure. One study found that fewer than 40% of lesbians who tried the procedure actually conceived compared with a reported conception rate of over 60% in lesbians who sought to become pregnant through intercourse with a man.

9. Do the development and awareness of sexual identity occur similarly for heterosexuals and lesbians?

Awareness of sexual orientation may occur as early as 10 years of age, with about 6 years elapsing before disclosure to another person. In addition, retrospective recall of age of first sexual or romantic attraction and of self-acknowledgment of sexual orientation was similar in heterosexual and lesbian subjects. Developmental precursors have not been clearly identified for lesbian identities.

BIBLIOGRAPHY

1. Bradford J. Ryan C: The National Lesbian Health Care Survey: Final Report. Washington, DC, National Lesbian and Gay Health Foundation, 1988.
2. Chu SY, Buehler JW, Fleming PL, Berkelman RL: Epidemiology of reported cases of AIDS in lesbians, United States 1980–89. Am J Public Health 80:1380–1381, 1992.
3. Deevy S: Older lesbian women: An invisible minority. J Gerontol Nurs 16:35–39, 1990.
4. Denenberg R: Report on lesbian health. Womens Health Issues 5(2):81–91, 1995.
5. Department of Health and Human Services: Healthy People 2010 Companion Document for Lesbian, Gay, Bisexual, and Transgender (LGBT) Health. Washington, DC, Government Printing Office, 2000.
6. Gay, Lesbian, Bisexual, and Transgender Health Access Project: Community Standards of Practice for Provision of Quality Health Care Services for Gay, Lesbian, Bisexual and Transgendered Clients. Boston, GLBT Health Access Project, 2000.
7. Good R: The gynecologist and the lesbian. Clin Obstet Gynecol 19:473–483, 1976.
8. Haas AP: Lesbian health issues: An overview. In Dan AJ (ed): Reframing Women's Health: Multidisciplinary Research and Practice. Thousand Oaks, CA, Sage Publications, 1994, pp 339–356 .
9. Pless B, Campbell P: Lesbian Focus Groups: [De]Constructing knowledge of lesbian health. Presented at the National Lesbian Health Care Conference, San Francisco, June, 2001.

10. Sadovsky R: Sexual orientation and associated health care risks. Am Fam Physician 15:201–210, 2000.
11. Solarz A (ed): Lesbian Health: Current Assessment and Directions for the Future, Institute of Medicine. Washington, DC, National Academy Press, 1999.
12. Stevens PE: Lesbian health care research: A review of the literature from 1970 to 1990. Health Care Women Int 13(2):91–120, 1992.
13. Turner CF, et al: Effects of mode administration and wording on reporting of drug use. In Turner CF, Lessler JT, Gfroerer JD (eds): Survey Measurement of Drug Use: Methodological Issues. DHHS Pub. No. 92-1929, Washington, DC, U.S. Government Printing Office, 1992.
14. White JC, Dull VT: Health risk factors and health-seeking behavior in lesbians. J Womens Health 6:103–112, 1997.
15. White J, Levinson W: Lesbian health care. What a primary care physician needs to know. West J Med 162:463–466, 1995.

28. BORDERLINE PERSONALITY DISORDER

Claudia R. Miller, MS, RN, NP

1. What is borderline personality disorder?

A personality disorder generally occurs when enduring patterns or personality traits become maladaptive, inflexible, and pervasive, causing subjective distress as well as significant impairment in functioning.

The term *borderline* originated in the psychoanalytic community in the 1930s to designate patients who did not quite fit into either the neurotic or psychotic category and, therefore, were considered to be on the borderline between neurosis and psychosis.

Borderline personality disorder (BPD) is characterized by extremes in emotion, thought, and behavior. People with BPD frequently complain of feeling empty and not knowing who they are. They have patterns of intense chaotic relationships; they fear abandonment and go to extremes to prevent significant others from leaving them. They also have affective instability, impulsivity, and self-destructive behaviors. Transient thought and sensory dysregulation, including depersonalization, dissociation, and delusions, may occur during times of stress and abate when the stressful situation ends.

The *Diagnostic and Statistical Manual of Mental Disorders, 4th ed.* (DSM IV), lists the nine criteria for BPD (patient must demonstrate at least five):

- Frantic efforts to avoid real or imagined abandonment. (Do not include suicidal or self-mutilating behavior covered in criterion 5.)
- A pattern of unstable and intense interpersonal relationships characterized by alternating extremes of idealization and devaluation
- Identity disturbance: markedly and persistently unstable self-image or sense of self
- Impulsivity in at least two potentially self-damaging practices, such as spending, sex, substance abuse, reckless driving, binge eating. (Do not include suicidal or self-mutilating behavior covered in criterion 5.)
- Recurrent suicidal behavior, gestures, or threats, or self-mutilating behavior
- Affective instability caused by a marked reactivity of mood (e.g., intense episodic dysphoria, irritability, or anxiety usually lasting a few hours and only rarely more than a few days)
- Chronic feelings of emptiness
- Inappropriate, intense anger or difficulty controlling anger (e.g., frequent displays of temper, constant anger, recurrent physical fights)
- Transient, stress-related paranoid ideation or severe dissociative symptoms

From the Diagnostic and Statistical Manual of Mental Disorders, 4th ed., revision. Washington, DC, American Psychiatric Association, 2000, with permission.

Studies indicate that 74% of people diagnosed with BPD are female. There are many theories as to why women seem to be more vulnerable to this diagnosis:

1. Depression is frequently a comorbid condition, and depression is more common in women.

2. Women make more suicide attempts and seek psychiatric care more often then men; thus, they are more likely to be diagnosed.

3. Women who have difficulty with regulating their emotions tend to internalize and self-direct their violent behaviors, whereas men tend to act out in more aggressive and antisocial behaviors.

2. How can I identify persons with BPD?

Comorbid conditions are often present with BPD. The nurse practitioner (NP) may initially see the patient because of depression, eating disorders, or substance abuse, but suspect BPD when quick and explosive mood changes disrupt the clinical relationship.

Patients can easily become dependent on caretakers, not only because of irrational fear of abandonment and inability to be alone, but also because of their tendency to split persons into good or bad objects. This cognitive style, labeled by psychoanalysts as "splitting," interferes with patients' ability to synthesize positive and negative feelings. Therefore, they may idealize a clinician until they perceive a real or imagined rejection and then quickly turn rageful, devaluing and dismissing one clinician after another.

When frustrated, borderline patients can be seen as manipulative, and make desperate attempts to have their needs met. Frequently, patients with BPD threaten suicide, because they lack coping skills.

3. What behaviors have been identified with BPD?

Self-mutilation is the hallmark of BPD. Razors, scissors, fingernails, and lit cigarettes are commonly used to inflict self- injury. Self-mutilation often begins as an impulsive, self-punishing act but over time may become ritualistic behavior. Self-inflicted pain may stem from a need to feel something, if the patient complains of feeling numb or empty. It also can be a distraction from emotional pain. Many borderline patients report a relief of tension, anger, or sadness after hurting themselves with a subsequent calm euphoria.

4. How do you assess the degree of danger from any self-mutilation?

Assessing the dangerousness of self-injury requires the NP to ask patients if they intended to kill themselves. It is a myth that asking about suicide may put the idea into the patient's head. If the NP says, "I'm concerned that you may be suicidal," the patient may feel safe enough to express the intentions of the self injurious behavior. The NP can utilize crisis intervention skills by providing support and an opportunity for ventilation to help put the patient's feelings into perspective.

5. If I suspect that a client has BPD, what history should I obtain to confirm or exclude my suspicions?

There is no quick assessment for BPD, because patient behaviors are based on responses to biologic, psychologic, and environmental factors. Indeed, it is not as important to diagnose BPD as it is to recognize maladaptive coping and to intervene appropriately. For instance, helping the patient with problem-solving often offers solutions that the patient did not know existed and thereby creates hope. Establishing the patient's other resources or social supports is important; a referral for mental health services may be indicated.

6. What are the objectives for managing patients with BPD?

The NP's first objective for the patient is safety. Suicidal threats and gestures reflect both overwhelming depression and hopelessness and attempts to manipulate others. Often these threats are not a wish to die but a means to communicate emotional pain and a plea for others to intervene. Unfortunately, repeated attempts can evoke complacency in significant others, which may result in more serious attempts by the borderline patient.

7. How do you respond if the patient threatens suicide?

All suicidal threats must be taken seriously, and assessing patients for plan, means, and intent is imperative. The initial question may be direct: "Do you have a plan to kill yourself?" If the patient has a plan, assessment of means is the next step: "Do you have pills? A gun?" Then assess the intent of acting on suicidal ideation by asking, "Are you concerned that you may act on your thoughts? If so,when?"

Determining whether the patient is able to cooperate in problem-solving can be assessed by offering to help, "Suicide is such a permanent solution to what is usually a temporary problem. Can we work together on another option?"

Questions such as, "You've been down before, what's helped?" or "What's prevented you from acting on these thoughts before?," may elicit prior strengths or support. Family and friends may be mobilized to provide support. The NP and the patient can come up with a safety plan that outlines what the patient can do or who the patient can call in times of distress. When danger appears imminent, the patient should be referred for emergency evaluation (see question 9).

8. What are the appropriate treatment or management strategies for patients with BPD?

Historically, intensive exploratory psychotherapy was the treatment of choice for patients with BPD. But this type of treatment is long-term and incompatible with current economic constraints in mental health care. Cognitive-behavioral therapy (CBT) in individual or group settings has proved to be effective and practical treatments for patients with BPD.

CBT focuses on thoughts or interpretation of events rather than the event that triggers extreme emotions and subsequent behaviors. Patients with BPD tend to think dichotomously. Dichotomous thinking plays an important role in the extreme reactions and abrupt mood swings characteristic ofh BPD. CBT helps patients with BPD to see the ambiguity in situations and people and thereby helps to regulate their emotions.

9. When and to whom should patients be referred?

Patients with BPD should be referred for therapy if their current crisis is beyond the scope of the NP. Of course, if danger is imminent, they should be referred to an emergency department for evaluation. Otherwise, the local community mental health services can provide appropriate referrals.

10. What types of medications are used to treat BPD?

Medications do not treat theBPD directly but rather symptoms of depression, anxiety, or psychosis. Selective serotonin reuptake inhibitors (SSRIs) are an effective and safe choice for treating depression and anxiety, whereas the tricyclic antidepressants can be lethal in suicidal patients. Benzodiazepines should be used cautiously, because substance abuse is common with BPD.

11. How does BPD influence health-seeking behaviors?

Patients with BPD may somatize their psychic pain and present frequently for medical care. As they focus on physical complaints, a secondary gain may be achieved through dependence on medical personnel. However, hypochondriacal patients tend to evoke helplessness and anger in caregivers, and if the patient perceives rejection, rage and desperation may ensue. The patient's hostile, angry demeanor may then present obstacles to health care management, because clinicians prefer to avoid such patients.

12. What specific strategies should I use for managing other health care problems in patients with BPD?

When determining the context of the visit, the NP can elicit the affective component and the coping skills of the patient with BPD by using the acronym **BATHE**, devised by Stuart and Lieberman (1993).

B = Background ("What is going on in your life right now?")
A = Affect ("How do you feel about that?")
T = Trouble ("What troubles you most about this situation?")
H = Handling ("How do you handle that?")
E = Empathy ("It must be very difficult for you.")

Confronting borderline patients about their behaviors is problematic, because the clinician fears their rageful reaction. However, a structured way of communicating with borderline patients was developed by the staff of the Comprehensive Treatment Unit of Saint John's

Mercy Medical Center in St. Louis. It is a three-part system of communication based on the acronym **SET**:

S = Support conveys concern (e.g., "I'm concerned about how you are feeling").
E = Empathy attempts to acknowledge the patient's feelings (e.g., "It must be very difficult for you").
T = Truth conveys the reality of the situation or consequences of the bahavior (e.g., "The truth of the matter is that I cannot prescribe you more medication"). Truth statements recognize that a problem exists but avoid blame.

It is important not to omit one of the SET stages. Omitting support may evoke charges that the clinician does not care. Omitting empathy leads to feelings of being misunderstood, and omitting truth does not call on the patient to solve problems.

The NP needs to be careful not to get caught up in the split between the good and the bad clinician. Consistency is important in working with borderline patients, and sometimes a written treatment plan tshared with the patient can ensure that all involved are aware of the expectations.

Focusing on patients' strengths helps them to focus on healthy resources. Finding something to admire in patients' attempt to master past pain can help them refocus on their ability to manage problems and relinquish dependency.

13. What controversies surround evaluation and treatment of BPD?

Patients with BPD historically have posed major therapeutic challenges for clinicians; consequently, the label BPD has negative connotations. Some controversy still surrounds the usefulness and validity of the diagnosis, because the prejudice against these difficult-to-treat patients may interfere with therapy. Unfortunately, the term is frequently associated with blaming the victim. Because of the prevalence of childhood sexual abuse in persons with BPD, some authorities assert that a traumatic diagnosis would be less pejorative.

Regardless of the label, the NP can benefit patients by being aware of their difficulties and potential behaviors, thereby taking a more proactive instead of a merely reactive approach.

BIBLIOGRAPHY

1. American Psychiatric Association: Diagnostic and Statistical Manual of Mental Disorders, 4th ed, Revision. Washington, DC, American Psychiatric Association, 2000.
2. Gunderson J: Borderline Personality Disorder: A Clinical Guide. Washington, DC, American Psychiatric Press, 2001.
3. Kreisman JJ, Straus H: I Hate You—Don't Leave Me. New York, Avon, 1989.
4. Linehan M: Cognitive-Behavioral Treatment of Borderline Personality Disorder. New York, Guilford Press, 1993.
5. Miller C, Eisner W, Allport C: Creative coping: A cognitive-behavioral group for borderline personality disorder. Arch Psychiatr Nurs 8:280–285, 1994.
6. Silk K, Nigg J, Westen D, Lohr, N: Severity of childhood sexual abuse, borderline symptoms, and familial environment. In Zanarini M (ed): The Role of Sexual Abuse in the Etiology of Borderline Personality Disorder. Washington, DC, American Psychiatric Press, 1994.
7. Stuart M, Lieberman J: The Fifteen Minute Hour. Norwalk, CT, Praeger, 1993.
8. Townsend M: Psychiatric Mental Health Nursing, 2nd ed. Philadelphia, F.A. Davis, 1996.
9. Vaillant G: The beginning of wisdom is never calling a patient a borderline. J Psychother Pract Res 1:117–134, 1992.

IV. Adjunctive and Complementary Measures

29. HERBAL AND NUTRITIONAL THERAPIES

Paula J. Watt, PhD, FNP, and Donna F. Haynes, PhD, RN, CS, WHNP, FNP

1. How common is the use of various herbal and nutritional supplements by the general public?

In 1993 Eisenberg and colleagues published a landmark study that shocked the traditional medical community because of the widespread use of alternative therapies in the U.S. In 1998, Eisenberg published an equally informative update of the dramatic changes between 1990 and 1997. The significant increase in alternative therapies led researchers to suggest more proactive research into methods, interactions, and standardization and to acknowledge the need to understand this phenomenon. Statistics about changes during the 7-year study period include the following:

- 47.3 % increase in total visits to alternative practitioners
- 629 million visits to alternative practitioners in 1997
- 18.4% of all prescriptions users took concurrent herbal and/or high-dose vitamins
- 45.2% increase in expenditure for alternative service
- $21.2 billion in 1997 with $12.2 billion out of pocket, exceeding expenditures for all U.S. hospitalizations
- Increased number of people seeking alternative therapies rather than an increased number of visits per person

2. What are the characteristics of persons who typically use herbal remedies/nutritional supplements?

- 49% have at least a college education
- 62% have an annual income > $20,000, 27% > $50,000
- 77% are Caucasian
- 68% are older than 35 years
- No significant difference between sexes
- Equal geographic distribution

3. What are the top four reasons for seeking treatment with these substances?

1. Back problems
2. Allergies
3. Fatigue
4. Arthritis

4. What questions should nurse practitioners (NPs) ask patients about herbal and nutritional therapy?

- What herbal products are they using?
- What other "alternative" methods are they using?
- What are the client's current medications?
- What results does the client expect to obtain from the product?
- What is the cost? If the product is expensive, can the claim be substantiated?

5. What information should NPs seek about each of the agents taken by their patients?

- Is the herb or product considered safe?
- What are the product claims? Any product that guarantees a "cure" should be approached with great caution or not recommended.

- Who reviewed the product for safety and effectiveness? What lab tests or research was performed and by whom? If the product was reviewed by a reputable committee, it is more likely to be represented correctly.
- Can the product be used safely with other medications?
- Do any of the herbs or products have major side effects or interactions with any of the patient's medications?
- If a client has an "unexplained" abnormal laboratory test, the practitioner needs to determine every herb or nutritional supplement the client is using. Herbs are frequently metabolized in the liver and may cause abnormal liver function tests or abnormal renal tests.

6. What are major classifications of the various substances in this broad category?

Before its official appointment as the National Center for Complementary and Alternative therapies, the Office of Complementary and Alternative medicine helped establish general categories of all alternative therapies to provide universal nomenclature to assist with understanding of the various therapies. Seven broad categories were identified to classify various therapies.

CLASSIFICATION	DEFINITION	EXAMPLE
Alternative systems of medical practice	Health care ranging from self-care according to folk principles to care rendered in organized health care system based on alternative traditions or practices.	Acupuncture, anthroscopically extended practice, ayurveda Community-based health care practices, homeopathic medicine Latin American rural practices/ Native American practices Natural products, naturopathic medicine, past life therapy Shamanism, Tibetan medicine, traditional Asian medicine
Bioelectromagnetic applications	Study of how living organisms interact with electromagnetic fields.	Blue light treatment, natural lighting, electro-acupuncture Electromagnetic fields, magnetoresonance spectroscopy Electrostimulation and neuromagnetic stimulation devices
Diet, nutrition, lifestyle changes	Knowledge of dietary or nutritional intervention to prevent illness, maintain health, and reverse effects of chronic disease	Changes in lifestyle/diet, Gerson therapy, macrobiotics Megavitamins, nutritional supplements
Herbal medicine	Using plant and plant products from folk medicine as pharmacologic agents	Echinacea, ginger rhizome, ginkgo biloba, ginseng root, Wild chrysanthemum flower, witch hazel, yellowdock
Manual healing	Using touch and manipulation with hands as diagnostic and therapeutic tool.	Acupressure, Alexander technique, biofield therapeutics, zone therapy Feldendrais method, massage therapy, osteopathy, reflexology, Rolfing Therapeutic touch, Trager method, chiropractic medicine

(Table continued on next page.)

CLASSIFICATION	DEFINITION	EXAMPLE
Mind/body control	Exploring the mind's capacity to affect the body, based on traditional medical systems that make use of interconnectedness of mind and body.	Art therapy, biofeedback counseling, dance therapy, guided imagery Humor therapy, hypnotherapy, meditation, music therapy, prayer therapy Psychotherapy, relaxation techniques, support groups, yoga
Pharmacologic and biologic treatments	Drugs and vaccines not yet accepted by mainstream medicine	Antioxidizing agents, cell treatment, chelation therapy Metabolic therapy, oxidizing agents (ozone, hydrogen peroxide)

7. What is the NP's role in relation to herbal and nutritional therapies?

According to Weil, early in this millennium 50% of all alternative therapies will be provided by members of the traditional medical community. As with any new treatment modality, the traditional health care provider is expected to learn as much as possible to assist clients in making sound health care decisions.

Only 38.5% of patients disclose voluntarily that they are using some form of alternative therapy. Clients are often hesitant to discuss "alternative practices." A common example is the use of herbal regimens to lose weight. These over-the-counter products often contain a potentially lethal combination of ephedra and ma haung, which can cause fatal cardiac arrythmias and death. They also increase blood pressure and heart rate. Caffeine, a key component of many of the "energy" and "diet" products, is contraindicated in people with high blood pressure, anxiety, mitral valve prolapse, and other disorders. The major roles of the provider include the following:
- Determining which therapies clients use
- Counseling patients about their use
- Becoming familiar with the common herbal combinations advertised in the community
- Keeping in mind that herbs are drugs, with great potential for side effects and dose-related problems
- Obtaining an objective reference on herbs and nutritional supplementation
- Becoming familiar with the most commonly used herbs that are considered safe
- Asking the questions listed in questions 4 and 5 for each alternative method that the client takes or considers

8. What are the common uses, doses, interactions, contraindications, and side effects of the most commonly used herbal and nutritional therapies?

Prescribing herb remedies is as complicated as pharmacologic interventions and should be done only when a provider has a complete understanding of the herb's usage, supposed indications, side effects, and interactions. Dosages must be individualized. The table on pages 188–189 summarizes the uses, drug–herb interactions, contraindications, and side effects for many frequently used remedies. The patient must be aware that these agents do not take the place of traditional medicine; they are complementary. Rare exceptions include the use of saw palmetto for benign prostatic hypertrophy.

9. How do you interpret the safety classification system for herbal products?

The American Herbal Products Association (AHPA) safety rating identifies four categories of herb safety:

Class 1: Can be safely consumed when used appropriately.

Class 2: Use restrictions apply, unless otherwise directed by an expert qualified in the use of the described substance:

Most Commonly Used Herbs in the United States

HERB	SAFETY RATING	COMMON USE	HERB–DRUG INTERACTIONS	CONTRAINDICATIONS	SIDE EFFECTS
Bilberry	1	Antioxidant, antidiarrhetic hypoglycemic astringent	None known	None known	Interferes with iron absorption
Black cohosh	2b/2c	Estrogen mimetic, uterine stimulant	Diabetic/hypertensive agents, HRT	May potential diabetic/hypertensive agents; pregnancy	
Chamomile	1	Anti-inflammatory, diuretic, antimicrobial, mild sedative	None known	None known	Potential ragweed allergy
Echinacea	1	Immune stimulant, antiviral, anti-inflammatory	None known	Not for progressive disease, diabetes; adverse effect on immunosuppressants	GI distress, headache
Ferverfew	2b	Anti-inflammatory for migraines, arthritis, tinnitus	None known	Pregnancy, arthritis without supervision	Oral ulcers, nausea, vomiting, sore/bitter tongue
Garlic	2c	Lipid reduction, blood thinner, hypoglycemic, anti-inflammatory	Increases anticlotting action of anti-inflammatory, synergistic with EPA oils	Anticlotting with hypoglycemic, anticoagulant; surgery	Flatulence, heartburn, nausea, vomiting, unpleasant oral sensations
Ginger	1/2b	Anti-inflammatory, antispasmodic, nausea, circulatory stimulant	May alter cardiac, diabetic, diabetic anticoagulant agents	Gallstones, high doses in pregnancy (abortefacient)	Heartburn
Gingko	2d	Memory, concentration, antioxidant, depression, vertigo, tinnitus, headache	May with MAO	Hypersensitivity	Nausea, headache, skin rash, stomach upset
Ginseng	2d	Energy, prevent illness, immune stimulant, hypertension, cholesterol, hypoglycemic	May potentiate MAO, increase phenelzine, acute illness; hemorrhage, thrombosis	Avoid in cardiac disease, diabetes, high or low blood pressure, steroids, anxiety, hyperactivity	None known
Gotu kola	1	Memory, circulation, diuretic, anti-inflammatory	Possibly with heparin	Epilepsy, pregnancy, breast-feeding	Photosensitivity, hives, contact dermatitis
Grape seed		Circulation, anti-inflammatory	None known	None known	None known

		Uses	Interactions	Contraindications	Side effects
Green tea	2d	Cholesterol, hypertension, diuretic; reduces platelet aggregation	None known	None known	Caffeine-related insomnia, anxiety, tachycardia
Hawthorn	1	Cardiac function, mild CNS depressant, antilipidemic	None known	Pregnancy, breast-feeding, hypertension, CHF	Nausea, fatigue, hand skin rash, perspiration
Horse chestnut	1	Circulation, analgesic, anti-inflammatory	Protein plasma-binding with pharmaceuticals	Pregnancy, breast-feeding, anticoagulant therapy, impaired kidney or liver function	GI irritant, shock, pseudo-lupus, toxic to liver and kidney
Kava	2d	Anxiety, analgesic, benzodiazepine withdrawal, muscle relaxant	Potentiates CNS effects of barbiturates, alcohol, antidepressants/antipsychotics	Endogenous depression, pregnancy, breast-feeding	Mild GI distress, yellow skin discoloration with long-term use
Milk thistle	1	Liver damage and disease, bile duct inflammation	None known	None known	Laxative effect (standardized formulations)
Saw palmetto	1	BPH symptom, diuretic, urinary antiseptic	None known	Pregnancy, breast-feeding	GI distress, diarrhea, headache, hormonal/endocrine effects
Siberian ginseng	1	Immunostimulant, hypotensive, hypoglycemic, chronic inflammation	Stimulants, antipsychotics, HRT, cardiac medications, anticoagulant, hypoglycemic, antihypetensives	Hypertension, pregnancy, breast-feeding; nervousness, anxiety, hyperactivity	Insomnia, anxiety, irritability, palpitations
St. John's wort	2d	Mild-to-moderate depression, external wounds and burns	Interacts with MAOs and antidepressants	MAO inhibitors, pregnancy, breast-feeding	Photosensitivity, delayed hypersensitivity
Valerian	1	Insomnia, nervousness, cramps, dysmenorrhea	Increases effects of sedatives and antidepressants	Only under supervision with sedatives and hypertension	Mild GI disturbance

CNS = central nervous system, BPH = benign prostatic hypertrophy, HRT = hormone replacement therapy, CHF = congestive heart failure, GI = gastrointestinal, MAO = monoamine oxidase.

- 2a: external use only
- 2b: not for use in pregnancy
- 2c: not for use in lactation
- 2d: other restrictions/professional guidance

Class 3: Significant data justify the following labeling "to be used only under supervision of an expert qualified in the appropriate use of the substance."

Class 4: Insufficient data are available for classification.

10. How can I stay current on information about herbal agents?

Several European and American organizations assist practitioners and consumers in understanding the growing body of herbal information:

- World Health Organization (WHO)
- German Commission E
- European Scientific Cooperative of Phytotherapy (ESCOP)
- American Herbal Products Association (AHPA)
- Herb Research Foundation

The German Commission E Monographs are the most comprehensive works published on the effects of various natural substances. The European text provides information about the appropriate use of herbs as well as what is currently known about interactions between herbs. Another excellent reference is *The Natural Medicines Comprehensive Database*. This reference is available by subscription in both book and e-mail forms. The e-mail version has continuous updates on herbs and current research data: http://www.naturaldatabase.com.

11. Which substances have been identified as potentially toxic?

According to the Natural Medicines Comprehensive Database, 12 substances have been identified as potentially toxic.

SUBSTANCE	TOXICITY
Blue cohosh	Induces inappropriate labor
Borage	Hepatocarcinogenic
Calamus	Malignant tumors in rats; should not be used chronically
Chaparral	Toxic to liver
Colt's foot	Carcinogenic, toxic to liver
Comfrey	Liver cancer in small animals, venocclusive disease in humans
Ephedra	Asphyxiation, heart failure
Germander	Toxic to liver
Licorice	Hyperaldosteronism, toxic to liver
Poke root	Poisonous, toxic lectins; mucus membraneirritating saponins
Sassafras	Liver cancer in animals
Wormwood	Contains toxic substances

12. What common problems are associated with herbal and nutritional therapies?

Three major issues apply to the use of herbal/nutritional therapies: lack of standardization among agents, risks of megavitamin use, and lack of educational standards.

13. Why is lack of standardization of the various agents a major problem?

Botanical medicines contain various substances as well as what is considered the biologically active ingredient. Actual amounts of these substances vary according to conditions in which the agents are grown, harvested, stored, and processed. Ensuring similarity among these substances is a daunting task. With no regulation of quality control, consumers cannot be assured they always receive the specified amounts of the active ingredient. Most credible manufacturers have internal quality standards to attempt batch-to-batch controls. Encourage clients to buy only from reputable sources and to stay with the same brand for each refill.

14. What is the rationale for megavitamin use?

When the Food and Drug Administration (FDA) made its dietary guidelines for various nutritional components, two issues were raised. First, the minimum daily requirements for supplements is based on the amount needed to prevent symptoms of deficiency. Theoretically, the overnutrition of the typical American should exceed these minimum requirements by far. However, early farming practices are believed to have drained necessary nutrients from the soil, preventing the transfer of vitamins and minerals into the produce. Therefore, even a nutritious diet may not include the necessary vitamins and minerals. Second, stressful demands on nutritional needs and the fast food craze, which can limit significantly the variety of nutritious foods necessary for proper metabolic processes, may have an impact on the dietary needs of the typical American. These solid arguments are a strong voice in the consumer, who heads to the health food store for megavitamin and mineral therapy. But as with herbs, these substances can be detrimental in high levels and should be evaluated carefully for safety and usefulness.

15. What educational issues are related to herbal and nutritional therapy?

No educational standards relate to recommending herbs to clients, but several questions should be asked before the client considers herbs. People recommending and selling herbal remedies and other alternative therapies often have no formal educational training.

16. What are the major specific interactions between herbal agents and prescribed or over-the-counter medications?

Currently 60 substances have been identified as interfering with commonly prescribed drugs. Most people think that herbs are safe because they are "natural"; they tend to forget that herbs are sources of biologically active substances. Appropriate utilization and maintenance of these substances are pharmacologic issues and should be taken seriously. If patients take the following herbs, consideration should be given to assessing the traditional medications that they take. Below is a *partial* list of the most common medications. For a complete list please refer to the current *The Prescriber's Letter—Natural Medicines Database* (1999).

HERB	POTENTIAL DRUG INTERACTION
5-HTP	Serotonin agonist, serotonin
Aloe latex	Antiarrhythmic, cardiac glycosides, corticosteroids, diuretics
Androstenendione	Estrogens
Brewer's yeast	Antifungals, monoamine oxidase inhibitors
Bromelain	Anticoagulants, antiplatelets
Buckthorn bark	Cardiac glycosides, corticosteroids, diuretics
Bugleweed	Thyroid hormones
Caffeine	Beta-adrenergic agents, central nervous system depressants, theophylline anhydrous (Theo-dur), multiple others
Calcium	Fluoride, fluoroquinolones, tetracyclines
Cascara	Cardiac glycosides, corticosteroids, laxatives, diuretics
Chasteberry	Dopamine D_2 antagonist, hormone therapy, metoclopramide (Reglan), oral contraceptive pills
Chromium	Insulin, zinc
Coffee	Antipsychotics, beta blockers
Danshen	Warfarin, antiplatelets

(Table continued on next page.)

HERB	POTENTIAL DRUG INTERACTION
Devil's claw	Antihyperglycemic agents, antihypertensives, cardiac drugs, warfarin
Digitalis	Cardiac drugs, digoxin (Lanoxin), macrolides, multiple others
Dong quai	Antiplatelet drugs, warfarin
Echinacea	Immunosuppressants
Ephedra	Antihyperglycemic agents, dexamethasone (Decadron), digoxin (Lanoxin), pitocin, theophylline
European mistletoe	Anticoagulants, antihypertensives, antidepressants
Evening primrose oil	Anesthestics, phenothiazines
Fenugreek	Anticoagulants, antihyperglycemic agents, steroids, hormone therapy
Feverfew	Anticoagulants, antiglycemics, antiplatelets, nonsteroidal anti-inflammatory drugs
Garlic	Warfarin, antiplatelets, antiglycemics
Ginger	Anticoagulants, antihypertensives, multiple others
Ginkgo biloba	Warfarin, antiplatelets, thiazides
Goldenseal	Antihypertensives, sedatives
Gossypol	Diuretics
Gotu kola	Antiglycemics, statins, sedatives
Grapefruit juice	Calcium channel blockers, carbamazepine (Tegretol), estrogens, statins, itraconazole (Sporonox), saquinavir, multiple others
Guar gum	Anticoagulants, antiglycemics, aspirin, glucophage, digoxin (Lanoxin), penicillin
Gurana	Theophylline anhydrous (Theo-dur), multiple others
Hawthorn	Cardiovascular agents
Horse chesnut	Anticoagulants, antiglycemics, protein-bound drugs
Horseradish	Thyroid agents
Kava	Alcohol, other sedatives
Licorice	Antihypertensives, multiple others
α-Lipoic acid	Antihyperglycemic agents
Panax ginseng	Multiple medications
Papain	Anticoagulants, antiplatelets
Passion flower	Hypnotics, sedatives
Pectin	Beta carotene, lovastatin, digoxin (Lanoxin), tetracyclines
Pysillium	Antiglycemics, carbamazepine (Tegretol), digoxin (Lanoxin), lithium
Red yeast	Statins, cytochrome P450-3A inhibitors, thyroid agents
Sage	Anticonvulsants
Saw palmetto	Hormones, oral contraceptives
Siberian ginseng	Sedatives, stimulants, antiglycemics
St. John's wort	Antidepressants, selective serotonin reuptake inhibitors, multiple others
Stinging nettle (above ground parts)	Anticoagulants, antihypertensives, antiglycemics, multiple others
Uva ursi	Urine acidfying agents
Valerian	Sedatives
Vitamin E	Bile acid sequestrants, warfarin
Yohimbe	Antihypertensives, multiple others

17. What patients are candidates for herbal or nutritional therapy?

Complementary health plans that integrate traditional and alternative therapies can vastly increase the efficacy of any treatment regimen. For example, we have long known that nutrition plays an important role in the treatment of many diseases. Belief in the system can play an important role in the body's response to any particular therapy. For health promotion and disease prevention, therefore, anyone can benefit from appropriate complementary and integrative therapies.

18. What risk of nutrient depletion is associated with any of the traditional medications?

One especially important consideration is the many classifications of drugs that can interfere with nutrient absorption or increase their utilization. This risk should be taken into consideration when prescribing and monitoring the effects of the medications, because nutritional supplementation may be indicated.

Common Drugs that Cause Nutrient Depletion

DRUG CLASS	NUTRIENT DISRUPTED
Colchicine	Vitamin B_{12}
Apresoline	Vitamin B_6
Digoxin (Lanoxin)	Magnesium
Statins	Coenzyme Q10
Questran, Colestid	Beta carotene, folic acid, vitamins A, D, E, and K
Loop diuretics	Calcium, magnesium, potassium, sodium, zinc
Thiazides	Magnesium, potassium, sodium, zinc
Potassium-sparing drugs	Folic acid
Anticonvulsants	Folic acid, vitamin D
Phenothiazines	Vitamin B_2
Glyburides	Coenzyme Q10
Glucophage	Vitamin B_{12}
Aluminum and magnesium salts	Calcium, phosphorus
H_2 blockers	Vitamin B_{12}
Bisacodyl	Potassium
Mineral oil	Vitamins A, E, D, and K, beta carotene, calcium
Stimulants	Calcium, sodium, potassium, vitamin D
Prokinetics	Vitamin B_2
Proton pump inhibitors	Vitamin B_{12}
Corticosteroids	Calcium; indirectly vitamin D
Estrogen	Vitamin B_6, magnesium
Oral contraceptives	Folic acid, vitamins B_2, B_6, and B_{12}, magnesium
Extended-release potassium	Vitamin B_{12}
Theophylline	Vitamin B_6
All antibiotics	Intestinal microflora, B vitamins, vitamin K
Tetracyclines	Calcium and iron
Sulfa drugs	Folic acid

19. What major controversies surround the use of nutritional and herbal substances?

Opponents of herbal therapy consider the lack of standardization as a major deterrent for its use, whereas proponents believe usage of the entire herb includes substances that are protective from side effects and offer benefits not fully understood. The content of herbal products varies widely depending on growing, harvesting, and storage conditions. Standardization identifies one or two components but is problematic without knowing which components in which amounts and in what combinations are important.

Herbal combinations can interact with one another and with medications. Caution should be exhibited with new combinations by even mainstream companies.

In 1975 The European Economic Community attempted to clarify distinctions between herbs and conventional drugs. They noted that consistent quality for products of vegetable origin can be ensured only if the starting materials are defined in a rigorous and detailed manner, including the specific botanical identification of the plant material and the geographical source and conditions under which the drug is obtained.

BIBLIOGRAPHY

1. Blumenthal M, Busses W, Goldberg A, et al: The Complete German Commission E Monographs—Therapeutic Guide to Herbal Medicines. Boston, Integrative Medicine Communications, 1998.
2. Eisenberg D, Davis R, Ettner S, et al: Trends in alternative medicine use in the United States, 1990–1997. JAMA 28:1569–1575, 1998.
3. Jellin MN, Batz F, Hichens K: Pharmacist's Letter/Prescriber's Letter, Natural Medicines Comprehensive Database. Stockton, CA., Therapeutic Research Faculty, 1999.
4. Lee R, Tyler V, Weart W: Herbal medicines you can recommend with confidence, Patient Care, Sept. 15:76–94, 1999.

30. MANUAL HEALING: THERAPEUTIC TOUCH

Carol E. Craig, PhD, FNP-C, RN

1. What is therapeutic touch?

Therapeutic touch (TT) is derived from a number of healing methods that involve moving the energy field that surrounds a body to balance energy and to promote healing. Methods range from massage therapy to "laying on of hands.".

2. What is the theory behind TT?

TT is one of a number of therapies that use the theory of a human energy field. This field surrounds the body and can be manipulated or moved to affect how a person feels and to promote healing. Some TT practitioners postulate that an energy exchange occurs between the client and the practitioner.

3. How is TT done?

Dolores Krieger, a nurse, was instrumental in the development of the original practice of TT, along with an unlicensed healer, Dora Kunz. Many TT therapists follow their guidelines. Most practitioners of TT do not actually touch the client but move the energy field by moving their hands a few inches above the body surface. The Krieger-Kunz technique involves five steps:

1. **Centering:** The first step is to center oneself before beginning therapy. The centering process involves becoming focused and attentive, rather like meditation. The practitioner becomes focused on the TT and lets all other thoughts leave the mind.

2. **Assessment:** The client's energy field is assessed by moving the hands a few inches above the client's body. Areas of differences or blockages in the energy flow are felt by the practitioner's hands as a difference in energy between the practitioner's two hands.

3. **Energy movement:** The practitioner moves his or her hands to sweep areas of energy that are blocked and to promote free flow of the body's energy.

4. **Repatterning:** The practitioner directs his or her own energy to assist the client to repattern energy, thereby promoting healing.

5. **Finishing:** The practitioner continues treatment until no sensory differences can be detected between the two hands.

4. How long does a therapeutic touch session take?

TT sessions have no set time frame, but frequently it takes between 20 and 30 minutes before the practitioner can detect no sensory differences between his or her hands.

5. How many sessions of therapeutic touch is a client likely to need?

It is hard to know. TT is considered a way of placing a client into a position to heal the self; healing may be rapid or slow. Published accounts of successful therapeutic touch interactions vary from one session to multiple sessions over several years. In general, people with minor ailments such as a headache may need a single session; those with severe physical and mental problems may ask for assistance over a long period.

6. What happens if I just move my hands over a client?

An important aspect of this technique is that the practitioner of TT must intend to help the client (intentionality). The practitioner of TT must be willing to share personal energy with the client and not simply make TT gestures in the client's energy field. Research studies have repeatedly demonstrated less therapeutic effect if the practitioner did "sham" movements, regardless of a client's belief or disbelief in the method.

7. Does the client need to believe that TT will help?

Most practitioners say that TT can be effective even if the client has no belief that TT will help. The intentionality of the practitioner to help is all that is necessary.

8. Can a practitioner harm a client's energy fields, either purposefully or inadvertently?

Little research has been done on potential harm to energy fields with the use of TT. Nelson stated, "What is the intention?—to help or to help heal; what motivates the intention? Compassion. Since the outcome is not in our hands, we are simply enhancing the person's own healing energies and, therefore, we cannot hurt anyone." Although this answer does not address a practitioner who may intend harm to a client, most TT practitioners seem to believe that the only effective TT is done with a helpful intention.

9. What is the difference between TT and massage therapies?

Most massage therapies concentrate on rubbing and/or exerting pressure on tensed muscles to promote stress reduction and healing. The general theory is that massage can loosen tight muscles, promote blood flow to an injured area and unblock energy fields to promote balance and harmony. Classic TT does not touch the body but works with the energy field that surrounds the body.

10. Does a person need to be licensed to do TT?

No. TT is not a licensed practice. TT has never been part of one particular profession's license to practice, although nurses have been instrumental in learning and using TT.

11. How does someone learn to do TT?

No certification programs exist for TT. Some nurses state that TT is simple to learn and teach it to family members who would like to learn to give TT treatments. Janet Quinn of the University of Colorado developed a series of three videotapes to teach TT. Many nurses learn TT at short workshops. Other nurses claim that TT is learned through apprenticeship and takes 1 or 2 years to do well.

12. How would a nurse find a competent TT practitioner?

Although the American Holistic Nurses Association does not certify TT practitioners, the association has courses in healing touch, which incorporates many of the principles of TT. The association can be found at www.ahna.org.

13. Is a physician's order necessary to do TT?

No, TT is considered a nursing intervention and does not require a physician's order.

14. When should someone consider using TT?

The technique assists the client in self-healing, and most practitioners claim no curative powers for TT. TT is never used for diagnosis but is an adjunct therapy to help the body to heal itself. Although research is equivocal, TT shows promise for pain and anxiety reduction. No evidence suggests that TT can be used to replace medications for surgical or burn pain, but it may enhance the effectiveness of medications. Clients need to be aware that TT is not touted as a curative treatment but as an adjunct to other modalities. Clients who want to have a treatment in which the body is brought into a condition for better self-healing are most comfortable with TT.

15. What client conditions respond best to TT?

Most practitioners use TT to help alleviate pain, reduce stress and anxiety, and promote wound healing.

16. Can I combine therapeutic touch with other therapies?

Yes. In fact, for some conditions TT is less effective than standard medical treatment but appears to be a good adjunct therapy. For example, TT has never been shown to be as effective for pain as narcotics, but TT plus narcotics appears to reduce client's perception of pain more than narcotics alone.

17. How can TT be incorporated into clinical practice?

TT can be used whenever a client needs help with pain, stress, or anxiety. Because sessions take about 30 minutes, TT is best done at specific appointments. Hospital-based nurses have an easier time incorporating a treatment with other care during an 8- or 12-hour shift, but TT can be used to help calm an anxious client or a client in pain at any time in a clinic setting.

18. What does research say about the efficacy of TT?

Research claims are equivocal, in part perhaps because of problems with standardization of TT techniques. Some studies use classic methods, whereas others involve actual touch. Further problems include the claim by some practitioners that TT is a holistic process and that the nurse-client relationship is essential to healing. Any studies, therefore, that separate the five steps and test only one aspect of the technique or that interfere with the relationship between practitioner and client violate the underlying assumptions of the theory. Some researchers state that equivocal or negative findings of TT are a result of this fragmentation.

19. Does research indicate that TT reduces pain?

TT was found to affect significantly subjective measures such as pain perception more frequently than it affects physiologic measures such as blood pressure and respiratory rate. Although many of these studies were small or lacked control groups, several reported interesting findings. Most studies found that people reported less pain or waited longer for pain medications when TT was used with pain medications than with pain medications alone.

20. Can TT reduce anxiety?

As with pain, TT has been demonstrated to be effective with subjective measures of anxiety but has not been demonstrated as effective with physiologic measures. Several studies found a reduction in anxiety and subjective stress with the use of TT.

21. Does TT effect immunity?

It is hard to say. A study of T-lymphocyte function and immunoglobin levels in students taking board examinations showed significant differences in IgA and IgM between TT and placebo groups. IgG differences were not found. This pilot study with only 20 subjects must be interpreted cautiously. Another pilot study found a trend in a subset of T cells for both practitioners and recipients of TT, but the significance of this finding is unknown.

22. What about wound healing?

Findings of the effects of TT on wound healing are equivocal. Studies of the effect of TT have included surgical wound healing, healing of burn wounds, and increased production of cells to promote healing. Studies by Wirth and colleagues demonstrated inconclusive results for wound healing, with significance for some variables and reverse significant findings for others. A study of in vitro erythropoiesis demonstrated no differences in hemoglobinization in TT groups from mimic or no treatment groups. Instead, three of the eight cultures showed reduced amounts of hemoglobin, which is opposite to the proposed theoretical direction.

23. Is TT safe?

TT has not been shown to be harmful to the client, and its safety is unquestioned. In a recent small study, Engle and Graney found vasoconstriction (a stress response) instead of vasodilation (a relaxation response) when TT was used, but the significance of this finding is unclear.

24. How is TT reimbursed?

Few insurance plans cover TT. Reimbursement is done by the client on an out-of-pocket basis.

25. What controversies surround TT?

TT may be the most controversial nursing intervention in the U.S.. The controversy stems from the failure of studies to demonstrate a "human energy field" and the inability of TT practitioners to detect the field. Others claim that TT has not established evidence of efficacy.

Although some researchers dismiss TT as "pseudoscience" and "fakery," others state that TT is a holistic process and cannot be tested when the relationship is removed from the process or when steps are tested separately.

Another controversy involves teaching TT within state or federally funded schools. Some people claim that TT is a religious practice and that teaching TT within any institution that accepts government funds violates the separation of church and state. Most practitioners agree, however, that TT does not require religious faith on either the client's or the practitioner's part; it is a broad, holistic therapy without specific religious content.

26. What research evidence is available about TT and pain?

Lin YS: Effects of therapeutic touch in reducing pain and anxiety in an elderly population. Dissert Abstr Int 59-07B:3349, 1998.

Meehan TC: Therapeutic touch and post-operative pain: A rogerian research study. Nurs Sci Q 6:69–78, 1993.

Muller-Hinze MLM: The effects of therapeutic touch and acupressure on experimentally-induced pain. Dissert Abstr Int 49-11B:4755, 1988.

Peck SD: The effect of therapeutic touch for improving functional ability in elders with degenerative arthritis. Nurs Sci Q 11:123–132, 1998.

Turner JG, Clark AJ, Gauthier DK, Williams M: The effect of therapeutic touch on pain and anxiety in burn patients. J Adv Nurs 28:10–20, 1998.

27. What research studies address TT and anxiety relief?

Gagne D, Toye RC: The effects of therapeutic touch and relaxation therapy in reducing anxiety. Arch Psychiatr Nurs 8:184–189, 1994.

Kramer NA: Comparison of therapeutic touch and casual touch in stress reduction of children. Pediatr Nurs 16:483–485, 1990.

Quinn J, Strelkauskas AJ: Psychoimmunilogic effects of therapeutic touch on practitioners and bereaved recipients: A pilot study. Adv Nurs Sci 15(4):13–26, 1993.

Snyder M, Egan EC, Burns KR: Interventions for decreasing agitation behaviors in persons with dementia. J Gerontol Nurs 21:34–40, 1995.

Olson M, Sneed N, LaVia M, et al: Stress-induced immunosuppression and therapeutic touch. Altern Thera Health Med 3:68–74, 1997.

28. What research studies discuss wound healing?

O'Manthuna DP: Evidence-based practice and reviews of therapeutic touch. J Nurs Scholar 32:279–285, 2000.

Wirth DP, Barrett MJ, Eidelman WS: Non-contact therapeutic touch and wound reepithelialization: an extension of previous research. Complement Ther Med 2:187–192, 1994.

Wirth DP: Complementary healing intervention and dermal wound reepithelialization: An overview. Int J Psychosom Med 42:48–53, 1995.

Wirth DP, Richardson VT, Martinez RD, et al: Non-contact therapeutic touch and full-thickness cutaneous wounds: A replication. Complement Ther Med 4:237–240, 1996.

BIBLIOGRAPHY

1. Bullough VL, Bullough B: Should nurses practice therapeutic touch? Should nursing schools teach therapeutic touch? J Profess Nurs 14:254–257, 1998.
2. Egan E: Therapeutic touch. In Snyder M, Lindquist R (eds): Complementary/Alternative Therapies in Nursing, 3rd ed. New York, Springer, 1998, pp 49–62.
3. Engle VF, Graney MJ: Biobehavioral effects of therapeutic touch. J Nurs Scholar 32(3):287–293, 2000.
4. Fontaine KL: Hand-mediated biofield therapies. In Fontaine KL (ed): Healing Practices: Alternative Therapies for Nursing. Upper Saddle River, NJ, Prentice-Hall, 2000, pp 220–232.
5. Krieger D: Therapeutic touch: How to Use Your Hands to Help or to Heal. Englewood Cliffs, NJ, Prentice-Hall, 1986.
6. Nelson L: Questions and answers about therapeutic touch. Available at http://www.therapeutictouch netwk.com.
7. Quinn J: Therapeutic touch as energy exchange: Replication and extension. Nurs Sci Q 2:79–89, 1989.
8. Rosa L, Rosa E, Sarner L, Barrett S: A close look at therapeutic touch. JAMA 279:1005–1010, 1998.
9. Seskevich J: Duke newspaper article and response, 1998 Available at http://www.voicenet.com/ ~eric/z/antiemly.txt.
10. Spence JE, Olson MA: Quantitative research on therapeutic touch: An integrative review of the literature 1985–1995. Scand J Caring Sci 11:183–190, 1997.

31. COLLABORATING WITH PHYSICAL, OCCUPATIONAL, AND SPEECH-LANGUAGE THERAPISTS

Laurie Grubbs, PhD, ARNP, ANP

1. What are the main differences between physical therapy, occupational therapy, and speech-language therapy?

As in the other health care disciplines, there are areas where all three disciplines overlap and areas where they are distinct. Recently, a physical therapist, occupational therapist, and speech therapist were asked how their roles differed. They jokingly replied, "Well, we're still trying to figure that out, but don't tell the insurance companies!" The aim of all three is to maximize function and return clients to their *prior* level of functioning. If a client is not an NFL football player before therapy, he probably will not be one after therapy!

PHYSICAL THERAPY

2. What is the main goal of physical therapy?

The main goal of physical therapy is to improve and maximize function whether it be at home, in the workplace or in the sports arena. Physical therapists (PTs) focus on improving gross motor movement (range of motion, strength and flexibility) in clients with musculoskeletal and neurologic problems such as cerebrovascular accident (CVA), traumatic brain injury (TBI), spinal cord injuries, burns, amputations, rheumatoid arthritis, cardiac dysfunction, back pain, orthopedic surgery, joint problems or injuries, and degenerative diseases of the central nervous system. They also assist clients in mobility and transfer, home management activities, and use of prosthetics and other assistive devices.

3. What treatment modalities are used by PTs?

MODALITY	ACTIVITY AND PURPOSE
Strength training	Begins with active range of motion (ROM) exercises, then advances to resistance/weight training; also includes balance and gait training, stair climbing, crutch walking, use of a walker, wheelchair and other transfer training.
Pool rehabilitation	Particularly helpful with joint problems; offers gentle resistance for increasing strength and flexibility.
Treadmill and stationary bicycles	Helpful for overall strengthening and conditioning, as well as balance.
Therapeutic balls	Therapeutic balls are used to increase strength of all muscle groups and to improve balance and coordination.
Medex machines	Increase strength and ROM of the back and neck. Many community gyms have taken up back rehabilitation as a money-making, marketing tool and have purchased Medex machines. With some luck, they are employing PTs or PT assistants to work with members on back- and neck-strengthening exercises. With the proper training, these machines can be quite helpful for mechanical low back pain.

(Continued on next page.)

MODALITY	ACTIVITY AND PURPOSE
Biodex machines	Increase strength and ROM of all joints. These expensive, sophisticated machines are entirely computerized and test all of the muscles surrounding a joint as well as all planes of joint movement; they also compare side-to-side performance and norms for age. Probably should be reserved for well-trained PTs, if for no other reason than safety.
Electrical stimulation	Used for pain control, muscle retraining, muscle relaxation, and reduction of inflammation. In pain control, the first step is to relax the muscle. Electrical stimulation causes the muscle to contract repeatedly until it fatigues and thus can relax.
Transcutaneous electrical nerve stimulation (TENS)	A portable unit that patients take home and wear all of the time. Delivers a lower level of current than electrical stimulation; used mostly for pain control. According to the gate theory, the brain receives the TENS signal, which blocks or masks the pain signal from reaching the brain.
Ultrasound	Increases the depth that heat can reach to the muscles, thus increasing blood flow to the injured muscle and reducing edema.

4. Is there a difference between outpatient and inpatient physical therapy?

The major difference between outpatient and inpatient physical therapy is the type of clients and problems seen. Obviously, inpatient PTs see clients in their more acute stage and focus on rendering them sufficiently functional to go home or to a rehabilitation or long-term care facility. Inpatient PTs see adult and pediatric clients with strokes, head injuries, spinal cord injuries, burns, and amputations and patients who have undergone orthopedic surgery. They work to improve strength, flexibility, and range of motion and to train clients for various activities of daily living (ADLs), such as crutch walking, stair climbing, transfer, and prosthetic training. PTs want to teach clients to be independent in their exercise regimen and to return clients to their previous level of functioning. Inpatient PTs also may work with terminal clients if for no other reason than to improve quality of life. For some clients, just to be able to sit on the side of the bed is a big step. It improves their psychological and physical functioning and gives the client and family an improved quality of life.

Outpatient PTs see a wide range of clients with joint and other musculoskeletal and neurologic problems, including ankle, knee, shoulder, back, and neck pain and injuries; capsulitis; bursitis; tendinitis, especially of the wrist, elbow, and ankle; joint instability; entrapment neuropathies; temporomandibular joint disorder; postoperative rehabilitation; chronic pain; incontinence; workers' compensation; and continuation of inpatient rehabilitation.

When considering referral to a PT, NPs should be aware of areas other than inpatient and outpatient clinics in which PTs work. A PT may be available in the school system for children with disabilities such as cerebral palsy, spina bifida, autism, and spinal cord injuries. Corporate PTs assist clients in "work-hardening" skills, which train them specifically for a certain job description. For example, people working in merchandise stocking may be trained by the PT in proper body mechanics and strengthening for lifting and moving heavy objects. Home health care PTs visit clients who are physically unable to come to the physical therapy facility. Home health PTs work with clients and their families to improve functional capacity in the home, specifically with ADLs such as bathing, cooking, stair climbing, crutch walking, and wheel chair transfer. Much, but not all, of this work is done with geriatric clients because they are often in need of this service.

5. What are the different specialties in physical therapy?

The many specialties include cardiology, orthopedics, neurology, ergonomics, electrophysiology, pediatrics, and geriatrics. Specialty certifications require additional years of experience and education in the specialty area, and PTs are required to pass a specialty examination to be certified.

6. What credentials are necessary for licensure as a PT?

Physical therapy education is experiencing some of the same growing pains as nurse practitioner education. Until recently, the minimal educational requirement was a 4-year baccalaureate degree from an accredited program. However, for all students currently entering PT programs, post-baccalaureate degrees will be required. PTs also must pass a state licensing exam in order to practice. All PTs who were licensed prior to 2002 will be grandfathered without additional formal education.

7. What is a physical therapy assistant (PTA)?

Whereas PTs have a bachelors or masters degree and are licensed, PTAs have a two-year associate degree and, in some states, also must be licensed, registered, or certified. PTAs cannot perform initial assessments, re-evaluations ,or discharges and are required to work under the supervision of a PT to perform the prescribed treatment regimen for a client.

8. At what point in the treatment plan should referral to a PT be made?

For clients with musculoskeletal problems or injuries who are not deemed to be immediate surgical candidates, it is generally standard practice to treat for 2–3 weeks with nonsteroidal anti-inflammatory drugs (NSAIDs), ice, heat, rest, and gentle stretching exercises. After 2–3 weeks, swelling and pain should be diminished and a more accurate assessment can be performed. If no improvement is seen, a referral to PT is advisable unless it is deemed a surgical problem. Even if surgery is likely, orthopedic surgeons often prescribe 6-8 weeks of PT before deciding on surgical intervention. If severe pain, swelling, limited ROM, or neurologic signs and symptoms are present, a referral to the orthopedist or neurosurgeon may be warranted and a computed tomography (CT) or magnetic resonance imaging (MRI) scan obtained.

OCCUPATIONAL THERAPY

9. What is the main goal of occupational therapy?

OTs have a wide scope of areas for practice. As with physical therapy, the main goal of occupational therapy is to improve and maximize function. Whereas PTs are generally concerned with gross motor movement, OTs are concerned with fine motor movement and cognitive tasks such as spatial and perceptual functions. Occupational therapists utilize a client's occupational and daily activities and movements as a basis for treatment rather than a preset group of exercises that may be hard for clients to remember and practice after discharge, especially if they have decreased cognitive functioning. The philosophy is that clients will improve more efficiently using movements with which they are already familiar and that they will continue to use in everyday life.

10. With what types of patients do OTs commonly work?

In conjunction with PTs, OTs assist all types of clients with strength, coordination, ROM, flexibility, and the endurance necessary to perform ADLs. OTs assist clients with stroke, spinal cord injuries, burns, amputations, rheumatoid arthritis, hand injuries, cardiac dysfunction, back pain, TBI, and degenerative diseases of the central nervous system in managing dressing, hygiene and grooming, eating, mobility and transfer, home management activities, and use of assistive devices and prosthetics.

11. What common areas or conditions are OTs likely to treat?

OTs work with hand and upper extremity injuries and problems. OTs are concerned with workplace rehabilitation, particularly for carpal tunnel syndrome and wrist tendinitis. They assist clients with work evaluation and work hardening.

OTs work cooperatively with speech therapists for the evaluation and treatment of dysphagia. Their goals in the treatment of dysphagia are to facilitate positioning during eating, to improve motor control of swallowing, to maintain adequate nutritional intake, to prevent aspiration, and to reestablish oral eating to the safest, optimal level.

OTs work with evaluation and treatment of visual defects, particularly visual perception, a process that integrates vision with other sensory input. They work specifically with visual attention, visual scanning, pattern recognition, visual memory, and visual cognition. In addition to vision, OTs rehabilitate other sensory dysfunctions such as light touch sensation, thermal sensation, superficial pain sensation, olfactory sensation, taste, position (proprioception), and motion sense (kinesthesia). A sensory retraining program focuses primarily on tactile and kinesthetic reeducation. OTs treat perceptual motor deficits by strengthening the discriminative skills of stereognosis and graphesthesia and improving problems with apraxia. They work with cognitive deficits in the areas of orientation and attention, memory, executive functions, reasoning and problem-solving skills, insight and awareness, and calculation abilities.

12. What modalities are used in occupational therapy?

The main principle of occupational therapy modalities is based on purposeful and functional activity training for specific tasks to reach neuromotor and cognitive goals. OTs are concerned with a goal, not just the activity surrounding a particular movement. Modalities include the following:

MODALITY	ACTIVITY AND PURPOSE
Biomechanic and sensorimotor exercises	Exercises to improve skills, strength, ROM, joint flexibility, endurance, coordination, and perceptual, cognitive, and social skills
Thermal modalities	Ultrasound, hot packs, and whirlpool are used to increase blood flow to the injured muscles and reduce edema as well as assist in the debridement of burns and wounds
Electrical modalities	TENS and electrical stimulation for pain reduction, muscle retraining, and muscle relaxation
Orthotics	Splinting is often used to prevent contractures and encourage proper alignment of weakened limbs.
Videofluoroscopy	Performed in conjunction with the radiologist to evaluate swallowing. This radiographic procedure uses a modified barium swallow recorded on videotape. It allows the therapist to see the client's jaw and tongue movements, to measure transit times, to see the swallow, and to detect any aspiration.
Strengthening exercises	Particularly to improve and strengthen swallowing mechanisms (e.g., head strength, tongue and jaw movement)

13. Describe the training of OTs.

Occupational therapy now requires a post-baccalaureate degree from an accredited program and state licensure. OTs can choose areas of specialization, but only hand therapy requires additional certification. Hand therapists treat orthopedic problems and injuries and must have 5 years of practice before they are eligible to sit for the hand therapy certification exam.

14. What is an occupational therapy assistant (OTA)?

Certified OTA education requires an associate degree and certification. As with PTAs, certified occupational therapy assistants (COTAs) cannot do initial evaluations or periodic assessments. They work with OTs in carrying out treatment plans. COTAs work in all areas, but less often in pediatrics because children change so rapidly and need frequent re-evaluation.

15. Describe the overlap between physical and occupational therapy.

Particularly with low-level functioning clients, PTs and OTs often begin cotreatment, working with the minimal skills necessary to perform ADLs. As the client improves, the treatments usually separate and become more specific, but attempts are made not to duplicate effort. In billing for Medicare, PTs can be more general and specify broader areas, such as increased ROM or increased pain control. OTs are required to specify exactly for which function the client is being prepared (e.g.,dressing, feeding) to ensure that duplication of effort does not occur.

16. How is a referral made to the PT or OT?

There are a variety of ways to order physical and occupational therapy. The main function of the health care provider is to deem the patient medically stable to undergo therapy. To be accepted into a rehabilitation center and qualify for Medicare, clients must be strong enough to tolerate physical and occupational therapy.

In the outpatient setting, verbal feedback and clarification are not immediately available; therefore, written prescriptions for referrals and treatment orders are necessary. A diagnosis must be provided by the NP with a request for evaluation and an indication of the intensity, frequency, and duration of therapy. Contraindications for certain interventions should be outlined. After initial referral for evaluation and treatment, extension of the treatment can be ordered if the client has not reached the treatment goal after the initial course of therapy. A written report is submitted from the PT covering goals, progress, and outcome measures and recommending any further treatment, which must be agreed upon by the NP.

17. How does a practitioner decide the quantity and quality of physical and occupational therapy?

The frequency and duration depend on many factors, including diagnosis, severity of the limitation, patient's motivation and tolerance, time constraints, and reimbursement constraints. Each patient must be managed individually. For outpatient physical and occupational therapy, the most popular regimen is 3 times per week for 2–4 weeks for adults. For children, therapy may continue for months or years, depending on the disability. Children have a potential for continued improvement as they grow and develop, whereas adults reach their maximal potential in a shorter period of time.

For home health care, clients may be sent home directly from the hospital and may need therapy 5 times per week for a few weeks until they can maneuver around their home setting (e.g., getting to the bathroom and shower, into bed, up the stairs, around the kitchen—anything that will assist their independence in ADLs). Inpatient clients are seen every day and often twice daily. Rather than see a client for an hour at a time, which many inpatients cannot tolerate, the time is broken up into two 30-minute sessions. This approach maximizes the effort that patients can put into the therapy, minimizes fatigue, and renders patients mobile twice rather than once daily.

18. Must the referring provider order specific modalities of treatment?

Specific treatment modalities can be ordered by the PT after the initial evaluation is performed and are based on which would be most helpful and appropriate for that particular client. After the initial assessment, the PT generally submits his or her findings, treatment goals, and an indication of the modalities planned for treatment.

19. Is physical therapy covered by insurance?

The various modalities are covered by insurance, and many are under one umbrella payment for physical therapy.

SPEECH-LANGUAGE THERAPY

20. What is the role of the speech-language therapist (SLT)?

SLTs evaluate and treat clients with both developmental and acquired communication disorders that result in difficulties in both the mechanical and cognitive aspects of speech (dysarthria, aphasia, disorders of phonation, language delays, stuttering or other disorders of language production). They also treat dysphagia, particularly in relation to stroke and other neurologic diseases. Specific functions of the SLT include the following:

- Diagnosis and treatment of speech and language disorders secondary to CVA, TBI, Parkinson's disease, or other central nervous system disturbances
- Diagnosis and treatment of functional or organic voice disorders
- Rehabilitation of laryngectimized patients
- Evaluation, educational planning, and speech and language habilitation of neurologic, developmental, cognitive, or emotional impairment in children.
- Evaluation and therapy for craniofacial disorders, including cleft lip and palate
- Speech and language evaluation and treatment for auditorially handicapped patients
- Evaluation and treatment of swallowing disorders

21. What types of patients do SLTs treat in the inpatient setting?

In the inpatient setting, SLTs assist clients who have had strokes or other muscular/neurological diseases that interfere with speech and swallowing. Along with OTs, they work with clients to increase chewing strength, and to develop facial muscles used for both speech and swallowing. SLTs work on expressive and receptive language skills for clients with aphasia. It is believed that cognition and language develop interactively and that this development continues into adulthood. When considering referrals, keep in mind that it is important to begin cognitive and speech therapy early for optimal relearning. Variables influencing recovery from aphasia include initial severity; age; type of aphasia (Broca's, Wernicke's, conduction, anomic, or global); etiology; premorbid intellectual level; personality variables such as motivation, insight, and self-corrective behavior; perseveration; and onset of therapy.

22. What types of patients do SLTs treat in the outpatient setting?

Clients who have not reached their maximal potential on discharge from an inpatient rehabilitation center may need continued outpatient speech therapy, especially those with expressive aphasia. Although a majority of the rehabilitation occurs early in the recovery period, an accurate prognosis often cannot be made until 1 year after the insult when the client's abilities in all areas have begun to stabilize. In the outpatient setting, a majority of speech-language therapy deals with articulation disorders and expressive aphasia.

Outpatient SLTs work in the school systems with congenital or acquired speech impediments. Chronic otitis media has increased significantly over the past decade because children enter daycare and preschool at an earlier age; as as result, conductive hearing loss is a common acquired articulation disorder. Stuttering is another problem frequently seen in the school systems. Because the exact cause of stuttering is unknown, it is one of the more difficult problems to treat and involves treating the whole family as well as the client.

Phonation disorders, which also come under the purview of outpatient speech-language therapy, may be due to physical problems or diseases, including paralysis, carcinoma, laryngeal tumors and lesions, infections, and papilloma. Speech therapy techniques are used to improve function of the vocal mechanism; when surgery removes laryngeal structures, new sources of phonation must be taught.

23. What modalities are used by SLTs?

MODALITY	ACTIVITY AND PURPOSE
Repetition	Exercises used in clients with aphasia as methods for retraining include auditory comprehension of spoken language, naming responses, phrases and sentences, pragmatic aspects of language, gestures paired with verbal expressions, writing and reading skills. Patients with stroke who have the potential to recover regain much of their speech within the first 12 weeks. This goal is accomplished through spontaneous recovery and repetition of language exercises.

(Continued on next page.)

MODALITY	ACTIVITY AND PURPOSE
Strengthening	Oral motor exercises for strengthening the muscles of speech and swallowing. Strengthening exercises may overlap with physical and occupational therapy.
Electrical stimulation	Particularly helpful in dysarthria for retraining the muscles of speech; may overlap with physical and occupational therapy.
Respiratory management	Retraining methods for clients with laryngeal resections include respiration training, muscular effort, esophageal speech, phonation with artificial larynx, altered head position, relaxation, and vocal rest. Used with neurogenic disorders, particularly for children with cerebral palsy. Examples include respiratory management, phonation, improved resonance, articulation, intelligibility, and prosody.
Retraining	Exercises for dysarthrias include appropriate posture and tone, muscle strength, respiratory management, phonation behaviors, articulatory skills, resonance characteristics, prosody, and nonverbal communication.
Language exercises	Exercises for the hearing-impaired patients include oral language, speech production, articulation, improved voice quality and prosody, and nonoral means of communication.

24. What information about referred patients is helpful for the SLT?

It is important to include the reason or cause for the referral, coexisting neurogenic diagnoses, coexisting major medical problems, complete diagnosis, localization of lesion (if present), presence of vision or hearing deficit, and signs of brainstem involvement, limb involvement, sensory deficit, or gait impairment. It is also important to include a history and physical exam (e.g., mental status, reflexes, laboratory findings, medications, and NP's estimate of language impairment). The SLT performs a complete assessment and makes recommendations for the treatment interval and duration. Speech therapy generally lasts several months, with re-evaluations at least every 6 months. Reports are sent to the health care provider after the initial evaluation, at 6 months, and at the termination of therapy.

25. What is the educational requirement for speech-language therapy?

A master's degree and certification by the American Speech and Hearing Association are currently required to be licensed as an SLT. With these credentials, SLTs can work in any area of speech therapy, but most select an area of specialty. A specialty license in speech-language therapy is not required, but during educational internships many SLTs become interested in an area and continue in that specialty after graduation. With a bachelor's degree in speech therapy, the practitioner may be licensed as a speech-language therapy assistant (SLTA), whose work is done mainly in outpatient settings and in school systems rather than in inpatient and rehabilitation hospitals.

26. How do PTs, OTs and SLTs get reimbursed?

Reimbursement varies among the three specialties. The variations depend on type of service, age of the client, diagnosis, and long-term prognosis. Reimbursement for pediatric clients is often more extensive and therapy more lengthy because children must continue therapy as long as they are developing to ensure that they reach their maximal potential. Maximal potential in adults is realized more quickly because they are developmentally stable when they begin therapy. For inpatient services, which are often covered by Medicare and Medicaid, reimbursement generally continues as long as the patient is making progress. For outpatient therapy, many managed care providers and insurance companies have a capitation on the number of PT, OT and SLT visits per year; therefore, patients must pay for any remaining therapy. If a client is insured through one of the more conscientious carriers, exceptions may be made on a case-by-case basis.

BIBLIOGRAPHY

1. DeLisa J (ed): Rehabilitation Medicine: Principles and Practice, 3rd ed. Philadelphia, Lippincott-Raven, 1998.
2. Hedge NM, Davis D: Clinical Methods and Practicum in Speech-Language Pathology, 3rd ed. San Diego, Singular Publishing, 1999.
3. O'Sullivan SB, Schmitz TJ: Physical Rehabilitation: Assessment and Treatment, 3rd ed. Philadelphia, F.A. Davis, 1994.
4. Pedretti LW: Occupational Therapy: Practice Skills for Physical Dysfunction. St. Louis, Mosby, 1996.

32. COLLABORATING WITH NUTRITIONISTS

Lisa Theriault, RN, MSN, CS

1. Why would a nurse practitioner (NP) want or need to refer to a nutritionist?

The U.S. Preventive Services Task Force recommends referral of clients to a registered dietitian or qualified nutritionist for further nutritional therapy and counseling if the clinician (1) is unable to perform a complete dietary history, (2) does not understand barriers to changes in eating, or (3) cannot offer individualized guidance on food selection and preparation.

In addition, clients may require more extensive counseling, monitoring, and nutritional therapy than a NP can provide in a limited amount of time. Examples include patients newly diagnosed with diabetes mellitus, undergoing chemotherapy, or diagnosed with an eating disorder such as anorexia nervosa. Evidence supports increased knowledge, increased long-term benefits, and improved eating behaviors associated with additional counseling provided by a nutritionist.

2. What is nutritional therapy (NT)?

NT consists of an assessment of the nutritional status of a client with a specific condition, illness, or injury, followed by the development of a treatment plan to monitor, administer, and evaluate specific nutritional needs. The assessment includes review and analysis of medical and diet history, blood chemistry values, and body composition measurements to determine nutritional status and treatment modalities.

3. What are the two major components of NT?

(1) Diet modifications and counseling and (2) specialized nutrition therapies.

4. Describe diet modification and counseling.

Diet modification and counseling include the development of a personalized diet plan to achieve medical goals such as improved blood glucose levels, reduced protein levels, or reduced caloric intake.

5. What is meant by specialized nutritional therapies?

Specialized nutritional therapies meet established nutritional needs through a variety of methods, including supplemental, enteral, or parenteral nutrition. Supplemental nutrition is appropriate for patients with pressure ulcers, chronic obstructive pulmonary disease, cerebral palsy, cystic fibrosis, muscular dystrophy, and inability to digest adequate nutrients through food intake. Enteral nutrition, delivered via tube, is appropriate for patients unable to ingest or digest food (e.g., stroke victims, clients with head or neck injuries). Parenteral nutrition, delivered via intravenous infusion, is appropriate for clients with severe burn injuries, in which hydration, electrolyte balance, and adequate caloric intake are vital to recovery and prevention of secondary infections, and for clients with gastrointestinal disorders that prevent normal absorption of nutrients.

6. Who provides NT?

Registered dietitians (RDs) or qualified nutritionists can provide a wide range of nutritional services. RD is a protected title given to providers meeting specific requirements, including (1) academic degree, such as bachelor of science; (2) approved internship or equivalent experience; and (3) successful completion of certification exam. In some states, RDs are licensed as nutritionists. In other states, no specific educational requirement is associated with the title of nutritionist, and no governing body qualifies the individual's ability. Reimbursement by third-party payors occurs only with RDs. For simplicity, the term *nutritionist* is broadly used in the following responses, to include both RDs and nutritionists; you should know whether in your state regarding "nutritionists" are actually RDs.

7. What are the benefits of NT?
- Increased rate of recovery
- Reduction in the incidence of complications
- Fewer hospitalizations
- Shorter hospital stays
- Reduction in drug, surgical, and other treatment needs
- Reduction of risks of diseases
- Improvement or maintenance of current health status
- Improvement in quality of life
- Reduction in health care costs
- Increased awareness of and responsibility for self-care

8. Which clients benefit from NT?
Acute nutritional needs
- Cancer
- Chemotherapy
- Eating disorders such as anorexia nervosa and bulimia nervosa
- Infectious process such as pneumonia
- Pediatric failure to thrive
- Pressure ulcers
- Trauma
- Postsurgical and other wound management

Complex nutritional needs
- Diabetes mellitus, types I and II
- Liver disease
- High risk of end-stage renal disease
- Inflammatory bowel syndrome
- Celiac disease
- HIV infection, AIDS
- Congestive heart failure
- Hypertension
- Obesity
- Hyperlipidemia
- Cystic fibrosis
- Chronic obstructive pulmonary disease
- Mental impairment (e.g., dementia, stroke)

Cultural/ethical needs: vegetarians
Preventative needs
- People with significant risk factors for cardiovascular disease, such as positive family history, obesity, elevated lipids, tobacco use, sedentary lifestyle, male gender, and advanced age
- People seeking guidance in relation to health promotion and maintenance
- Athletes

9. What is the role of the nutritionist?
- Screen individual nutritional risk.
- Collect pertinent information for comprehensive nutrition assessment.
- Assess nutritional status of a patient with complex medical conditions.
- Manage the normal nutritional needs of people across the lifespan, including infants through geriatrics and a diversity of culture and religions.
- Calculate and/or define diets for common conditions such as health promotion or disease prevention or chronic diseases.
- Design and implement nutrition care plans as indicated by the client's health status.
- Measure, calculate, and interpret body composition data.

- Develop and implement transitional feeding plans, such as conversion from one form of nutrition support to another.
- Conduct the nutritional care component of an interdisciplinary team conference to discuss client treatment and discharge planning.

10. What type of nutritional interventions should one expect for specific health problems?

CATEGORY	NUTRITIONAL INTERVENTIONS
Cardiovascular diseases	Assess current dietary intake (saturated fat, cholesterol, sodium, fiber)
	Assess nutritional needs (e.g., low saturated fat, low cholesterol, low sodium, high fiber)
	Measure and calculate body composition
	Develop dietary plan to lower lipids, blood pressure, weight
	Counsel about importance of lifestyle modifications to maintain current cardiovascular function and prevent further complications
	Monitor progress (e.g., lipid levels, blood pressure, weight)
Eating disorders	Assess current dietary intake (number of meals/day, calories, protein, carbohydrate, fat, empty calorie foods, laxative use, purging)
	Assess nutritional needs (e.g., increasing caloric count, high nutrient-rich content)
	Measure and calculate body composition
	Develop dietary plan to maintain or increase weight, specific nutrient content
	Counsel about importance of maintaining caloric intake and nutritional level to stabilize weight
	Monitor progress (e.g., weight, nutrient status)
	Initiate supplemental, enteral, or parenteral therapy as necessary
Gastrointestinal disorders	Assess current dietary intake (e.g., fiber, gluten, calories, fat, lactose)
	Assess nutritional needs (e.g., increased soluble fiber, increased insoluble fiber, decreased saturated fats, gluten-free, lactose-free)
	Develop dietary plan to maintain weight, normal bowel status, specific nutrient content
	Counsel about importance of maintaining appropriate nutritional intake to stabilize bowel function
	Monitor progress (e.g., weight, bowel status, nutrient status)
	Initiate supplemental, enteral, or parenteral therapy as necessary
Renal disorders	Assess current dietary intake (e.g., protein, fluid, sodium)
	Assess nutritional needs (e.g., protein, fluid, and sodium restriction)
	Develop dietary plan to maintain kidney function, weight, specific nutrient content
	Counsel about importance of maintaining appropriate nutritional intake and fluid intake to stabilize renal function
	Monitor progress (e.g., urinary output, weight, blood pressure, electrolytes, blood urea nitrogen, creatinine)
	Initiate supplemental, enteral, or parenteral therapy as necessary
Post-surgical and wound management	Assess current dietary intake (malnutrition, decreased intake, NPO status, protein, fluids)
	Assess dietary needs (e.g., increased protein, increased calories, increased nutrient content)
	Develop dietary plan to achieve normal wound healing
	Counsel about importance of maintaining appropriate nutritional intake to facilitate the healing process
	Monitor progress (e.g., wound status, weight)
	Initiate supplemental, enteral, or parenteral therapy as necessary

(Table ontinued on next page.)

CATEGORY	NUTRITIONAL INTERVENTIONS
Respiratory disorders	Assess current dietary intake (e.g., calories, fluid, protein, fats) Assess nutritional needs (e.g., increased or decreased caloric intake, decreased fats, increased proteins, increased fluid) Develop dietary plan to maintain energy level and appropriate weight Monitor progress (e.g., weight, respiratory status) Initiate supplemental, enteral, or parenteral therapy as necessary
Cancer	Assess current dietary intake (calories, protein, fat, fluids) Assess nutritional needs (e.g., increased calories, increased protein, increased fluids) Develop dietary plan to maintain weight and immune status, specific nutrient level Counsel about importance of maintaining appropriate nutritional intake to maintain function of immune system Monitor progress (e.g., weight, white blood cell count, temperature, specific nutrient level) Initiate supplemental, enteral, or parenteral therapy as necessary
Diabetes mellitus, types 1 and 2	Assess current dietary intake (e.g., calories, simple and complex carbohydrates, fats, protein) Assess nutritional needs (e.g., decreased calories, limiting carbohydrates and fats) Develop dietary plan to maintain glucose level and weight Counsel about importance of maintaining appropriate nutritional intake to stabilize blood glucose levels and prevent complications Monitor progress (e.g., blood glucose levels, weight)
Pediatric failure to thrive	Assess current dietary intake (e.g., calories, protein, carbohydrates, fats) Assess nutritional needs (e.g., increased calories, increased protein, increased carbohydrates, increased fats, nutrient content) Develop dietary plan to maintain weight and height Counsel about importance of maintaining appropriate nutritional intake to stabilize weight, height Monitor progress (e.g., weight, nutrient level) Initiate supplemental, enteral, or parenteral therapy as necessary
Infectious process	Assess current dietary intake (calories, protein, fluids) Assess nutritional needs (e.g., increased calories, protein, and fluids) Develop dietary plan to maintain immune status, weight, specific nutrient level Counsel about importance of maintaining appropriate nutritional intake to stabilize and improve immune status Monitor progress (e.g., weight, nutrient level) Initiate supplemental, enteral, or parenteral therapy as necessary
Liver or biliary disorders	Assess current dietary intake (e.g., calories, protein, carbohydrates, fluid, sodium) Assess nutritional needs (e.g., increased calories, increased carbohydrates, decreased protein, decreased sodium, limit fluids) Develop dietary plan to maintain weight, specific nutrient level Counsel about importance of maintaining appropriate nutritional intake to stabilize liver function Monitor progress (e.g., weight, cognitive functioning) Initiate supplemental, enteral, or parenteral therapy as necessary

11. Can NT be included in a patient's plan of care only in select health care settings?

No. NT is available and can benefit patients in just about any health care setting, including the following:

- Inpatient care
- Mental health services
- Primary care
- Ambulatory care
- Nursing home care
- Home health care

- Community health services
- Hospice care
- Subacute care
- Rehabilitation services
- Assisted living centers
- Day care

12. What types of insurance covers NT?

- Medicare Part A and Part B: see table.
- Medicare + Choice: plans in HMOs may reimburse dietitians directly.
- Medicaid: no federal criteria specifically related to nutrition services. Programs vary from state to state; many states cover nutrition services as part of prenatal/child care.
- Managed care organizations: services vary from plan to plan. Most require referral from primary care provider and cover only medically necessary nutrition therapy; weight control frequently is excluded.
- Military health care system: TRICARE/managed care provides services in military facilities. No nutritional services provided to beneficiaries remotely located from military facilities.
- Federal employees health benefits program: most coverage determinations made by Office of Personnel Management (OPM) in coordination with the private health plans that contract with it to provide care.

Coverage continues to evolve with policy changes at both state and federal levels.

Medicare Coverage of Nutrition Services

SETTING	COVERAGE OF NUTRITION SERVICES
Medicare Part A	
Inpatient hospital services	Hospitals must provide nutrition services and must retain dietitian as employee or independent contractor. Nutrition services as not reimbursed as separate charge.
Skilled nursing facility services	Skilled nursing facilities must use services of qualified dietitian. Nutrition services are typically included as part of administrative costs and not reimbursed as separate charge.
End-stage renal disease facilities	Required to provide dietary services from qualified dietitian. Nutrition services are not reimbursed as separate charge.
Home health care services	Specialized nutrition expertise must be available within home health agency to be Medicare-certified. Dietitians are currently not eligible for separate per-visit reimbursement; services are covered by agency's administrative costs.
Hospice service	Dietary counseling is covered service for hospices that are Medicare-certified. Reimbursement for dietary counseling is included in flat-rate payment and not provided as separate charge.
Medicare Part B*	
Inpatient hospital services	Only hospital-based diabetic education programs are covered.
Physician-based or physician group-based practice	Nutrition services may be covered if they are reasonable and medically necessary. These services must be provided by employee of physician-based practice and must be directly supervised by physician.
Ambulatory surgical clinics	Nutrition services may be covered if they are reasonable and medically necessary. Clinic employee must provide these services.
Ambulatory clinics	Nutrition services may be covered if they are reasonable and medically necessary. Clinic employee must provide these services.
Rural health clinics	Nutrition services may be covered if they are reasonable and medically necessary. Clinic employee must provide these services.

* Requires referral from primary care provider

13. If I refer a patient, how long should I expect the patient and nutritionist to work together?

The duration of the relationship between the nutritionist and client varies, depending on a number of factors: (1) complexity of the problem(s), (2) client's cognitive and physical abilities, and (3) client's progress during therapy. Clients with multiple health problems often require a greater number of interventions and closer monitoring, which necessitate greater supervision by the nutritionist. Clients with cognitive and/or physical limitation(s) may require more intensive consultation. Clients who have difficulty with progressing (i.e., demonstrating benefits such as improved blood sugars) usually require more intensive consultation. Aelected programs (e.g., diabetic education) that cover the nutritional aspect of the specified disease typically have a pre-established duration.

14. What type of feedback should I expect after an NT consultation or referral?

Expect an initial consultation report, either verbal or written, within the first several weeks of the visit. Subsequent follow-up reports may vary, depending on the institution or nutritionist. Professional courtesy suggests periodic documentation in lengthy cases with a final report when the relationship is terminated.

15. How do you select an appropriate nutritionist?

Determine whether all nutritionists in your area are RDs or whether other persons use the title. It is best to refer to a RD so that the patient's nutrition consultation will be covered by third-party payors. You should be able to identify specific RDs who provide nutrition care related to your patient's problem(s). If you are not familiar with the local nutritionists/RDs and their areas of expertise (e.g., eating disorders, athletics, diabetes), ask for recommendations from valued colleagues. Referral lists are often available at local health care institutions and through the American Dietetic Association (800-366-1655) or at http://www.eatright.org. It is ideal to call RDs identified through referral lists and to verify that they accept consultations related to your patient's needs.

BIBLIOGRAPHY

1. American Dietetic Association: Medical nutrition therapy protocols: An introduction. J Am Diet Assoc 99:351, 1995.
2. American Dietetic Association website: http://www.eatright.org.
3. Carey M, Gillespie S: Position of the American Dietetic Association: Cost effectiveness of medical nutrition therapy. J Am Diet Assoc 95(1): 88–91, 1995.
4. Klein S, et al: Nutrition support in clinical practice: A review of published data and recommendations for future research directions. Am J Clin Nutr 66(3): 683–706, 1997.
5. Laramee S: Position of the American Dietetic Association: Nutrition services in managed care organization. J Am Diet Assoc 96:391–395, 1996.
6. Pfau PR, Rombeau JL: Nutrition. Med Clin North Am 84:1209–1230, 2000.
7. Shikany JM, White GL: Dietary guidelines for chronic disease prevention. South Med J 93:1157–1161, 2000.
8. Thompson RL, et al: Dietary advice given by a dietitian versus other health professional or self-help resources to reduce blood cholesterol. Oxford, Cochrane Library, 2001.
9. U.S. Preventive Services Task Force: Guide to Clinical Services: An Assessment of the Effectiveness of 169 Interventions. Baltimore, Williams & Wilkins, 1995.

INDEX

Page numbers in **boldface type** indicate complete chapters.